The Duke University Medical Center Book of Diet and Fitness

The Duke University Medical Center Book of Diet and Fitness

Developed by the Duke Diet and Fitness Center

Michael Hamilton, M.D., M.P.H.
Ronette L. Kolotkin, Ph.D.
Dianne F. Cogburn, M.P.H., R.D.
D. T. Moore, M.S.
with Kathryn Watterson

FAWCETT COLUMBINE

NEW YORK

WE DEDICATE THIS BOOK TO

E. HARVEY ESTES, M.D.
Distinguished Service Professor,
Department of Community and Family Medicine
Duke University Medical Center

AND

SIEGFRIED HEYDEN, M.D.
Professor,
Department of Community and Family Medicine
Duke University Medical Center

both of whom had the wisdom
to recognize the power of diet and fitness
in achieving health and well-being
long before it was popular.

Contents

Acknowledgments

It is difficult if not impossible to acknowledge all those who have contributed to this book. Certain people stand out, however, because of their involvement in helping to make it possible.

First, we wish to thank the many participants in the Duke Diet and Fitness Center program. Their successes (and failures) have helped us to learn what works and what doesn't. Their support and enthusiasm created the demand for this book.

We also wish to thank Dr. George Parkerson, chairman of the Department of Community and Family Medicine at Duke Medical Center, for his commitment to the basic concept of this book—that sensible nutrition and fitness are essential to optimal health and well-being.

For his careful review of countless manuscripts and his suggestions for improvements, we thank Jon Carmel, administrative director of the Diet and Fitness Center. His input made him, in effect, a "silent author."

We appreciate the role of our New York contingent in making this book a reality—Kitsi Watterson, Sydelle Engel, Mort Engel, Joëlle Delbourgo, Betsy Rapoport, and Judy Knipe. Also thanks to Dr. Richard Atkinson for his helpful suggestions.

The staff of the Diet and Fitness Center deserves major credit: Franca Alphin, Phillis Byrd, Barbara Dean, JoAnn Fafrowicz, Sue Forbes, Olga Hamilton, Kim Helmink, Dody Holt, Michele Hudgins, Vanessa Lipscomb, Laura McLeod, Amy Moyer, Nancy Proia, Shelton Spicer, Donna Yates, and our chefs, Michael Eddins and Patricia Woods. Their team spirit and sense of humor allowed us to look back at our efforts and say, "It was hard work but fun."

Finally, our families have our deep appreciation for their willingness to review our drafts and to listen (probably more than they really wanted) to our ideas on diet and fitness.

Foreword

The Duke University Diet and Fitness Center program has been helping people understand and manage their weight problems for many years. Although thousands have benefited from direct involvement in the program, they represent only a few of the millions of people in our society who need help. This book extends the expertise of the Duke Diet and Fitness Center program to this larger group, which may include you or someone you love. Now you, your friends and family can enjoy the benefits of this sensible weight management program that is based upon cutting-edge scientific knowledge and which you can accomplish at home.

Diet has become increasingly important in our society because food is the focus of much of our everyday mental, physical, and social activity. Instead of facing the problem of obtaining enough food to survive, most of us have an overabundance. Our only problems are which foods to select and how much to eat. These problems are magnified into major dilemmas for those of us who become overweight.

As a family physician with additional training in epidemiology, and as a person who has experienced some personal weight problems over the years, I sincerely endorse the Duke Diet and Fitness Center program and this book. The authors are the very people who are responsible for planning and conducting the program at Duke University Medical Center. What they say in the book is what they say every day to people who attend the Diet and Fitness Center in Durham. Now, through this book, they are sharing it with you.

The advice of these experts is medically sound. It is effective because it is sensible, doable, and suitable for the needs of most people with a weight management problem. These experts recognize the importance of a nutritionally sound diet, regular physical exercise, attention to emotional factors, and special care for medical problems that may be associated with overweight. They understand the difficulties involved with personal life change, and that quality of life must be maintained and elevated whenever lifestyle is modified. To them each person is more important than how much that person weighs.

It is my belief that the Duke Diet and Fitness Center program as detailed for you in this book will be of special value as you, and those who are important to you, seek improved health and well-being through better weight management.

George R. Parkerson, Jr., M.D., M.P.H.
Professor and Chairman
DEPARTMENT OF COMMUNITY AND FAMILY MEDICINE
DUKE UNIVERSITY MEDICAL CENTER

The Duke University Medical Center Book of Diet and Fitness

1

The Duke University Diet and Fitness Center Program: Who We Are and What We Do

This is not a typical diet book. It offers no gimmick, quick fix, or guaranteed cure. What it does offer is a practical, livable program which thousands of people have followed to lose weight—and keep it off. If you follow our program, you'll be able to control your weight for the rest of your life, without feeling deprived, hungry, or locked into ineffective yo-yo diet cycles.

With this book, you will learn how to make choices about your exercise and eating patterns that will benefit you both physically and psychologically. This practical approach will put *you* in control and enable you to feel confident about managing your weight.

Within days of beginning this program, we believe you will begin to feel better, more energetic and alive. You'll be surprised that this low-calorie diet will not give you between-meal hunger. In a one-year follow-up survey of our clients, about 70 percent reported that they continued to feel good and had maintained the weight that they had lost on the program or had lost more weight during the year.

While weight loss is the gold standard of success for most people who

3

diet, it is only one of the benefits of the Duke University Diet and Fitness Center program. Along with weight loss, many of our clients also enjoy reductions in their blood pressure, blood glucose levels, and blood cholesterol. They report that in addition to feeling better physically, they know themselves better, take greater responsibility for themselves, and feel more hopeful and optimistic about life.

For many years, Duke University has been a leader in medical research and has provided a wide variety of programs for improving health. Since its inception more than sixteen years ago, the Duke Diet and Fitness Center (DFC) has become a recognized leader in weight management. With a success rate of 70 percent, the center has helped many thousands of people achieve better health through sustained weight loss and lifestyle change.

The DFC approach differs greatly from quick-fix, radical diets—ranging from fasting to diets consisting of liquid protein. Some fad diets have serious side effects, including malnutrition, abdominal pain, decreased renal function, depression, weakness, electrolyte losses, anemia, rapid pulse, even death. Moreover, the overwhelming evidence is that fad diets just don't work. What counts most in dieting is long-term results—how long the pounds stay off—and analysis of the long-term results of these diets shows that most people regain the weight they lost within a year. If you follow these diets, you're going to experience long-term frustration.

At the Duke Diet and Fitness Center, we believe that the best approach is a nutritionally sound diet, restricted in calories to produce a gradual weight loss, and a sensible exercise program that fits naturally into your lifestyle. Our experience is that for weight loss to be lasting, it must occur in response to specific lifestyle changes that are reasonable and realistic so that they can be practiced on a permanent basis. A new awareness of nutritional choices, emotional motivations for eating, fitness, and health, combined with strategies that help you practice new patterns of thinking, eating, and physical activity will be most effective on a long-term basis.

How We Do It: A Positive Approach to Losing Weight

The Duke University Diet and Fitness Center program is based on the following principles:

Self-Awareness
With self-awareness, you will be able to set realistic and achievable goals.

Education
You will learn how to make choices about what you eat based on sound information about foods, nutrients, and calories. We will assist you in designing exercise programs that meet your individual needs. You will learn that weight loss may be slower than you might wish, but that through lifestyle change, it can be *permanent*.

Realistic Goals
You will develop your own individualized short- and long-term goals that are realistic and *attainable*.

Development of Strategies
You will learn strategies for planning and monitoring your actions and activities that help you to achieve the goals you have set for yourself.

Advance Planning
You will learn to make your choices about what to eat in advance instead of leaving selections to chance at the last minute. The same is true for your decisions about physical activity and exercise.

Monitoring
You will learn to record daily events, what you eat, when and how you exercise, how you feel, and what you weigh to serve as a visible reminder of what you do. Keeping records will discourage you from straying from your intended nutrition and exercise plan, increase your awareness of the relationship between your moods, eating, exercising, and the events in your life, and prepare you to cope with similar—and often difficult—situations in the future. Additionally, a written record is a good way to measure your accomplishments and to chart your progress.

Maximizing Success
You will learn practical methods to support the maintenance of your diet and exercise program to ensure your continued progress.

Finally, we will ask you to recognize and acknowledge your success on many levels. Remember that the scale is only one measure. We'll help you to notice changes in how you look and how you feel, and to celebrate if you have reductions in the levels of your blood pressure, cholesterol, or blood sugar. You'll learn to appreciate improvements in your fitness and general well-being that enhance the quality of your life. You'll be rewarded with a sense of accomplishment and confidence in your ability to make changes. You will have made a new beginning.

Success Through Small Changes

Willpower and desire are not enough to make you change your life. You must also develop and practice skills that will make change happen. This book will teach you how to develop those skills through a better understanding of how and why you eat and careful practice of basic principles of diet and fitness.

In fact, a new and healthy lifestyle can become so much a part of you that you'll want to stay with the DFC program simply because it helps you feel your best. You will quickly appreciate something that you've always known, but perhaps have forgotten: small changes in your life can make a tremendous difference in the way you feel. Even small changes can improve your health and the way your body functions and help you to feel better about yourself.

If you learn to view positive health habits as a gift to yourself rather than as a necessary evil or a punishment for being overweight, you will feel better about making these changes. With practice and a positive attitude, you can look forward to regular exercise and a healthy diet as a normal, everyday part of your life.

We will help you learn, as our clients at the Diet and Fitness Center have learned, how to create success on a day-to-day basis. With a series of accomplishments, one step at a time, you will soon be successful in reaching your goals. The small changes count; if you eat fewer calories than you normally eat each day, if you make an appointment with yourself to exercise five minutes more than the day before and keep it up, or if you love chocolate or pepperoni but learn to incorporate these foods into your meal plan and control the portions that you eat, you'll be well on your way to reaching larger goals.

Who Benefits From DFC's Program?

Our clients are a diverse group from every walk of life. They work, run businesses, industries, and families. Many of them are achievers in almost every area except one: when it comes to eating food, they lack control. Like some of you, many DFC graduates began this program because they reached a turning point in their lives that made them want to do something for themselves. Sometimes the catalyst was the beginning of a new relationship or marriage, a promotion, a career change, a new job, or retirement. For others, the decision to change was triggered by a personal crisis, such as the end of a relationship or the death of a loved one. Others were motivated by the recognition that being overweight was jeopardizing their health. For a great number, there was no sudden clap of thunder; their revelations were slow and gradual. They simply decided they wanted to get back into smaller clothes again, improve their health, feel more energetic, begin an exercise program, or regain their self-confidence.

Some of the people who have benefited from the DFC program will become familiar to you as you undergo many of the same experiences they have had in learning about themselves and changing their eating and exercise patterns.*

Nina Halloran, thirty-one, woke up one morning with a hollow, unhappy feeling. As she watched the changing patterns of light through the leaves of a tree outside her window, she thought about her encounter the day before with an old friend who couldn't hide his shock at the twenty-five pounds Nina had gradually gained in the six years since her first child was born. Lying there, she realized that while she had been taking good care of her husband, her two children, and her co-workers, she had been neglecting herself. Her main treats were the chocolate chip cookies or bowls of ice cream she ate when she felt depleted at the end of the day. Two months after beginning the Diet and Fitness Center program, Nina had assessed her own wants and dreams for the first time in her life. With the help of a support group, she realized how heavily she relied on other people's opinions, and she began to address some of the issues that made her overeat. Today, she is twenty-two pounds lighter than she was that morning she woke up

*The case histories in this book are composites based on the stories and situations of actual people who have participated in the Duke University Diet and Fitness program. All client names are fictitious.

feeling so unhappy. She goes to aerobics classes four times a week and cooks healthy, low-calorie meals that keep her in good shape. She has tremendous energy again, and has found that her husband and children are happier too.

At the age of fifty-five, John Larsen was named president of an international corporation. Shortly after he was promoted, the hours he had reserved for squash games with his old college buddy got squeezed out by the demands of his schedule. John enjoyed the challenge and the excitement of his work so much that he wasn't aware of any strain, nor was he particularly bothered by the extra twenty pounds he slowly gained. His fun-loving and attractive wife, Lily, however, noticed that particularly when they were entertaining, John ate too much and drank too much. At first she made jokes about his stress levels and his need to purchase new shirts and suits. But finally she got worried that he was going to do physical as well as emotional damage to himself if he didn't slow down. "Look," she said to him one night, "I'm serious about this. Your blue eyes are still as wonderful as they ever were, but twenty pounds extra is twenty pounds too many. So stop already." John looked at her and in his forthright way declared that he would confront the problem directly. On the DFC program, he lost twenty pounds and changed his patterns of eating. Although his work demands are still intense, John is much more relaxed than he was before. He works out daily at the corporate gym, plays squash whenever he can, and maintains a healthy diet despite his corporate travels and numerous meals out.

Forty-eight-year-old Rita Caparelli rarely left her house because staying on her feet for more than half an hour made her uncomfortable. Abandoned by her husband when she was in her twenties, Rita had raised four active children who always vied with her for their share of potato chips, soft drinks, Oreo cookies, and Twinkies. Somehow Rita also had managed to run a successful mail-order business from a beat-up desk in the foyer of her home. Although she never talked much about it, she took daily doses of insulin for her diabetes. And while her doctor urged her to lose weight, her afternoon snacks soothed her growing fear of leaving her house. She thought that she "needed" her Popsicles and chocolate bars, and felt hopeless about changing anything. The turning point for Rita came when the last of her children moved away from home, and she found herself wandering around the house wondering what her life meant, and why she felt so useless. She had never realized how fat she had become over the years. After two and a half weeks at the Diet and Fitness Center, Rita Caparelli had lost nearly ten pounds and was exercising every day. She was able to stop taking insulin completely. She decided to lose another thirty-five pounds, which she did, but she lost them gradually as a part of her ongoing lifestyle change.

For eighteen-year-old Nathan Bennett, the catalyst for beginning the DFC program was the promise of a fresh start as a college freshman. Since the third grade, Nathan had been the butt of "fat boy" jokes. While he was a good sport about the razzing, inside he hated being called "Blubber Bennett." Over the years, none of Nathan's secret summer plans to lose weight had ever materialized, but he decided that this summer was his last-ditch chance to make it happen. He also figured that once he lost weight, it might be easier to maintain new patterns in a new environment, away from old friends and old habits. At the same time, he was nervous about dating and making good grades—and he wanted to be prepared for being successful both socially and academically. Through strategies he learned at DFC, Nathan lost the weight; now he looks like a lifeguard who could be in the movies. His college life has been more fun than he ever would have imagined, and he still enjoys the shock effect he creates when he sees old high school friends during college vacations at home.

The first thing you will experience with the Diet and Fitness Center program is a sense of relief at having decided to make a change in your life. You'll begin to feel hopeful and confident as you learn that changing unhealthy habits is not simply a matter of willpower. A desire to become slim and healthy will be translated into tangible steps—a road map with clear directions, and a variety of different routes from which you, the individual traveler, can choose. The road begins here.

2

What It Means to Be Overweight: The Medical and Social Consequences

If you're overweight, you're not alone. At least thirty-four million people in the United States are in the same condition.

Overweight and obesity are terms often used interchangeably, but they are different. *Overweight* simply means what it says—an excess of body weight. Excess body weight, however, doesn't always mean excess fat. For example, football players are often overweight, but their "overweight" may consist primarily of increased muscle tissue.

The term *obesity* specifically refers to an overabundance of fat tissue. While the exact measurement of body fat requires sophisticated laboratory procedures that are generally unavailable in the usual medical setting, most experts agree that obesity exists when actual body weight exceeds desirable body weight by 20 percent or more.

Desirable Body Weight

The phrase "desirable body weight" was coined by the Metropolitan Life Insurance Company, which developed tables based on records of life insurance policyholders that projected the appropriate weight for a given height that would promote the longest life span.

For many years, these tables have been considered the standard for people who want to maintain a healthy weight. Assumptions based on these tables have been challenged, however, because holders of insurance policies may not be typical of the general population. Furthermore, a feature of the tables that divides body types into frame sizes of small, medium, or large was never consistently measured. Also, the Metropolitan Life Insurance tables do not adjust for age. These criticisms led to a downplaying of the title of the original 1942 tables ("ideal" body weight) to "desirable" weight in 1959, and simply to "height–weight" tables for those published in 1983 (see table 1).

Table 1.

1983 Metropolitan Height–Weight Table

Height	Small Frame	Medium Frame	Large Frame	
	◄——————— lb ———————►			
men*				
5'2"	128–134	131–141	138–150	*Weights at ages
5'3"	130–136	133–143	140–153	twenty-five to
5'4"	132–138	135–145	142–156	fifty-nine based on
5'5"	134–140	137–148	144–160	lowest mortality.
5'6"	136–142	139–151	146–164	Weight in pounds
5'7"	138–145	142–154	149–168	according to frame
5'8"	140–148	145–157	152–172	(in indoor clothing
5'9"	142–151	148–160	155–176	weighing five pounds,
5'10"	144–154	151–163	158–180	shoes with one-inch
5'11"	146–157	154–166	161–184	heels).
6'0"	149–160	157–170	164–188	
6'1"	152–164	160–174	168–192	
6'2"	155–168	164–178	172–197	†Weights at ages
6'3"	158–172	167–182	176–202	twenty-five to
6'4"	162–176	171–187	181–207	fifty-nine based on
				lowest mortality.
women†				Weight in pounds
4'10"	102–111	109–121	118–131	according to frame
4'11"	103–113	111–123	120–134	(in indoor clothing
5'0"	104–115	113–126	122–137	weighing three
5'1"	106–118	115–129	125–140	pounds, shoes with
5'2"	108–121	118–132	128–143	one-inch heels).
5'3"	111–124	121–135	131–147	
5'4"	114–127	124–138	134–151	
5'5"	117–130	127–141	137–155	
5'6"	120–133	130–144	140–159	
5'7"	123–136	133–147	143–163	
5'8"	126–139	136–150	146–167	
5'9"	129–142	139–153	149–170	
5'10"	132–145	142–156	152–173	
5'11"	135–148	145–159	155–176	Courtesy of Metropolitan
6'0"	138–151	148–162	158–179	Life Insurance Company.

Because of the large number of people studied and the length of follow-up, the Metropolitan Life Insurance tables are, in spite of these criticisms, the best information we have on the relationship between weight and longevity.

Selecting Your Desirable Weight

As you can see, the height–weight table is organized according to frame size, with a range of weights allowed for each height within a frame-size category. We suggest you follow the directions in Table 2 to estimate your frame size, then select the suggested weight in the frame size for your height. For example, the desirable weight for a 5′5″ woman with a medium frame would be approximately 134 pounds.

Table 2.

Estimating Your Frame Size

To make a simple approximation of your frame size:

Extend your arm and bend the forearm upwards at a 90-degree angle. Keep the fingers straight and turn the inside of your wrist toward the body. Place the thumb and index finger of your other hand on the two prominent bones on either side of your elbow. Measure the space between your fingers against a ruler or a tape measure. Compare this measurement with the measurements shown below.

This table lists the elbow measurements for men and women of medium frame at various heights. Measurements lower than those listed indicate that you have a small frame, while higher measurements indicate a large frame.

Height (in 1″ Heels)	Elbow Breadth (in Inches)
men	
5′2″–5′3″	2½–2⅞
5′4″–5′7″	2⅝–2⅞
5′8″–5′11″	2¾–3
6′0″–6′3″	2¼–3⅛
6′4″	2⅞–3¼
women	
4′10″–4′11″	2¼–2½
5′0″–5′3″	2¼–2½
5′4″–5′7″	2⅜–2⅝
5′8″–5′11″	2⅜–2⅝
6′0″	2½–2¾

*Source of basic data: Data tape, HANES I.

Courtesy of Metropolitan Life Insurance Company.

Calculating Your Percent Overweight (or Underweight)

To determine your percent over or under desirable weight, calculate the difference between your actual weight and the desirable weight you selected and divide the difference of these two weights by your desirable weight and multiply the result by 100. This will give you your percent over or under your desirable weight.

Why We Get Fat

Body fatness results from a prolonged imbalance between energy intake (the food one eats) and energy expenditure (the amount of energy expended by the body). Excess food that is not needed by the body to maintain its physiologic functions and physical activities is stored as fat in the cells of adipose tissue. These cells lie beneath the skin in the subcutaneous tissues, but they are also found in tissues deeper within the body. When excess energy is stored as fat in the cells of adipose tissue, we become "fat." If all the adipose cells are filled to capacity with fat, new cells are created, which then allows an even greater level of obesity—one which may be even more difficult to reduce over time.

A Biological Basis of Fat

There is a practical, natural, and biological reason for our capacity to develop fat. Without the ability to store fat, we wouldn't have fuel to burn in times of food scarcity. It's easy to see that an animal's ability to eat beyond its immediate energy needs allows it to store excess energy as fat for use during periods when it is unable to find food.

Our taste for fatty foods may also have a biological usefulness. Fatty foods offer an energy advantage because fat contains more than two times as many calories per gram as protein or carbohydrate (fat contains nine calories per gram and protein or carbohydrate four calories per gram). Dietary fat is lighter in weight for its energy content than protein or carbohydrates, and therefore less work to carry as we move about from place to place. Dietary fat is also converted to body fat more efficiently than protein or carbohydrate.

In the absence of a food shortage, however, most of us don't have the same need our primitive human ancestors had to overeat or store body fat for survival. Today, excess body fat represents a natural process that is not only maladaptive but hazardous in terms of health and longevity.

The Genetic Blueprint for Overweight

While body weight seems to depend on a complex interaction of several factors, medical studies have shown that inheritance plays a far more important role in weight than was previously understood.

We now know that someone whose parents are overweight or obese has a greater chance of being overweight too. A person with thin parents is less likely to be overweight. But don't be discouraged. Studies indicate that about 30 percent of the variability in weight between individuals is accounted for by inheritance. That leaves room for lifestyle to play a significant and important role.

While you may have been born with an inherited tendency that influences the direction of your weight upwards, remember, that tendency can be modified by your eating habits and your level of physical activity.

Hazards for the Unwary

Environmental influences also can be extremely powerful in determining body weight. For example, studies of women in our society show that overweight is more prevalent among those with low socioeconomic status, but that the reverse tends to be true among men.

Obviously, environment can be a help or a hindrance to managing weight. Unfortunately, our food-oriented society sets many traps for the unwary, and getting through an ordinary day means encountering a succession of temptations.

- Each checkout counter at the grocery store tempts us with attractive displays of candy.
- Foods high in fat and calories are served in restaurants and many public places.
- The friends we visit set out chips and cheese and offer high-calorie drinks.
- Social and business interactions take place over food, often because mealtime is the most convenient time to meet.
- Intimate relationships center on food—going out to dinner, cooking together, snacking together.

- Emotions—including a desire for love or comfort, anxiety, anger, and happiness—tend to be soothed by eating.

Our society's advances in technology also contribute to excess body weight by encouraging a sedentary lifestyle. The pace and demands of our lives are such that we arrange our schedules to save time and avoid movement.

- We ride on escalators and in elevators instead of using stairs.
- We use garage door openers rather than getting out of the car and lifting the door by hand.
- The electric typewriter or computer reduces the small amount of energy we used to spend at the old manual typewriter.
- Dishwashers and other home convenience items such as garbage disposals reduce the energy we use in maintaining our homes.
- We take taxis instead of walking from one destination to the next.
- Even for short distances, we drive to do our errands instead of walking or riding a bicycle.
- When we go shopping, we park as close as we can to our destination to save steps.
- There are even devices that automatically switch off household lights at night, thus saving us the effort of walking from room to room!

The Medical Consequences of Overweight

Excess body fat is a fertile subsoil for many illnesses that can have a profound effect on our quality of life and reduce our chances for living productively into old age. Studies indicate that people who are 20 percent or more over desirable body weight are more likely than lean people to develop

- Coronary artery disease (heart attack and angina)
- Hypertension (high blood pressure)
- Type II (adult-onset) diabetes
- Hyperlipidemia (elevated cholesterol levels)
- Respiratory dysfunction
- Gallstones
- Abnormal tests of liver function due to infiltration of liver cells by fat

• Certain skin disorders
• Certain cancers, particularly cancer of the cervix and endometrium in women, and cancer of the colon, rectum, and prostate in men

The distribution of body fat is also important. People with potbellies seem more predisposed to diabetes, hyperlipidemia, high blood pressure, and coronary artery disease than those people whose excess weight is primarily situated in the hips and thighs.

The role of excess fat in the development of these disorders is not fully understood. It's evident, however, that being 20 percent or more overweight is a risk factor for their onset. The statistics that link obesity to disease are so overwhelming that in 1985, the National Institutes of Health Consensus Development Conference declared obesity to be a disease in its own right.

Being slightly overweight doesn't lead to such dire consequences but can contribute to feelings of fatigue or breathlessness when walking short distances or climbing stairs. If you're overweight, these and other everyday difficulties can decrease the quality of your life and limit your choices.

Social and Psychological Consequences of Overweight

Beginning with childhood, the social and psychological consequences of being overweight can be overwhelming. Children like Nathan Bennett who are overweight are often labeled with degrading nicknames such as "Fatty," "Lardo," or "Tubby." As a result, their strengths and talents are often neglected, and their self-esteem suffers. Studies have shown that the fat child is the least desirable friend among classmates. Shown pictures of handicapped children, fat children, and deformed children, and asked to choose among them, most school children in one classic study chose the fat child last. In another study of six-year-olds, the youngsters characterized the fat child as a liar, as well as being lazy, stupid, and dirty.

Adults who are very overweight may also suffer from prejudice and discrimination, and have restrictions placed on their opportunities in life. Studies have shown that fat people have more difficulty getting into college, and getting jobs and promotions in the business world. One study showed that American executives lose $1,000 per year in income for every ten pounds that they are overweight. In addition to peer disapproval, overweight people often view themselves in disparaging ways, compounding the problems of low self-esteem.

Only six months after she began to lose weight, Nina Halloran was made supervisor of her division in the computer company for which she worked. Previously, she hadn't been aware of any discrimination, but afterwards she felt that the promotion came both because of her weight loss and because she simply felt better about herself and was more outgoing with her colleagues. In addition, she realized that being overweight had limited her versatility and her enjoyment of many simple pleasures she could share with her husband and kids. She loved to swim, for instance, but because she felt embarrassed about the way she looked in a bathing suit, she had stopped swimming. She never wore shorts in the summer, and she wore loose dresses with no waist rather than the tailored and fitted clothing which previously had looked best on her. She confided to her support group that when she was feeling heavy, she didn't have the confidence to approach her husband sexually as often as she might otherwise have done.

For Nathan, of course, a whole new world opened up when he lost weight before his freshman year of college. He was amazed the second week of school when his roommate told him that a girl he had met the night before was interested in going out with him. At first he thought that the girl must have him confused with someone else, but when she called him up and asked him out, he happily accepted.

As we'll see later, some people use being overweight as a way of masking personal issues and not getting to the root of problems. For instance, for someone who is nervous about dating and afraid of rejection, being overweight can be a good defense against facing that possibility.

Following the DFC Program at Home

If you were to come to the Diet and Fitness Center in Durham, North Carolina, we would ask you to stay at the center for at least one week, preferably for four. It takes that amount of time, we believe, for you to achieve the greatest benefits and to develop new habits of eating, exercising, and thinking.

With this book, you can now be a successful DFC client at home. In

the four one-week sections that follow, each of them devoted to a particular aspect of the DFC plan, we will take you through our program step
by step.

In *Week One: Getting Started,* you'll learn more about yourself and how
your lifestyle affects your patterns of eating and physical activity. With
the aid of a number of quizzes, you will make discoveries about yourself
and your present habits that will lay the groundwork for making permanent changes. Later in the program, as you look back to see your original
answers, you will be pleasantly surprised at the transformation in your
attitudes and self-esteem.

Week Two: The DFC Nutritional Plan provides everything essential for
making the right dietary choices, including how to determine the number of daily calories you should eat in order to lose weight, sample
menus in several calorie ranges, a discussion of the six food groups, and
tempting recipes developed at the Diet and Fitness Center. Best of all,
our plan allows you to tailor your menus to suit your individual taste and
circumstance. A Daily Food Diary will encourage you to keep records of
the foods you eat.

Fitness is fundamental for weight management. *Week Three: The DFC
Fitness Program* tells you how to get into shape while you are implementing the nutritional program. The photographs will help you follow the
exercises easily, and you'll learn how to keep a Daily Exercise Log to
monitor your progress.

The theme of *Week Four: How to Be a Success Forever* is enjoying being
a thinner, healthier person. Have you eaten more than you'd planned to
at a party? Do some of your friends think you look *too* good? In this
crucial section, DFC strategies for dealing with temporary setbacks—and
even with success—will show you how to employ the tactics and re-
sources you've already developed to achieve your goals.

You have already begun to work toward a physical and psychological
transformation. Remember to look for improvement, not perfection.
Every accomplishment, no matter how small or large, will be exciting
and will help you on your journey to better health and fitness. The next
leg of that journey is self-discovery.

WEEK ONE

Getting Started

3

Getting to Know Yourself

Self-awareness is an important first step in the process of change. Like most people, you are probably able to initiate a diet and exercise program that will lead to weight loss. But, to be truly successful and to be motivated to maintain such a program, we believe that you must be as knowledgeable as possible about

- Your health and how it is influenced by your weight
- Your eating patterns and the nutritional consequences of these patterns
- Your physical activity and its effect on your health
- Your emotions and the psychological factors that contribute to your particular eating or exercise patterns

Armed with this knowledge, you can change your thinking and establish healthier patterns that eventually will become second nature.

Self-Awareness Through Assessment

At the Diet and Fitness Center, the first few days of each person's program are dedicated to a comprehensive assessment by a physician, dietitian, exercise physiologist, and psychologist. Through these assessments, each client gains greater self-awareness and is better able to structure an individual plan that is appropriate and realistic.

After Rita Caparelli's self-assessment, she began to understand what a significant impact her excess weight had made on her life. She also realized that when she had first developed diabetes, she hadn't ques-

21

tioned whether she could do anything to reduce or eliminate her reliance on daily doses of insulin. Nor had she faced up to why she was spending most of her time at home. She recognized that her attitude had been one of hopelessness. She simply had not believed that she could be successful in changing long-standing patterns. As a result of her self-assessment, Rita began to confront these uncomfortable truths: she was terribly overweight; she was endangering her health and perhaps shortening her life. Moreover, she wasn't having any fun. Step by step, as she began to make specific changes that improved her health, she began to feel better and to enjoy herself.

Nina Halloran's self-assessment led her to realize that what she really wanted was a chance to be herself without being so concerned about pleasing everyone else. She saw that she didn't have to continue overeating as long as she was willing to meet her needs in other ways. She felt that she was beginning to rediscover herself as a woman and that the good feelings she had about herself spilled over into good mothering.

During his self-assessment, John Larsen was able to pinpoint ways in which his job as a corporation president interfered with his squash games and a healthy diet. A perfectionist who had difficulty delegating responsibilities, John realized that he spent more time than necessary on the details of various projects. As a result of his revelations, John made changes in his work schedule that helped him to relax. He built in time for daily workouts that further reduced his stress level. He felt better about himself and found that healthy eating was a natural extension of his new sense of well-being.

In the questionnaires that follow, we ask you to assess the attitudes, habits, preferences, and feelings associated with your weight. We will also ask you to examine the ways in which your weight has affected your life.

Answer these questions honestly, but if you find yourself "cheating," don't be upset. Those little white lies may indicate that you need to take an even deeper look at yourself. These tests are designed to be completed in the book and to be kept as a record for your future reference. Six months from now, you may want to take some of these tests again and congratulate yourself on your progress.

Assessing Your Physical Health

Your physician's assessment of the safety of any health program, including this one, is extremely important. If you decide to embark on our program, we feel it's important that you involve your physician as a partner in your efforts. Your doctor can suggest modifications of the diet and exercise program that may be indicated because of your health. A doctor can also monitor the levels of your blood pressure, cholesterol, uric acid, and blood sugar. We suggest that your doctor measure these values before you start and, depending on your health, at periodic intervals after that. Even if you're in a low-risk category, your blood pressure and cholesterol levels will probably improve as you proceed with this program. Your doctor also may wish to monitor and adjust your medication requirements, which may change as a result of this program.

Your Weight as a Health Factor

If you have avoided knowing exactly what you weigh, then it's time to get on the scale.

1. What is your current weight? _____
2. What do you want to weigh (your goal weight)? Think about your answer, and write down the weight at which you believe you would look and feel your best. _____
3. Have you ever weighed that amount in your adult life? _____
4. How many years ago? _____

Comments
Turn to the chart on page 11 to determine your "desirable" body weight and to page 12 to calculate your percent of desirable weight. (For consistency we will use the term *desirable weight* throughout this book.)

Now, consider the following:

• 10 percent over desirable body weight, with no known medical problems (particularly hypertension, diabetes, coronary artery disease, or high cholesterol): Losing weight at this time may not be essential to your physical health. However, this book will help you to lose excess fat and to become physically fit, both of which may improve your appearance.

- 20 percent to 40 percent over desirable body weight: You are more likely to have some of the medical problems listed below, or are at greater risk of developing them in the future.
- 40 percent to 99 percent over desirable body weight: You are moderately to severely obese. Consult a physician because you are medically at risk.
- 100 pounds or more, or 100 percent over desirable body weight: You are dangerously obese, and your health is at severe risk. Use this book in working with your physician and other health professionals. You also may need a more intensive medical setting to initiate the weight loss your condition requires.

Selecting a Goal Weight

Don't be embarrassed if you selected a goal weight that is higher than your desirable weight. It's probably a more realistic weight to strive for than your desirable body weight. We believe that your goal weight is extremely important to your success because it is *your* goal, not someone else's. If you select a reasonable goal weight—one that you have previously attained and maintained as an adult—and that goal is attainable within a reasonable time frame, you are more likely to be successful.

Answer true or false to the following to determine possible medical problems associated with being overweight.

Medical Problems Associated with Being Overweight

T F I have coronary artery disease (usually manifested by angina or heart attack).

T F I have diabetes.

T F My ankles and legs are frequently swollen.

T F I have high blood pressure.

T F I have high cholesterol.

T F I have difficulty breathing.

T F I often fall asleep during the day, even in meetings or when talking to people.

T F I often have painfully stiff joints, and my hips and knees often hurt.

T F I have gallstones.

Comments

If you answered *true* (T) to any of these items, you have a medical problem commonly associated with being overweight, and you need to see your physician before starting this program. Many of these conditions may improve with weight loss and physical conditioning.

Symptoms that May Indicate Health Risks

If you are unaware of any specific health problems that affect you, the following items may uncover one or more reasons for caution.

Cardiac Symptoms

T   F   I often feel tired, even after a good night's sleep and a relaxing day.

T   F   I have discomfort in my chest, jaw, or arms when I walk, climb stairs, or get excited.

T   F   I wake up at night because I am short of breath.

T   F   I periodically have palpitations or an irregular heartbeat.

T   F   I get lightheaded when I exercise.

Comments

If you answered *true* (T) to any of these items, it is possible that you have a cardiac problem that needs medical attention, especially if you are a smoker. Obtain a health checkup immediately, and have your physician monitor you closely while you follow the DFC program.

Diabetes Symptoms

T   F   I often feel tired even after a good night's sleep and a relaxing day.

T   F   My vision becomes blurred off and on during the day.

T   F   I get frequent skin infections.

T   F   After I have gone to bed, I usually get up at least twice during the night to urinate.

T   F   (For women) I have frequent vaginal infections and discharge.

Comments

If you answered *true* (T) to any of these items, it is possible that you have diabetes mellitus and therefore need medical attention.

Arthritis Symptoms

T F I regularly have pain and stiffness in my hips, knees, and ankles.

T F I often have pain in the joints of my hands and fingers.

T F I have had severe attacks of pain in one joint such as the big toe or ankle.

Comments

If you answered *true* (T) to any of these items, you may have one or more types of arthritis and should see your physician.

Your Potential Health Risks Based on Family History

Many illnesses seem to run in families. If you know about specific diseases that have affected other members of your family, you may be able to take preventive health measures to avert the onset of these diseases or to enable their early detection.

Members of my immediate family (parents, grandparents, or siblings) have or have been treated for

coronary artery disease before the age of sixty
diabetes
high cholesterol level
high blood pressure
cancer of the colon, breast, uterus, or rectum

Comments

If any members of your immediate family have had these conditions, it is important that you see your physician at periodic intervals to screen for them. If you are overweight, you are at additional risk, so it's especially important that you have periodic screening examinations.

Assessing Psychological Aspects of Your Weight and Lifestyle

How Being Overweight Has Affected Your Life

Being overweight can significantly affect your self-esteem, your relationships, and the way you function on a day-to-day basis. How much your weight affects your life varies dramatically from person to person. Although you may think that very obese individuals are more disturbed by their weight than slightly overweight people, this is not necessarily true.

Very strong negative feelings about being overweight can trigger a vicious cycle: Being overweight lowers self-esteem and personal effectiveness, leading to social withdrawal, more overeating, and further weight gain, which leads again to more bad feelings, and back around the circle again.

T F   I avoid social gatherings because I am self-conscious about my appearance.

T F   Because of the way my body looks, I'm afraid of getting too close to anyone.

T F   I avoid sexual encounters because of my weight.

T F   I don't want anyone to see my body because of my weight.

T F   My decisions about where I go and what I do are affected by my weight.

T F   I have stopped swimming and wearing shorts because of my weight.

T F   I wouldn't feel confident going for a job interview at my current weight.

T F   I don't like myself because of my weight.

Comments

Total the number of items that you answered *true* (T), then read the appropriate evaluation.

0–2: Being overweight has very little, if any, impact on your everyday life. Because of this, you are not very likely to start a diet and exercise program, and should you do so, you might lose interest in it within a short period of time.

3–5: Your weight has a moderate impact on your life. Being aware of limitations associated with being overweight can help you feel motivated to change. Set realistic goals for yourself and notice the ways in which your life improves as you achieve these goals.

6–8: Your weight has a significant impact on many aspects of your life. You probably spend a lot of time wishing that your weight wasn't such a problem. Sometimes it may frighten you to admit that your weight is out of control. You may feel hopeless about ever being able to lose weight and get into shape. To help you feel more optimistic about your prospects for change, you may want to consider counseling.

Your Attitudes Toward Change

Have you ever been able to make changes in your eating and activity patterns, only to go back to old patterns and to regain the weight you lost? If so, particularly if this is a habitual pattern, you may have a problem with your attitudes toward change. The following items were designed to assess your attitudes toward change and to identify your particular areas of difficulty.

T F Once I reach my goal weight, my problems will vanish and my life will be completely different.

T F When I diet, I look forward to the foods I can eat once I'm off the diet.

T F After I eat something that's not on my diet, I feel like a failure. I tell myself, "I've blown it already, now I can eat whatever I want."

T F I feel successful at dieting only if I reach my goal weight.

T F Even when I eat well and exercise regularly, I feel frustrated if the scale doesn't show that I've lost weight.

T F I plan to save my large-size clothes just in case I need them again.

T F It's terribly unfair that other people eat as much as I do and don't have a weight problem.

T F Someday there will be a way I can lose weight without having to eat smaller portions of food.

T F I go on a diet to lose weight every year even though I know I will probably regain the weight.

T F I want to lose weight, but I have great difficulty making a daily effort to change my behavior.

T F I believe that eating wisely and counting calories dooms you to a life of misery.

T F It's hard to believe that what I eat and whether I exercise have much effect on my health.

T F Because I have a family history of obesity, there is nothing I can do about being overweight.

Comments

Total the number of items that you answered *true* (T), then read the appropriate evaluation.

0–2: You have realistic attitudes toward weight management and are not apt to sabotage your own plans. You expect to be successful at weight reduction and habit change even though you know that change is difficult and often frustrating.

3–8: Some of your attitudes are unrealistic and may stand in the way of your success. Identify which attitudes are self-defeating, and keep them in mind when you begin to set goals for yourself.

9–13: Your beliefs, attitudes, and expectations are unrealistic and self-destructive. You are also easily discouraged and have great difficulty with motivation. In order to achieve long-term success, you must identify and change these self-defeating patterns. Some of the goals that you set for yourself should address your attitudes. See "Strategies for Changing Destructive Attitudes and Thoughts" on page 66.

Your Emotional Eating Patterns

For some overweight people, eating is simply a love affair with food. For others, however, overeating has a strong emotional basis, and may be a way of dealing with stress, anger, anxiety, and boredom. Often such people feel controlled and obsessed by food.

T F If someone hurts me or makes me angry, I feel better if I eat something.

T F When I feel that my friends or family are disappointed in me, I turn to food for comfort.

T F When I have a lot of work pressure, I find myself eating.

T F I often find myself eating because I don't have anything else to do.

T F I only eat fattening food when I'm alone and others can't see me.

T F I overeat when I'm feeling lonely.

T F I overeat after an argument with my mate or my boss.

T F Sometimes I don't stop eating even though I feel nauseous or I can't breathe.

T F I feel very guilty and ashamed when I overeat.

T F I become panicky if food is not available when I want it.

T F I'm always thinking about food.

T F Once I start eating, I can't stop until I've finished whatever is in front of me.

T F My eating is always extreme; either I'm perfectly in control or completely out of control.

Comments

Total the number of items that you answered *true* (T), then read the appropriate evaluation.

0–2: For the most part, your eating patterns are unrelated to your emotional state. On your weight-reducing program, you need to pay particular attention to calories, portions, food preferences, eating habits, and exercise.

3–6: You have some emotional overeating tendencies that need to be addressed. Begin to pay attention to the relationship between your emotional needs and your eating patterns. See chapter 11 for a more complete discussion of emotional eating.

7–13: Food plays a central role in your emotional life. There is a strong relationship between how you feel and how much or what kinds of food you eat. Simply going on a diet does not address emotional eating tendencies. You must learn to (1) better recognize your feelings, (2) separate feelings from food, and (3) find other coping mechanisms besides eating. See chapter 11 for a complete discussion of emotional eating.

Your Personal Body Image

Often your perception of the way you look does not correspond with the way you *actually* appear.

Look at the drawings that follow and identify which of these looks like you right now.

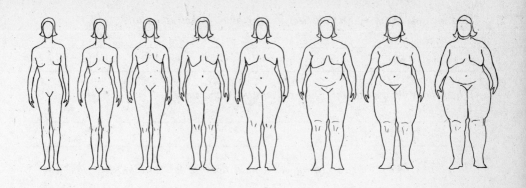

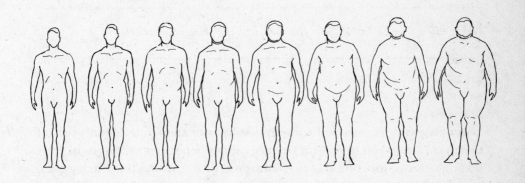

How do you feel as you look at the image you have chosen?

_____

_____

Would others agree with your self-appraisal?

_____

_____

Which body image looks the way you would like to look if you could?

_____

_____

Have you ever looked that way before?

_____

_____

How do you think you would feel if your body looked like that?

_____

_____

Which body image do you want six months from now?

_____

_____

How many pounds do you think you would have to lose to look this way?

_____

_____

How will you be different once you look like the image you selected?

_____

_____

Comments

You may perceive yourself to be much heavier than you actually are. If that is the case, you may tend to have difficulty noticing changes in your body as you reduce, or you may continue to see yourself as heavy even after you lose weight. On the other hand, you may think of yourself as thin but feel shocked when you see yourself in a photograph. If that is the case, you will probably wait too long to begin a weight reduction program because you don't realize how heavy you are. It will be very important as you change to modify your self-image as well as your behavior.

While you may never have *exactly* the body shape that you desire, it is possible to lose fat and tone muscles so that your body is much more to your liking. Visualize yourself becoming more and more like the image you have chosen, and practice good habits which will help you to reach your goals.

Assessing Your Nutritional Preferences and Habits

Promotion of overall health is a priority at the DFC. For the average person, it's sensible to eat a diet that reduces fats and simple sugars and increases complex carbohydrates and fiber. Studies indicate that such a diet combined with weight control may help to reduce the risk of certain chronic diseases.

How Your Diet Adds Up

Fat Preferences

T F I regularly eat potato chips, crackers, or cheese.

T F I often eat foods that are cooked in butter or oil or covered in rich sauces.

T F I usually eat fried foods instead of broiled or baked foods.

T F I drink several glasses of whole milk each day.

T F I eat more than one egg a day.

T F I usually put generous amounts of butter or margarine on vegetables, dinner rolls or toast, and on baked or mashed potatoes.

T F I usually eat meats such as bacon, sausage, luncheon meats, roasts, and heavily marbled steaks instead of fish and poultry.

T F I frequently eat whipped cream, heavy cream, sour cream, cream cheese, and ice cream.

Comments

Total the number of items that you answered *true* (T), then read the appropriate evaluation.

0: Your diet is probably low in fat.

1–4: Your diet, like that of many Americans, is probably too high in fat or cholesterol. You can learn simple but effective strategies for reducing your intake of fat and cholesterol.

5–8: Your diet is high in fat and cholesterol. By modifying a few food choices and habits, you can significantly decrease the amount of fat and cholesterol in your diet, which will reduce your caloric intake and lead to weight loss.

Fiber Preferences

T F I rarely eat several servings of vegetables in a day.

T F I rarely eat whole fruits with skins and/or seeds (berries, apples, pears) in a day.

T F I rarely eat food made with beans and peas more often than once or twice a week.

T F I rarely eat more than one serving of whole wheat bread and/or high-fiber cereal in a day.

Comments

Total the number of items that you answered *true* (T), then read the appropriate evaluation.

    0: You are making some good fiber choices.

    1–4: Your diet is probably low in fiber. You can improve your health by adding fresh fruits and vegetables, whole wheat breads, and high-fiber cereals to your diet.

Sugar Preferences

T F   I usually finish my meals with a dessert such as pie, ice cream, cookies, or candy.

T F   I rarely choose a piece of fruit for dessert.

T F   When I snack, I usually choose something sweet over something salty.

T F   Instead of drinking water, I usually have a soft drink or fruit juice.

Comments

Total the number of items that you answered *true* (T), then read the appropriate evaluation.

    0: Your intake of simple sugars is probably appropriate.

    1–4: Soft drinks, desserts, and other high-sugar foods provide "empty calories" and are not a good nutritional purchase. In addition, many sugar-laden foods come packaged with saturated fat. If you are interested in calorie control, you may need to spend your calories more wisely on foods that have greater nutritional value. Substitute more fruits and lower calorie beverages for sugar-laden foods.

Your Eating Patterns

To lose weight and keep it off permanently, you need to examine the ways in which you eat. As you answer these items, make a list of the problem areas. The problems are described in the paragraph following each series of items. In chapters 4 and 5, you can create specific goals and learn strategies to deal with your individual problem areas.

T F   I go to drive-up windows at fast food restaurants so that people won't be able to watch what I eat.

T F I wait until others are not around so that I can indulge in high-calorie foods.

Problem: *Closet eating.* You are self-conscious about your weight and what you eat in front of people. You fear other people's judgment. Because you believe that you are not allowed to eat certain foods, you tend to "sneak" them.

T F I never have leftovers because I eat them as I clean up after the meal.

T F I eat constantly when I'm preparing food.

Problem: *Eating during food preparation and cleanup.* You are making the mistake of eating two meals for every one you prepare. Remember, every nibble adds calories to your intake and can result in unwanted excess weight.

T F I always go back for seconds.

T F I never leave anything on my plate.

T F I prefer all-you-can-eat restaurants to restaurants where the food is served in single portions.

T F I often eat so much at night that I'm too uncomfortable to fall asleep.

Problem: *Portion control.* You are a member of the Clean Plate Club. In the chapters on nutrition, you will learn how to make appropriate choices with regard to portion sizes.

T F I eat so often that I don't know what it means to feel hungry.

T F I usually eat food when I'm watching television.

T F It is difficult to get through the night without snacking.

Problem: *Snacking between meals.* You are making the mistake of using food and habitual snacking as a way of providing yourself with an activity. It will be easier for you to control your weight once you stop snacking between meals.

T F I eat so quickly and automatically that sometimes I'm unaware of what I eat.

T F I am always the first person to finish my meal.

Problem: *Rapid eating.* You are not taking time to enjoy your meal. Slow down and learn how to give your brain enough time to signal you that you are no longer hungry.

T F   I'm usually so busy at work that I don't take time to eat lunch.

T F   I never know when I'm going to eat. Often it just depends on my mood.

T F   More often than not, I skip breakfast and lunch and begin snacking when I get home.

Problem: *Irregular meal pattern.* You have a habit that creates a chain of problems. You probably are consuming more calories than you would if you distributed your calories into three separate meals. Some structure and scheduling of meals will make a big difference in your weight control.

T F   I often eat a very large quantity of food in a short time. I know what I'm doing, but I can't stop.

T F   I often feel completely out of control when I eat.

Problem: *Binging.* You eat to satisfy emotional needs, and you are surprised, and sometimes disgusted, when you think about the quantity of food you just consumed. You can set goals and learn strategies to control your binges.

T F   I usually go to the grocery store without a shopping list.

T F   I buy whatever looks good to me.

Problem: *Lack of advance planning.* Buying whatever foods appeal to you at the moment, without a plan in mind, sets you up for overeating when you get home. Advance planning is a strategy that will help you to successfully control your weight.

T F   I never read nutrition labels on the foods that I consume on a daily basis.

Problem: *Lack of nutritional awareness.* You are not making informed food choices. Your diet may be unhealthy because of this. See the section in chapter 7 on how to read nutrition labels.

Assessing the Impact of Your Physical Condition on Your Life

What's Your Physical Condition?

Being able to perform everyday activities without undue fatigue is important. In many ways, the negative effects of inactivity are insidious and subtle. Answer true or false to the following statements which are designed to help you become aware of the possible negative impact your physical condition has on your life.

T F I avoid social or recreational settings that involve physical exertion.

T F I avoid going out or going to special events if I have to walk far to get there.

T F I avoid going shopping or going out with friends because keeping up with them leaves me short of breath.

T F I limit my activities because I feel clumsy and uncomfortable with my physical capabilities.

T F I have difficulty walking up or down a flight of stairs.

T F My sexual activity is affected by my physical condition.

T F I have difficulty bending over to tie my shoes because of my weight.

Comments

If you answered *false* to all of the preceding statements, then your physical condition allows you to lead a normally active life. If you answered *true* to four or fewer statements, then your physical condition has a moderate impact on your life. If you answered *true* to five or more of these statements, then your physical condition has a significant impact on your life and day-to-day activities. Your social and intimate relationships appear to be suffering due to your limitations. Your lack of physical ability is playing a central role in your daily life, and you are probably missing much of what life has to offer. In addition to the help this book can provide, consider seeking professional assistance for help in changing your situation.

Your Attitudes Toward Exercise

Your attitudes about exercise determine, to a large extent, whether you exercise correctly, consistently, or even whether you exercise at all. Understanding your feelings about exercise, whether they're positive or negative, can go a long way toward shaping your behavior in a constructive manner. Answer true or false to the following statements.

T   F   Making the time to exercise is a low priority.

T   F   I believe that once I've lost weight, I won't have to exercise anymore.

T   F   Once I begin exercising and I miss a day, I feel I've blown it and I quit.

T   F   I think exercise is punishment.

T   F   I am intimidated and angered by joggers, walkers, and other exercisers.

T   F   I avoid exercising because I hate to sweat.

T   F   I secretly rejoice when my doctor tells me to "take it easy" because then I have an excuse not to exercise.

Comments

If you answered *false* to all of the preceding statements, then your attitudes toward exercise are positive. If you answered *true* to any four questions, then your attitudes may be limiting your chances of viewing exercise in a positive light and reaping its many benefits. If you answered *true* to five or more of these statements, then you can assume that your negative attitudes about exercise are a limiting factor in your ability to set up a regular exercise habit. Your fear and loathing of exercise will make long-term adherence to any program a difficult task. Nevertheless, if you are willing to learn about the benefits of exercise and if you are willing to try, many of your attitudes can be overcome.

Keep Your Assessment in Mind

Now that you have completed these questionnaires, you should have a better understanding of yourself and your habits. It's time to look at your motivation and to set goals for yourself. Keep your problem areas in mind as you proceed through this book. If you forget how you fared in these quizzes, refer to them to remind yourself of some of the obstacles that may stand in your way as you work successfully to change your lifestyle. Remember that all of the areas that you have identified as problems can be addressed and changed. Four or five months, or even a year from now, take these quizzes again to see how you have changed.

4

How to Set Achievable Goals

Now that you've gained a new awareness of yourself, you can begin to set some realistic goals for making changes in your life. We will help you to make a list of goals that are positive, personal, and practical. At the DFC, we call this process of writing out lists a "strategy." As you'll see, some strategies involve several steps. Together, they provide a proven blueprint that will help you to set goals you *can* attain. As you formulate these objectives, you will better understand your motivation, as well as your ambivalence, and begin to take positive steps toward making changes you have thought about for years.

Strategy 1. Identify Your Reasons to Change

Take a hard look at the questionnaires you completed in chapter 3 and begin to identify your immediate reasons for wanting to change.

Understanding these concrete reasons can help you to stay motivated for a long period of time—perhaps for the rest of your life. Louise Borngard, thirty-eight, creative director for a large ad agency, wanted to shed the twenty-six excess pounds that had slowly crept up on her. While stylish clothes and her trademark of fabulous scarves made her look dramatic and fashionable, Louise had grown more and more uncomfortable with her weight. Her business lunches, dinners, and dates "kept" her heavy, and she didn't like the loose-fitting clothing she felt she needed to wear as a result. In quiet moments with herself, she began to notice the flab on her arms and to pinch the roll of flesh that had accumulated around her waist. Because she was a great cook and loved to eat as well as entertain, she couldn't imagine how to go about losing weight. Louise's list of immediate reasons for wanting to change included

1. I don't like having a fat stomach!
2. I want to wear the fitted clothes that make me look the most attractive.
3. I hate being overweight.

Mark Loomis, on the other hand, hadn't been terribly bothered by his weight because he was a successful businessman who was well adjusted to being 6'1″ and weighing 240 pounds. His employees worshiped him and were thrilled when he was named by *Black Enterprise* as one of the top twenty black executives in New York City. Mark had close friends and enjoyed an active social life. Nevertheless, he began to feel worn out, even exhausted, at the end of the business day. He developed high blood pressure and was put on a hypertensive medication that interfered with his sexual performance. His doctor told him that he should lose weight because his heart was under too much stress. Mark's immediate reasons for wanting to change included

1. I don't have enough energy.
2. I want to have a happier sex life.
3. I don't want to have a heart attack or a stroke.

Make a list of your own immediate reasons for wanting to change.

My Reasons to Change

1. _____

   _____

2. _____

   _____

3. _____

   _____

4. _____

   _____

5. _____

   _____

Strategy 2. Plan Your Long-Term Goals

Now, imagine where you would like to be if you could snap your fingers and magically achieve all your ultimate goals by tomorrow.

Your long-term goals may seem almost impossible to reach, but it's important to imagine the treasure at the end of the rainbow. The process of setting and visualizing these long-term goals will help you to maintain your long-term motivation. Without them, you are likely to quit too soon—reaching some of your goals, but falling short of what you really want to achieve.

Louise's long-term goals were

1. I want to wear size 8 clothing for the rest of my life.
2. I want to look smashing for the rest of my life.
3. I want to be physically fit for the rest of my life.

Mark's long-term goals were

1. I want to lower my blood pressure and eliminate the need for medication.
2. I want to enjoy sex for the rest of my life.
3. I want to increase my energy and stamina.
4. I want to live to be 104!

In making your own lists, most of you will have weight loss as your first goal, but don't forget the goals of fitness, better self-image, and a healthier lifestyle as well.

Long-term goals may be modified as your needs and desires change. For example, once you have lost twenty-five pounds, your new long-term goal may be to maintain your weight and never to gain back excess weight. If your goal, like Mark's, is to stop taking hypertensive medicine, your new list of long-term goals may include the following:

1. I'll stay off blood pressure medication.
2. I'll continue an active and pleasurable sex life.
3. I'll learn how to play tennis.

Visualize your goals and think in terms of six months from now, one or two years from now, even ten or twenty years from now. Make the list as long and as complicated as you'd like.

My Long-Term Goals

1. _____

   _____

2. _____

   _____

3. _____

   _____

4. _____

   _____

5. _____

   _____

6. _____

   _____

7. _____

   _____

Strategy 3. Plan Your Short-Term Goals

Step 1. Set Goals for Yourself, Not for Others

Learn to be the center of your own life. Don't try to lose weight to please or impress others. Taking care of yourself—looking better and feeling better—will also benefit the people who love and care about you. You may feel uncomfortable and selfish at first, but with practice, you will be able to put your own needs first without sacrificing those of others.

It's important to acknowledge this principle and keep it in mind when setting any goals.

Step 2. Set Small Goals

Small, practical goals that you can accomplish in a short period of time are often the easiest approach to major transformations. Sometimes long-term goals seem overwhelming. That's why it's so important to break them down into smaller tasks that you can accomplish one day and one week at a time so you won't feel defeated before you start. As you incorporate these small changes into your life, you can gradually add new short-term goals.

If your long-term aim is to improve your cardiovascular system and avoid heart surgery, for instance, start by setting a short-term goal of exercising at an appropriate level for your fitness, perhaps ten to fifteen minutes a day. Although your long-term goal may be to exercise for forty-five minutes five days a week, you need to start slowly and add time as you progress.

Louise Borngard is a good example of how these gradual changes can work. Louise determined to lose a total of twenty-six pounds—which would put her weight back to where it was in her twenties. When she first began, she was used to having a glass of wine at lunch and two cocktails before dinner, followed by wine with her meal. Setting only small goals at first, she begin drinking wine spritzers with lunch. After three weeks, she began to drink only one spritzer at lunch. As she made each change, she thought of it as permanent, and it became so. Eventually she had only an occasional cocktail and one glass of wine with dinner.

Louise also happened to be a gourmet cook who viewed butter as an essential ingredient. She eliminated excess fat from her cooking in small steps. First she started cooking with small, measured amounts of olive oil instead of butter. After a couple of months, she began to alternate olive oil with a no-stick spray that contained no oil and no calories. She also began steaming, baking, and broiling more of her food. She followed a caloric regime that started at 1,200 calories a day and eventually rose to 1,500. In addition, she began exercising by walking around her neighborhood a few times a week until she was walking forty-five to sixty minutes five or six times a week. She added a block each week.

Step 3. Transform Bad Habits into a Series of Manageable Tasks

Deeply ingrained habits are hard to stop, and you can't just wish them away. Breaking them down into smaller, more easy-to-accomplish goals makes your task simpler. John Larsen had trouble with nighttime snacking, so he started with a plan to limit his snack to 150 calories. The second week, he limited it to 100 calories, and the third week, to 50. To help him avoid temptation, he played squash, went for walks with his wife, played bridge, or talked to friends on the phone. After a few weeks, he was able to completely stop snacking at night without even missing it. Like John, when you succeed at accomplishing smaller goals, you'll gradually break deeply ingrained habits that aren't good for your health or your weight.

Step 4. Make Your Goals Realistic

The danger in perfectionism and unrealistic commitments is that they simply don't work.

Unrealistic Goals
1. I'll walk one hour a day and do aerobics six days a week.
2. I'll stick with a 1,000-calorie diet for the rest of my life.
3. I'm going on vacation for three weeks and I will come back five pounds thinner.
4. I'm going trick-or-treating with the kids at Halloween and I won't have any candy.
5. I'm baking cookies for the church bake sale and I won't eat any of them!

In order to achieve long-term success, you need to find goals that you can live with and incorporate into your daily schedule.

Realistic Goals
1. I'll start my exercise program by walking fifteen minutes four mornings a week.
2. I'll eat 1,200 calories a day for the next two weeks.
3. On vacation, I'll eat well-balanced meals, limit the portions of the foods I want, and maintain my current weight without gaining.
4. On Halloween, I'll allow myself two or three pieces of candy that I'll eat at the end of the evening.
5. I'll buy cookies for the church bake sale and deliver them directly to the church from the store so that I won't be tempted to eat any of them.

Remember, if your goals are not realistic, you are setting yourself up for failure.

Step 5. Set Specific, Concrete Goals

If your goal is to "stop cheating," and you plan to have two scoops of ice cream on Friday night, you may still feel that you cheated, when in fact you succeeded at planning and controlling what you ate. Vague, unspecified goals aren't helpful. Instead, specify exactly what you plan to do.

Don'ts
- I'm going to be good this week.
- I'm going to exercise this week.
- I'm going to stop cheating.

Dos
- This week, I'm going to eat 1,200 calories a day.
- I'm going to walk for twenty-five minutes after dinner every evening this week.
- I'm going to plan my meals two days in advance and stick with the plan.

Step 6. Set Positive, Not Negative, Goals

Negative goals make you feel deprived instead of making you feel good about your accomplishments.

Negative
- I won't have any high-calorie drinks this week.
- No more pigging out while I watch TV!

Positive
- I'll choose club soda with a twist of lime this week.
- I'll play the piano for one hour at night. After that, I'll read.

Step 7. Avoid All-Or-Nothing Thinking

Don't set all-or-nothing goals and then expect perfection. If your goals make you feel deprived, you'll be set up to go overboard and then quit after having "failed" to achieve impossible goals. If you know that you're going to have particular cravings and can plan for them and limit your portions, you won't feel that you have to be perfect or punished.

Don't Say:
- I'll *never* eat butter again!
- I will *never* eat another sweet thing!
- I'm *never* going to watch TV again because it gives me too many food cues.

Do Say:
- This week I'm not going to eat butter on my toast.
- Today I'm going to eat fruit to satisfy my craving for something sweet.

By eliminating all-or-nothing thinking, you'll avoid a sense of failure if you achieve only part of your goal.

It was natural for Nina Halloran to set up no-win situations for herself. When her children were young, Nina periodically would decide she *had* to do something about her weight. She'd vow never again to eat ice cream, candy, or desserts. "Some people live their whole lives without sweet stuff," she would tell herself. "You can do it! It's just mind over matter!" She usually succeeded for about three weeks. Then she would have a major binge on candy, cookies, and ice cream. She admitted that during those binges it wasn't unusual for her to consume two candy bars, half a bag of cookies, and a pint of ice cream in one evening.

Through the DFC program, Nina learned how to set more practical, less perfect goals. Now, she plans to have a favorite dessert every Friday. She eats it in a controlled fashion and doesn't feel guilty or deprived. She still has an occasional binge, which she has learned to control by purchasing smaller quantities than previously. She no longer blames herself or feels like a failure. Instead, she acknowledges that she has deviated from her plan, accepts that she doesn't have to be perfect to succeed, and continues with her daily change-of-habits program.

Step 8. Establish Fall-Back Positions

Set up a series of choices in your goals that lie between perfection and failure. Your first aim may be not to eat any desserts this week. A second aim could be a low-calorie dessert. That way, even if you don't stick to your main plan, the caloric content will be low. A second fall-back position would be to eat the dessert you want, but to limit the portion.

Step 9. Praise Yourself for Reaching Small Goals

It's extremely important to recognize and appreciate each small accomplishment. They are your building blocks for long-term success.

Here's how Louise dealt with her goals. Although she wondered whether the changes she was making were large enough to reach her ultimate desires, she took our advice and congratulated herself on small changes. Each time she drank a spritzer for lunch, she told herself she was doing a great job. After she had cooked with olive oil instead of butter for a week, she treated herself to a manicure. When she went out to an elaborate dinner party and controlled what she ate, she congratulated herself by going to a movie she had wanted to see. When Louise had total lapses or used a fall-back position that didn't meet her goal, she reminded herself not to feel guilty, that everyone slips up every now and then. It wasn't long before she realized that this was exactly the right way to approach her long-term goals. After the first year of her program, Louise had lost sixteen pounds. The second year, she lost an additional ten pounds.

By taking a series of small steps, and by praising yourself for each goal that you reach, no matter how small, you, like Louise, can make a transformation that will endure.

Step 10. Don't Use the Scale as Your Only Measure of Success

The scale is only one indicator of success—and not a very reliable one at that. Even though you've been achieving your short-term goals of eating better and exercising, *the scale does not necessarily respond consistently to the changes you have made or the work you have accomplished.* Don't you remember times that you've eaten to excess for several days or a week and not had any weight gain? During those times you may have believed that you could get away with eating everything you wanted to eat, but then suddenly, the scale jumped five pounds!

In the same way, you can watch your food intake carefully for several days, or even for a week or more, without the scale reflecting any weight loss. Many people give up at this point because the scale doesn't show what they expect. Don't let this happen to you. The scale will eventually catch up with your habit changes. Don't allow the numbers on the scale to interfere with your progress.

Step 11. Write Down Your Short-Term Goals

Use the following sample lists of short-term goals as a guide for creating your own goals. Notice that even though these are short-term goals, which can be set for one day, one week, or one month, they could also be goals that you will want to maintain on a long-term basis. Which ones would you be willing to set for yourself now? After you read the lists, write down your own short-term goals. Make daily and weekly goals.

Include a variety of objectives—not just weight—and list as many as you think you can realistically accomplish. Be as specific as you can. These are the goals you propose to achieve. They suit *you* and will work for you. They are your framework for success.

Remember to work on only a few goals at a time. As you accomplish them, you can gradually add new goals to your list. Over a period of time, as you are setting up new goals, you can refer to this list for ideas.

Weight
I will lose _____ pounds this week.
I will weigh myself two times this week and record the weight.
I will measure my hips and begin to chart my progress.

Food Intake (See pages 84–85 for calculating your calorie intake.)
I will limit my calorie intake to _____ calories a day.
I will plan my meals one day in advance.
I will write down the calories I eat after every meal.
I will keep my food diary up to date.
I will plan my meals to avoid leftovers.

Nutritional Goals
I will eat three well-balanced meals a day.
I will eat a variety of foods that are good for me and that are
  within my caloric budget for the day.
If I am tempted to have a snack between meals, I will drink seltzer
  with a twist of lime in it.
I will avoid foods that are high in fat and sugar.
I will eat fresh and nutritious foods.

Exercise (See page 290 for determining your exercise prescription.)
I will plan my exercise and keep a record to measure my progress.
I will walk _____ minutes a day.
I will ride my exercise bike _____ minutes when I can't walk
  outside because of the weather.

Appearance
I will look in the mirror every day and notice changes.
I will try a new hairstyle this week.
I will try wearing a new color tie or scarf today.
I will take time to dress especially well for work tomorrow.

Health

I will decrease my stress this week by doing deep relaxation exercises for twenty minutes a day after work.

I will get the sleep I need this week so that I will feel better and have more energy during the day.

I will have my cholesterol and blood pressure checked on a regular basis.

Self-Esteem

I will write down my feelings every day in my journal.

Today and every day for the rest of this week, I will think positive thoughts about myself when I wake up in the morning, even if I feel I'm making them up.

I will decrease negative thoughts about myself.

I will try to make one new social contact this week.

This week, I will try to think about how other people feel instead of thinking about how nervous I am or how I appear to them.

Attitude

I will feel good about all of my accomplishments, no matter how insignificant they may seem.

I will view food planning as a gift to myself rather than as a punishment.

I will recognize my resentment about needing to lose weight and reduce those feelings.

I will tell myself that my weight is not my identity!

I will say every day, "It's never too late for changes!"

I will embrace the idea that it's good to do these things for myself, and that I will feel happier and look better as a result of doing them.

12. Review and Reevaluate Your Goals

All goals need to be reevaluated and revised over time.

Reasons to Change a Goal

• You have achieved the goal, and you are ready to add new or more challenging goals.

• You have recognized that a particular goal you set was unrealistic or didn't fit into your lifestyle.

• You have become aware of an obstacle to a goal which makes that goal unattainable.

Following a setback, it's especially important to revise your short-term goals. Establish small, simple goals that you can easily accomplish. These will rebuild your motivation and commitment. For example, if you were walking forty-five minutes five days a week, and you stopped walking because you got sick, revise your exercise goals. Your new goal might be to walk at a comfortable pace for twenty minutes. Add five minutes each week, and in a short while you will be up to your previous level without getting discouraged along the way.

Strategy 4. Assess Your Motivation

Maintaining the focus to accomplish a goal—any goal—requires long-term motivation. This means that you need to value the goal and expect to achieve it. You need motivation to make plans, to take deliberate actions, to endure discomfort in getting through challenging times, and to maintain your resolve. Motivation is key to your long-term weight control. At first, change may be difficult and awkward. But eventually, new habits become old and familiar, and you take them in stride as part of your life.

Step 1. Consider Your Feelings about Your Weight

At the DFC, we have found that a person's level of discomfort with appearance and weight affects motivation to achieve a goal of weight reduction.

If you are experiencing

- *Moderate discomfort,* your motivation to change is probably high because your discomfort isn't overwhelming but is sufficient to motivate you to do what is necessary.
- *Very little discomfort,* your motivation to change your eating or exercise habits may be low because being overweight doesn't adversely affect your life on a day-to-day basis.
- *Extremely disturbed and troubled,* you may lack motivation because you feel overwhelmed by what is required of you or you are too anxious to begin changing your habits.

It's interesting that your own feelings of dissatisfaction about your weight don't necessarily correspond to how overweight you are. You might think, for instance, that a woman who is 5′4″ and weighs 125 pounds feels great about herself, and that any man or woman who weighs 320 pounds is miserable, but that's not necessarily so. We've seen people who are 100 pounds overweight who are not consciously miserable, and we've seen men and women who are only ten or twenty pounds overweight who *are* miserable—and everything in between.

What does being overweight mean to you? Do you hate your weight on a daily basis, or is your weight a concern only when you shop for clothes or go on vacation? Can you visualize yourself as a person who is fit and thin? Even if you have difficulties with your motivation, don't be discouraged. You can strengthen and reinforce your motivation by following the steps we're presenting here.

Step 2. Consider Your Belief in Yourself

Believing that you can change is a positive factor in achieving change. If you hate the way you look, but lack faith in your ability to change, you may want to see a therapist or a counselor to help you deal with your feelings of hopelessness *before* you start trying to manage your weight. Gaining insight into your feelings and becoming aware of your options can give you confidence in your ability to set and achieve long-term goals. Once you believe you can change, then your motivation to work at modifying your habits and reaching your objectives will increase.

Step 3. Think about Your Ambivalence Toward Change

Everyone has feelings of ambivalence. This doesn't apply only to weight control; it applies to many areas of life. You may want to stop smoking, change jobs, lose weight, leave a bad relationship, or develop your muscles. You may want to do these things but not get around to them because of conflicting feelings about change.

Fear

Fear is a major reason for not making changes. No matter how eager you are to be thinner, healthier, and more beautiful, actually achieving these goals can trigger new, strange, and unpredictable feelings—even if you've been thin sometime earlier in your life. You know what to expect from yourself as you are now. Even if you're miserable, it's easier to stay the same because changing and doing things differently require effort, thought, and commitment, which may frighten you. Thinness may bring new expectations, from yourself and others.

Pleasure in Eating

Another reason you may want to stay the same is because you get gratification from eating. You don't want to give up your snacks or your daily dish of ice cream!

Hating Physical Exercise

You have the pleasure of not being physically active. You can sleep in rather than getting up for an early morning walk or sit down for a snack instead of going for a swim.

Weight as an Excuse

You can blame your failures and difficulties on being overweight without looking at any other possible reasons. If you didn't get a job promotion, for example, you can blame it on your weight. If you don't date, you can attribute it to being heavy without looking for other possible explanations.

Stalling for Time

You can put off doing things that you have associated with being thinner. You don't have to seek a job promotion, meet new friends, or buy new clothes as long as you are heavy. You can "save" these things for when you lose weight.

Step 4. Evaluate the Pros and Cons of Change

Write down your positive and negative feelings about exercising, eating nutritiously, losing weight, and becoming healthier and more attractive.

The following lists, created by Rita Caparelli and Mark Loomis, include the pros and cons of short- and long-term goals.

Rita Caparelli's Pros and Cons of Change

Pro

1. My sister will stop nagging me.
2. I hate the way I look now; maybe I will look and feel better!
3. Maybe I will get off insulin and control my diabetes.
4. I can buy pretty clothes.
5. I'll feel great about myself!

Con

1. I'm terrified of feeling deprived!
2. I hate exercise!
3. My kids will expect me to get out of the house and get a better job.
4. I won't be able to eat ice cream, chocolate candy, and cookies every day!
5. Everyone will fuss over me if I lose weight! But I'll be the same person that I am now! I'm scared of what I'll be like thin!

Mark Loomis's Pros and Cons of Change

Pro

1. I'll feel good doing what is best for my health.
2. My heart condition will improve!
3. My doctor will be pleased.
4. My sex life will improve.
5. I'll look more athletic.

Con

1. I hate limiting my portions! I won't be able to eat what I want!
2. I won't be able to drink as much as I want to.
3. Planning meals and exercising will take time away from my business.
4. I've always been big. I'll feel silly and weak when my body is smaller.
5. Will people like me just as much if I'm different?

Now make your own list. Be as honest as you can in evaluating your motivation. Think about what you have just learned about your dissatisfaction with your weight, as well as your motivation, belief in yourself, and ambivalence. Write down what you have to gain and what you have to lose if you achieve your short- and long-term goals.

My Pros and Cons of Change

Pro

1. _____

2. _____

3. _____

4. _____

5. _____

Con

1. _____

2. _____

3. _____

4. _____

5. _____

Compare your pros and cons. By looking at the positive consequences, you'll see the ways in which you are motivated to achieve your goals. By looking at the negative consequences, you'll see some of the obstacles in your path and understand changes that you need to make in your attitude. This list also will give you a sense of what you have to look forward to, and strengthen the short- and long-term goals that you want to achieve.

Step 5. Accentuate the Positive

If you've failed at dieting before, you may worry that you won't be able to maintain your motivation on this health plan for a long time. Bolster your confidence by thinking about past successes you've had. Certainly you needed long-term motivation to get through college or to finish a big project at work. You were successful when you learned a new job skill or went after something else that was important to you. Now you take those accomplishments for granted because you've already achieved them and because they're part of your life.

Someday you will also be able to take being healthier and thinner for granted. You'll be used to healthy habits, and they will be natural and comfortable to maintain on a day-to-day basis. You'll be amazed to look back at the changes that you have made.

You have already begun working toward being a more healthy and fit person. Now you can begin implementing strategies that will help you achieve your goals. Remember to give yourself credit for each goal that you reach, and congratulate yourself often.

5

Strategies for Reaching Your Goals

We believe that most inappropriate eating and activity patterns are learned habits. While you may view yourself as a "compulsive eater," for instance, very few overweight people have a truly compulsive eating disorder. Instead, it's likely that you eat in response to certain cues, such as the sight and smell of food, social pressure, feelings that are hard to deal with, or thoughts about personal weaknesses. Unlearning these old habits requires active problem solving and behavior change, rather than reliance on willpower.

At the DFC, we teach you how to achieve your goals through a variety of *strategies* that you can utilize for the rest of your life. Strategies are specific plans or tools for success. Many people rely on willpower and the excitement of a new diet program to achieve weight control, only to discover that these quickly fade and weight control becomes a struggle once more. Permanent weight control requires long-term planning and application of strategies.

In this chapter, you will learn strategies for changing any unwanted habits, as well as strategies for continuing your progress. Some of these strategies relate directly to your personal weight control goals (for example, how to decrease caloric intake by preplanning in a diary, or how to avoid the temptation of high-calorie foods), and others address issues that may indirectly influence your ability to control your weight (for example, how to change destructive thought patterns, obtain social support, change body image, and decrease stress). Keep these strategies in mind as you embark on your lifestyle change program.

Strategies for Changing Your Habits

Step 1. Identify and Interrupt Ingrained Habits That Cause You Problems

You may shower *after* breakfast and read your mail *before* cooking dinner because that's the way you've always done it. These habits, just like many of your eating and activity patterns, are second nature to you. To change such deeply ingrained habits, you must

1. Identify a habit you want to change
2. Observe the sequence of events leading up to the behavior
3. Implement a plan of action that interrupts the sequence of events and leads to achieving more positive behavior

To begin with, let's look at an example of a habit that does not involve eating. Mark Loomis never remembered to use his seat belt, and he wanted to use it regularly. Calling upon a DFC strategy, he identified the sequence of events leading up to the behavior. He found that normally he unlocked the car door, got in, adjusted the mirror, turned on the ignition, backed out of the driveway, and drove off. The plan of action he decided on was to unlock the car door, get into the car, see a large plastic trash bag on the steering wheel that he placed there the night before, which reminds him to put on the seat belt. Then he removes the trash bag, adjusts the mirror, starts the car, backs out, and drives off. The trash bag doesn't make him change his behavior, but it serves as a reminder that interrupts his usual habits. Once he is reminded, he can choose what to do. For the strategy to be effective, he needs to be motivated and willing to make the decision to put on his seat belt. The same applies to the following examples about food and exercise.

Problem: Nina Halloran eats a snack around 10:30 every evening.
   Goal: to break the habit.
   Sequence of events:
1. Sits in the den, watching the late news on television with her husband.
2. After the news, husband fixes two bowls of ice cream.
3. They eat the ice cream in the den.

Strategy:

1. Nina watches the late news in the upstairs bedroom.
2. Asks husband not to offer and not to bring her a bowl of ice cream, but to bring her a glass of ice water instead.
3. Asks husband to eat his ice cream downstairs, not in front of her.
4. Reads a book before her husband comes to bed.

Result: This strategy worked for Nina. When she changed her usual sequence of events, her urge to eat ice cream was not as strong as it had been previously.

Mark Loomis dealt with his exercise problem by using the same technique he used to solve his seat belt problem.

Problem: "forgetting" to exercise.

Goal: to exercise five days a week.

Sequence of events:

1. At the end of the day, Mark gets his mail out of the mailbox.
2. Goes into his house.
3. Has a soft drink.
4. Reads his mail.
5. Fixes dinner.
6. Eats and cleans up.
7. Talks on the phone and takes care of leftover business.
8. At bedtime, he is too tired to work out on his rowing machine but remembers that he has forgotten to do it.

Strategy:

1. Puts a red piece of paper in his mailbox that serves as an exercise reminder when he picks up his mail after work.
2. Goes into his house.
3. Immediately changes into his sweat suit.
4. Rows for half an hour.
5. Continues with his evening activities.

Result: It was easier for Mark than he imagined it would be to break his habit of forgetting to exercise. He found that he enjoyed his new routine so much that he looked forward to it.

Make your own diagrams of the problem, the goal, and the sequence of events which lead up to a certain habit of your own that inhibits your progress toward your goal. Begin with one or two automatic or predictable reactions. Next to each sequence, write in the strategies that will help you to develop new and productive habits.

Step 2. Understand the Concept of Food Cues

Stimuli in your environment that are associated with eating or that trigger overeating are called "food cues." It's important to understand how different situations trigger repeated behavior that ends up boosting your consumption of excess calories even when you are not particularly hungry.

External food cues may be
- the time of day (the 10:30 P.M. snack)
- location (in the den or some other specific place you associate with eating)
- the situation (you nibble while you're preparing dinner)
- the smell or the sight of food (a dish of candy that's sitting on a table or a food advertisement in a magazine or on television)

Social food cues stem from
- celebrations that are associated with eating and camaraderie
- finding it difficult not to eat when you see others eating
- recreational eating

Physiological food cues can include
- hunger
- fatigue
- a desire for increased energy

Psychological food cues happen
- when the antecedent to eating is a feeling—such as anger, anxiety, loneliness, or sadness
- as a result of habit
- from ambivalent feelings about losing weight
- food preparation that is a source of pleasure and gratification
- eating as a source of pleasure, reward, and self-esteem

Step 3. Identify Your Own Food Cues

A major strategy for breaking habits that sabotage your efforts to lose weight is to identify the food cues associated with your eating behavior. This strategy allows you to anticipate times when you will be vulnerable and plan for them.

Sometimes identifying food cues can be confusing because the process actually involves a complex chain of stimuli and responses. When people are trying to lose weight, they often put all of their energy into changing the final response in a behavior chain through the strategy of willpower—for example, they see the cookies and try *not* to eat them. Although willpower is an option, there are a number of other strategies to implement at an earlier stage. The earlier you intervene in a chain of events that lead to overeating, the easier it is for you to resist temptation.

After Nathan Bennett ate a number of cookies, for instance, he tried to figure out what food cues were involved. He was surprised at the lengthy chain of cues and responses that had led to his overeating. Nathan figured out that

a. he had been anxious about the load of work he had to do, which
b. contributed to an argument with his brother.
c. Later on, when watching television, he
d. saw a commercial for chocolate cake and
e. thought, "That looks great! I'm feeling hungry."
f. He decided to take a walk, with no particular destination in mind.
g. On the walk, he noticed a convenience store and
h. went in, theoretically to buy a quart of milk.
i. He spotted the cookie aisle and
j. bought chocolate chip cookies.
k. He got home and
l. put the cookies in the cookie jar on the counter.
m. Later, he caught sight of the cookies in the jar and
n. ate the cookies.

In Nathan's case, a number of strategies might have worked to intervene or to break the cycle of events. Knowing that anxiety about his work often predisposes him toward irritability with others and a desire to eat, he could have decreased his stress by

1. Doing relaxation exercises.
2. Staying late at the school library to catch up on his work.
3. Talking to his brother about their argument and attempting to resolve their differences.
4. Walking in the other direction (away from the store), or making sure not to bring any money with him on his walk.

5. Having walked past the store, he could have told himself that even though he had run out of milk, it would be better not to go into a food store in his present state of mind. He could do without milk, or his mother could get some later.
6. If he did go into the convenience store, he could avoid walking down the cookie aisle since he knows it will tempt him.
7. He could see the cookies at the grocery store but decide to buy fruit or a lower-calorie snack instead of cookies.

Once you recognize the feelings, the physiological states, the social or environmental situations, and the times of day that have become established as your "food cues," you can plan to break those automatic associations that you have traditionally responded to by eating.

List your major food cues here.

External/Social	Physiological/Psychological
1. Tempting food at party	1. Test anxiety
2. _____	2. _____
3. _____	3. _____
4. _____	4. _____
5. _____	5. _____

Focus on what strategy you can set up for yourself to offset ingrained habits and associations. List the proposed strategies that will interrupt the sequence of events that triggers your eating.

External/Social	Physiological/Psychological
1. Socialize away from food table	1. Do relaxation exercises
2. _____	2. _____
3. _____	3. _____
4. _____	4. _____
5. _____	5. _____

Step 4. Anticipate Breaking the Chain. Imagine Yourself Using a Strategy at a Vulnerable Time Rather Than Eating

Visualize difficult situations that tempt you and then picture your success in choosing an option other than eating. This will help you practice these strategies when you have the opportunity.

Step 5. Plan Ahead! Don't Wait Until You're Overtaken by Events and Have an Overwhelming Urge to Eat

For instance, you know that you always eat too much on Friday nights. Ask a friend to go to the movies with you or plan to go to a social function or a concert. Anticipate these occasions so you won't have to rely on willpower because you will have given yourself options much earlier in the process.

Remember that the goal is not to develop willpower, but to succeed at better eating and health habits that will lead to weight loss. For example,

- If pastries drive you wild, don't go into the bakery.
- If you are a chocoholic, don't volunteer to make fudge and brownies for the school bake sale.
- Don't buy a dozen donuts or bagels for your office staff if you can't resist two or three for yourself. Bring strawberries or flowers instead.
- Don't buy candy for your secretary or for the grandchildren if it will tempt you.
- Don't think it's "silly and childish" not to have enough control to keep sweets in the house and not eat them. It's *smart* not to have sweets in the house, because that's what works!

Strategies for Continuing Progress: Record Keeping

Step 1. Record Changes in Your Weight

Weigh yourself once or twice a week and record your weight in the weight loss chart at the end of this section (see page 76).

Remember that you will need to recalculate your rate of weight loss as you make progress (see page 75 for instructions on calculating weight loss). When you are the heaviest, you will be able to lose weight more rapidly. As you lose weight, however, your rate of weight loss will slow down. Expect some plateaus and periods in which your weight loss will be almost imperceptible. Don't be discouraged!

Step 2. Record Changes in Your Measurements

Every month, record the measurements that are the most important to you, such as those of your waist, hips, thighs, arms, chest, and calves. Sometimes even when the scale doesn't reflect changes, you will see your measurements decrease due to the exercise you've been doing. This will encourage you to continue your good work. (See the chart on page 77.)

Step 3. Record What You Eat in a Food Diary

At the DFC, we use a small diary that lists the portion, the food, and its total calories, with a place to record the number of foods you eat from each food group.

In your own diary (see page 136 for sample), you should write down exactly what you eat during the day. At the end of the day, total the calories and notice how many items you have checked off from each food group. (For more on the checking system, see chapter 6.) Do weekly totals as well. This system will help you to limit what you eat and drink.

Step 4. Record Your Exercise

Keep an exercise log (see page 310 for sample). Plan and record each walk, workout, or exercise session. At the end of the week, review your exercise record and see what you've accomplished. (For more on setting up your exercise prescription, see page 290.)

Step 5. Record and Review the Goals You Have Reached

Recording the goals that you reach on a daily or weekly basis can give you a real sense of accomplishment. By keeping a daily record, you'll be able to see the progress you're making toward your short- and long-term goals.

Review and evaluate your progress at the same time each week, perhaps on Sunday night. Evaluate the progress you've made toward your larger goals on a monthly basis as well. When you are feeling low and like an underachiever, get out your weight and measurement charts and graphs. These records will remind you of how far you've come.

Step 6. Reward Yourself for Progress

If you have set four short-term goals for yourself for the day, and you have achieved three of them, praise yourself out loud. You may feel silly hearing yourself say: "Good job! I'm doing well. I deserve to feel good about myself and what I am doing. I'm doing what I've set out to do! I'm on my way to success." It's important to take credit for what you've accomplished and to *hear* the praise.

Reward yourself by taking time to do something pleasurable that you wouldn't normally do. Make a long-distance telephone call to a friend or take time to soak in a hot bath before going to bed.

When you've achieved your goals for a week or two, buy yourself flowers or a book. Give yourself a new shirt or a music tape. Schedule some luxury: get a stylish new haircut, a massage, a facial, a manicure, whatever makes you feel pampered.

After the first or second month, buy tickets for a special event. Ask your spouse or a friend to go out with you for the evening and celebrate. Or have a weekend vacation. You are making progress and you deserve rewards!

Step 7. Update Your Goals

As you begin accomplishing your short-term goals, you may begin losing some of your motivation to continue. If, for instance, you wanted to lose weight so you'd look good at your cousin's wedding, and you did that, then you will no longer have that goal. When your clothes become looser, you will lose your inspiration to get into them. When you can breathe more easily and feel better about your body, you will have lost two more reasons for continuing to utilize the new behavior habits you have learned.

Recognize the progress you've made and gradually update your goals. Add new and different ones. An essential strategy in your continuing effort is to be realistic about what is possible on a daily basis. Keep setting goals that you can accomplish. Remember that each small step adds up. Before you realize it, you will have accomplished a great deal. You will feel so good about yourself that those feelings will further stimulate your progress.

Strategies for Changing Destructive Attitudes and Thoughts

If you can develop and maintain a positive and realistic attitude toward weight loss and exercise, you will stand a good chance of reaching your goals. Negative thoughts weaken your motivation and impede your progress. Changing these attitudes is not always easy, but you can do it!

Step 1. Identify and Change Your Destructive Attitudes

Identify which of the following destructive patterns apply to you:

Expecting immediate results. Most problems do not disappear overnight, but if you remember that any progress is better than none, ultimately you will be successful.

Expecting yourself to be perfect. When you deviate from your food or exercise plan, forgive yourself and tell yourself it's progress you're seeking, not perfection. You can reach your goals without setting impossibly high standards.

Being overly critical of yourself. Practice saying positive things about yourself. Instead of saying, "I was bad!" say, "It was a bad choice to buy those cookies." Feeling guilty and calling yourself names is destructive rather than constructive.

Expecting change to occur magically. Change requires thought, action, and commitment, not magic or wishful thinking.

Getting discouraged or easily frustrated. If you expect setbacks and uneven progress, you will not be so easily discouraged or frustrated. Long-term success is a gradual process. As long as you're making gradual changes in your habits, you'll be successful.

Expecting yourself to fail. Expecting failure often leads to failure because you're likely to stop trying when you reach an obstacle. Believe in yourself and you won't be as likely to quit when you experience a setback.

Seeing catastrophes where there are merely difficulties. Difficulties are inevitable in life. Learn to regard them as obstacles that can be overcome.

Feeling resentful about having to change. Remember that resentment only stands in the way of progress. Practice letting it go. Put your resentment in an imaginary garbage bag and throw it out with the trash.

Expecting your problems to disappear when you've lost weight. If you believe this, you are bound to be disappointed. Weight reduction does not guarantee a happier life, a new romance, or a job promotion.

Expecting no pain, no gain. There is no virtue in deprivation. You need not punish yourself to be successful.

Being preoccupied with food. Redirect your thoughts away from food. Avoid looking at food spreads in magazines, and limit discussion of recipes and restaurants. Discover other pleasures and interests besides food. Direct your thoughts in other ways. Think about the interesting people that you met, the great discussion that you had, the unusual movie that you saw, or the new art gallery that is opening.

Step 2. Give Yourself Positive Reinforcement for the Things You Do Well

When you're having a problem remaining motivated, praising yourself for past accomplishments will help you deal with your present difficulties in a more realistic manner. Tell yourself that you are a terrific person and that every day you are getting closer to your goals. Be sure to congratulate yourself for every one of your accomplishments, even if they seem small.

Step 3. Practice Taking Responsibility for Yourself Today

Start with positive messages, such as, "Today I am in charge of my life. Today I will be good to myself. I deserve what's good for me."

Step 4. Accept Compliments from Others

If you are like Rita Caparelli, you may have difficulty accepting compliments. Whenever someone told her how great she was looking, she got angry and thought, "It was horrible of me to have let myself get so fat! I don't deserve a compliment for becoming normal again!" Enjoy the fact that others are appreciating you and telling you when they notice changes.

Step 5. Maintain a Positive Attitude

Don't be cynical about your ability to change. Give yourself positive reinforcement about using these strategies and anticipate success!

Strategies for Obtaining Social Support

You are ultimately responsible for your actions, but it's important to realize what a strong influence family and friends can have on your efforts to control your weight. Making long-term change is usually easier when you can do it within a supportive environment.

Exactly what constitutes "support" depends on you. Direct praise and recognition for your accomplishments might be supportive or not, depending on how you feel about attention being focused on your efforts. Indirect encouragement, such as suggesting a walk instead of a rich dessert after dinner, or talking about going to a new art gallery instead of an all-you-can-eat buffet, is usually welcome and helpful.

Step 1. Learn How to Ask for Support

Many people find it difficult to ask for support.

- You may believe you don't deserve support and have no right to ask for it.
- You're embarrassed about exposing your needs or experiencing possible rejection.
- You see yourself as autonomous and independent of others, so you equate asking for assistance with being weak and inadequate.
- You erroneously believe that if others really cared enough, they would automatically provide the support needed.
- You use the lack of a loved one's reinforcement as an excuse for your own lack of success.
- You see yourself as totally responsible for your problems, and therefore you do not expect anyone to help you solve them.

Step 2. Make Requests of Family and Friends

Whatever problems you may have in asking for the responses you need, it's to your advantage to understand and overcome them. Other people rarely provide automatic support. More often than not, you need to make specific requests of them. For instance, tell them: "I'd appreciate it if you would ask me how I'm feeling rather than how many pounds I've lost." Or, simply say: "Tell me when you think I look good or when you notice a difference." To someone who isn't helpful, but who is willing, you might say: "Would you please snack in the kitchen rather than in the bedroom in front of me?"

Also ask your family or close friends
- to avoid bringing snacks or high-calorie foods into the house.
- to help you with after-meal cleanup, if that's a time you usually nibble.
- not to offer you food and to avoid suggesting going out to eat pizza.
- not to "police" your behavior. Suggestions may be helpful, but you are responsible for what you eat.

Let your friends and family know that you will be showing them your love in ways other than those involving food.

Step 3. Join Support Groups

Groups like Overeaters Anonymous or Weight Watchers can be extremely helpful. If you don't like organized groups, find one or two other friends who are also trying to lose weight. Call each other every day or two to share support and stories of small victories. (For more on identifying and dealing with unsupportive behavior, see chapter 14.)

Strategies for Changing Body Image

Adjusting the image you have of your body to fit reality is an important component of permanent weight loss. If you have been overweight for many years, you may continue to think of yourself as fat, clumsy, awkward, obese, and unathletic even after your body has become trim and firm.

People often become heavy in the first place because they are unaware of the changes taking place in their bodies. On the other side of the coin, even when they have lost a significant amount of weight, they are unable to see or feel the transformation they've gone through. They look in the mirror and still see a fat person.

Rita Caparelli remembers that when she previously had lost fifteen pounds, she hadn't felt any thinner. When she had gone to buy clothes, she had tried on dresses that seemed to be the right size for her, but the salesperson had told her they were too big. Rita had been used to wearing tent dresses and oversized blouses, so she had never had an accurate idea of how her body really looked. She also had never examined herself in the mirror, except to put on makeup or adjust a hemline, and she had avoided being photographed.

Since she hadn't felt any slimmer to herself after her fifteen-pound weight loss, it had been easy for her to regain all of her weight. Now, following the DFC program, Rita has come to understand how body changes happen slowly and gradually, and that often it takes six months to a year or more before her self-image matches how she looks to others. Rita also has learned to make a conscious effort to change how she thinks about her body image.

There are many strategies you can use to help develop a realistic and positive image of yourself.

Step 1. Take Monthly Pictures of Yourself As You Lose Weight

Compare "before" and "after" pictures and look for specific differences. Is your waist smaller? Is your stomach flatter? Do your arms look thinner? Congratulate yourself on each small change that you notice.

Step 2. Look at Your Body, Preferably in the Nude, Every Day in a Full-Length Mirror

Become fully aware of your body size and shape, your waist, arms, hips, and legs, and notice changes as they occur.

Step 3. Look at Yourself in a Three-Way, Full-Length Mirror at Least Once a Month

If you don't have a three-way mirror, go to a regular clothing store. Look for changes in the front view, side view, and back view of your body since the last time and try to observe yourself objectively.

Step 4. Go Shopping and Try On Sizes That You Used to Wear, As Well As Those That Fit You Now

Ask a salesperson or a friend to help you determine how the new sizes are fitting. Don't be discouraged if you expected to be able to wear a certain new size that doesn't fit yet. Go back to the store in a few weeks and try again. Make sure to try on clothing made by several different manufacturers since sizes often differ from one label to the next.

Step 5. Keep Your Wardrobe Current

Don't wait until you're at goal weight before buying new clothes. Choose new styles that are relatively formfitting even if you are still overweight. Unlike loose, oversized garments, those that conform to your body help you visualize and adjust to your changing image.

Step 6. Give Away Your Old Clothes

When you buy new clothes, give away your "fat clothes." If you keep them around, you are telling yourself that someday you will be fatter again; you are making a commitment to failure. Keep only one item of "fat clothing" to remind yourself of the progress you have made.

Step 7. Touch and Feel Your Body

Become aware of the changes. Does your stomach protrude as much as it used to? Do your hips feel smaller or less flabby? Do your thighs feel firmer when you touch them?

Step 8. Ask People You Trust to Give You Feedback About Your Appearance

Ask good friends to tell you when they notice changes or improvements.

Step 9. Experiment with Your New Appearance

Get suggestions on new clothing styles you never thought you could wear, but that you would look wonderful in now. You might want to go to an image consultant, a clothes buyer, or a color analysis expert to give you advice about clothes styles, hairstyles, and colors that are flattering for you. Get dressed up, go out, and enjoy the way you look and feel.

Step 10. Participate in New Physical Activities

You may have avoided many activities in the past because you felt that you were too clumsy or because you didn't want anyone to notice how you looked in shorts or a leotard or sweatpants. New experiences will give you a sense of your options and a more accurate perception of your body. Remember that any new strenuous physical activity should be started gradually. It may be prudent to check with your physician just before beginning.

Step 11. Don't Let an Occasional Food Binge Distort Your Image of Yourself

You may look worse to yourself after a food binge simply because of your humiliation and embarrassment about your loss of control. For example, you may think, "I'm grotesque," or "I look terrible! My hips are monstrous," when in fact your body has not changed size or shape.

Strategies for Reducing Stress

Stress in its various forms often leads to overeating. While a certain amount of stress can motivate and challenge you to perform at peak efficiency, an excess can take a toll on your health, particularly when that stress is chronic and you take no time to unwind.

Eating Patterns in Response to Stress
- Overeating during and/or between meals
- Feeling preoccupied with eating and food
- Going for long periods of time without thinking about food and then gorging
- Skipping meals, particularly breakfast or lunch
- Eating erratically during hectic periods

If you have developed such eating habits in response to the tension you're experiencing, you are using an ineffective method of coping with stress. By learning strategies for reducing stress, you will probably find the task of weight control to be much easier than you thought.

Step 1. Identify the Stress In Your Life

In order to control your weight and reduce the stress in your life, it's essential to identify the sources of strain.

Potential Sources of Stress

Minor hassles, such as getting stuck in traffic, choosing the wrong line at the supermarket checkout counter, or getting charged for a bill already paid, are unavoidable.

Major life changes, such as divorce, death of a loved one, a geographic move, a job change, or retirement, are undeniably stressful.

Conflict in relationships, at home, in friendship, or on the job, can create a tremendous amount of tension in your life.

Poor time management, having too much to do and too little time to do it, makes anyone anxious.

Personality type affects the way you experience stress. Controlling, perfectionist, nonassertive, approval-seeking, and pessimistic personalities are associated with excessive stress.

Step 2. Utilize Accessible Methods for Reducing Stress

No matter what stress you have in your life, you can learn to manage it in a more constructive way. You don't need to eat when you're tense; you need to know how to relax. The following methods will help you to relieve tension and anxiety, and to achieve a deeper level of personal comfort.

Progressive relaxation. For the first week or two of practice, use the tension-release method described here. Find a quiet place where you will not be interrupted for at least ten to twenty minutes. Sit in a comfortable chair, lie down with your head propped up (lying flat tends to encourage sleep), sit cross-legged on the floor—whatever feels most restful.

Relax your muscles in an order that you will remember—from head to toe or toe to head. Use the same order on a daily basis, and be consistent about your practice. Begin by taking a deep breath and holding it while you tense the muscle for five seconds. Then exhale slowly and keep the muscle relaxed for thirty seconds. Repeat this tension-release cycle for each muscle.

After mastering the tension-release approach to relaxation, shift to a release-only technique in which you exhale and relax each muscle without prior tension.

Finally, you will be ready for mini-sessions. These are five-minute periods that will help you to relax no matter where you are or what time of day you feel the need.

Breathing exercises can help you to increase general body awareness and aid you in releasing tension.

1. *Deep breathing.* Either lie down flat on the floor or stand up straight and breathe in deeply to a count of eight. Then exhale slowly to a count of ten. Repeat this exercise ten times.

2. *Purposeful sighing.* Sit or stand up straight. Sigh loudly, as if you had just been relieved of a great burden, and let the air rush out of your lungs, making a noise as it escapes. Don't think about inhaling; just let the air come in naturally. Repeat this exercise ten times.

3. *Alternate breathing.* Sit comfortably. Rest the index and second fingers of your right hand on your forehead. Close your right nostril with your thumb. Inhale slowly through your left nostril. Close your left nostril with your ring finger and simultaneously open your right nostril by removing your thumb. Exhale slowly and fully through your right nostril. Inhale slowly through your right nostril and continue to do this ten more times, alternating sides.

Biofeedback can train your body to respond differently to stress. Many hospitals and clinics offer training in biofeedback. Using sophisticated equipment, you can be taught to monitor and control physiological activities, such as heart rate, blood pressure, and muscle tension.

Deep massage is very soothing, restoring circulation to tense muscle groups. Ask a massage therapist to concentrate on the area where you feel the most tension.

Yoga can help you to relax and control your breathing. Many good classes and books are available to teach you various techniques.

Meditation can lower your blood pressure, relax your entire body, and give you a sense of inner peace. It takes time to learn how to meditate, but there are many books and classes available.

Hearty laughter gives a good workout to the diaphragm, lungs, and circulatory system, and helps you to relax. Go to a funny movie, or rent a comedy and play it on your video cassette recorder. Laughter contributes to an overall sense of well-being as well as to a release of tension.

A hot bath can be very calming. Fill the bathtub with bubble bath, or add bath oil or powders and luxuriate. Salt baths, steam baths, and saunas are pleasant means of winding down and getting a better perspective on the issues at hand.

Recreational activities can be a wonderful diversion from troubles and tension. Think about what you enjoy the most. Organize a softball game, go bowling, or play volleyball, golf, or tennis with your friends. Time out for Trivial Pursuit, bridge, bingo, or other games is time well spent.

So far, you have assessed your medical history, attitudes, and motivation. You have set short- and long-term goals and have learned strategies for changing habits and solving problems that interfere with achieving your goals. Now that you have a better understanding of the importance of behavioral strategies to the DFC program, you are ready to progress to Week Two and learn our nutritional strategies.

This chart will enable you to graph your weight over a one-month period. On the vertical axis toward the top of the chart, write your present weight rounded to the nearest 10 pounds. For example, if your weight is 186 pounds, you would write 190, using one of the lines with a 0. Then fill in the lines below by 5-pound decrements. For example:

190
185
180
175
170

Next, write the date you wish to begin recording your weight on the horizontal axis above "Day 1" and the subsequent dates by one-day increments, for example, 6/23, 6/24, 6/25, 6/26, 6/27, 6/28, 6/29, 6/30, 7/1, 7/2, 7/3, 7/4, 7/5, etc.

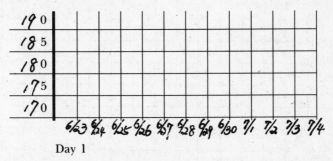

Day 1

Now plot your weight, 186 pounds, on Day 1 of your diet and subsequently on the days when you weigh yourself.

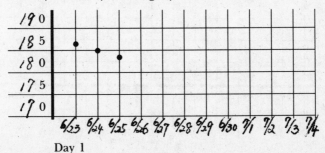

Day 1

Chart For Recording Your Weight

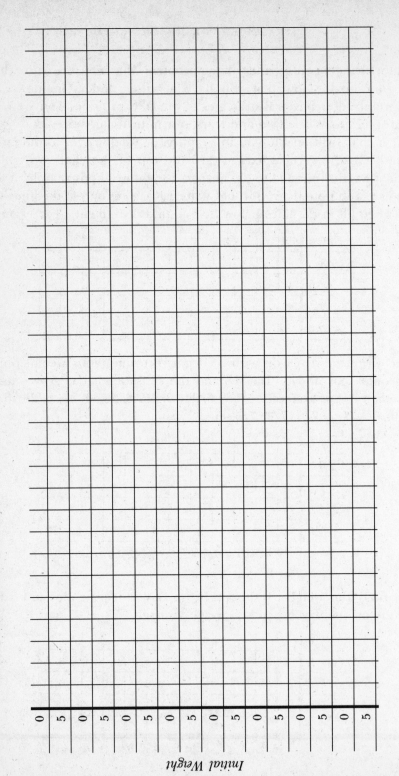

Initial Weight

Chart for Recording Your Measurements

Body Circumference* (Inches)	Date	Date	Date	Date	Date
Arm					
Chest					
Waist					
Abdomen					
Hips					
Thigh					

*It is helpful to select some easily identified body landmarks so that you can measure the same place each time. For example, measure next to a mole on your arm or thigh. Your belly button is a made-to-order landmark for measuring your abdomen.

The DFC Nutritional Plan

6

A Good Diet Makes Sense: The DFC Approach

The DFC diet doesn't depend on pills, powdered or liquid supplements, or mysterious food combinations. There's no list of "forbidden" or "diet" foods that are difficult to find in ordinary food stores.

Instead, ours is a sensible, practical, and healthy diet that can be followed for a lifetime. Bagels, pita pizzas, muffins, beef stir-fry, and flank steak, as well as other easily purchased foods, are included. It is an appropriate diet for adults of any shape, weight, or age, and you can take its dietary principles with you to restaurants, parties, and vacations.

We believe that a realistic and workable diet is one that can be modified to fit individual taste and lifestyle. Instead of thinking, "I can't wait until I go off this diet so I can eat my favorite dessert again," you will learn to design meal plans that include your favorite foods, but in portions that are calorie controlled and provide nutritionally balanced meals.

Major Features of the DFC Diet

The DFC diet is low in calories, fat, and cholesterol, high in dietary fiber, moderate in sodium, low in simple and added sugars, and high in complex and natural carbohydrates. Its major features include

1. A healthy distribution of fats, proteins, and carbohydrates
2. Attention to calorie and portion control
3. Meal planning
4. Nutritional balance through the use of the six food groups
5. Variety in foods and menus

Calorie Control on the DFC Diet

Estimating Your Daily Caloric Requirements

Before you go any further, review the assessments you made in chapter 3 about your nutritional habits, your desirable weight, your goal weight, and your overall shape.

Daily caloric requirements vary among individuals and depend on inheritance, age, sex, body weight, and physical activity level. At a stable weight, the calories you eat are balanced by those your body uses to maintain its physiologic functions and those that are burned to provide energy for physical activity. When you eat more calories than are needed to maintain your body weight, an imbalance occurs and the excess calories are stored as fat. On the other hand, when you eat fewer calories than needed to maintain body weight, a caloric deficit occurs, and your body burns some of the excess calories it has stored as fat, which then causes you to lose weight. When you weigh less, you'll need fewer calories to maintain that weight, and your daily caloric requirements will decrease accordingly.

Therefore, in choosing the caloric level of your diet it is helpful to have an estimate of your metabolic rate, that is, the number of calories you require each day to maintain your present weight at your current level of physiologic function and physical activity.

Your daily metabolic rate is simply the number of calories you burn in a day—your body's expenditure of energy over twenty-four hours. There are three major components of daily metabolic rate: (1) the energy expended at rest, (2) the energy expended during physical activity, and (3) the energy expended in processing the food we eat (called the thermic effect of food, or TEF).

Resting metabolic rate (RMR) is the energy (calories) expended to maintain your normal physiologic functions (breathing, circulation of blood, disposal of waste products through the kidneys, etc.) when your body is at rest. Resting metabolic rate is fairly constant and represents an obligatory expenditure of calories by the body under resting conditions, much like the amount of gas that would be required for your car to remain in the garage with the motor idling for twenty-four hours. Resting metabolic rate generally utilizes about 65 percent to 70 percent of the total calories burned each day.

The energy expended due to physical activity in sedentary persons accounts for about 15 percent to 20 percent of the calories burned each day, but in highly active people it can be as high as 40 percent. Clearly, this component of daily energy expenditure is one over which you have significant control.

The third component of daily energy expenditure, the thermic effect of food (TEF) accounts for proportionally fewer calories (10 percent to 15 percent) of the body's total daily energy expenditure and is less well understood. TEF is influenced by the energy costs of digesting, absorbing, and processing food.

Table 3.

Estimating Your Level of Physical Activity

Level	Description of Activities
Low	Sedentary, with very little walking or climbing of stairs. Most work or home activity is done while seated. No regular physical activity.
Moderate	Physical activity level is somewhere between "low" and "high," with sporadic exercise lasting 30 minutes or less two or three times a week.
High	Daily strenuous manual activity either at home or at work. Daily exercise lasting at least 30 minutes.

To make a rough calculation of your total daily energy expenditure or metabolic rate, first estimate your level of physical activity by consulting table 3, then use the metabolic rate tables (tables 4 and 5) that follow. (These tables are based on the work of Dr. Oliver Owens, chairman of the Department of Medicine at Southern Illinois University School of Medicine.)

Examples: A man who weighs 220 pounds and exhibits a medium level of physical activity would require 2,660 calories a day to maintain his current weight. A 140-pound woman exhibiting a low level of physical activity would require 1,494 calories daily to maintain her weight. Both persons, then, would want to reduce their daily intake of calories in order to lose weight.

Table 4.

Daily Metabolic Rate Table for Men Based on Weight and Physical Activity by Five-Pound Increments (125–350 Lbs.)

Weight (in Pounds)	Level of Physical Activity		
	Low	Moderate	High
125	1,762	2,055	2,349
130	1,789	2,087	2,386
135	1,817	2,120	2,422
140	1,843	2,150	2,458
145	1,871	2,183	2,494
150	1,898	2,215	2,531
155	1,926	2,247	2,568
160	1,952	2,278	2,603
165	1,980	2,310	2,640
170	2,008	2,342	2,677
175	2,034	2,373	2,712
180	2,062	2,405	2,749
185	2,089	2,437	2,786
190	2,117	2,470	2,822
195	2,143	2,500	2,858
200	2,171	2,533	2,894
205	2,198	2,565	2,931
210	2,226	2,597	2,968
215	2,252	2,628	3,003
220	2,280	2,660	3,040
225	2,308	2,692	3,077
230	2,334	2,723	3,112
235	2,362	2,755	3,149
240	2,389	2,787	3,186
245	2,417	2,820	3,222
250	2,443	2,850	3,258
255	2,471	2,883	3,294
260	2,498	2,915	3,331
265	2,526	2,947	3,368
270	2,552	2,978	3,403
275	2,580	3,010	3,440
280	2,608	3,042	3,477
285	2,634	3,073	3,512
290	2,662	3,105	3,549
295	2,689	3,137	3,586
300	2,717	3,170	3,622
305	2,743	3,200	3,658
310	2,771	3,233	3,694
315	2,798	3,265	3,731
320	2,826	3,297	3,768
325	2,852	3,328	3,803
330	2,880	3,360	3,840
335	2,908	3,392	3,877
340	2,934	3,423	3,912
345	2,962	3,455	3,949
350	2,989	3,487	3,986

Table 5.

Daily Metabolic Rate Table for Women Based on Weight and Physical Activity by Five-Pound Increments (100–300 Lbs.)

Weight (in Pounds)	Level of Physical Activity		
	Low	Moderate	High
100	1,342	1,565	1,789
105	1,361	1,588	1,814
110	1,380	1,610	1,840
115	1,399	1,632	1,866
120	1,418	1,655	1,891
125	1,438	1,677	1,917
130	1,457	1,700	1,942
135	1,476	1,722	1,968
140	1,494	1,743	1,992
145	1,513	1,765	2,018
150	1,532	1,788	2,043
155	1,552	1,810	2,069
160	1,571	1,833	2,094
165	1,590	1,855	2,120
170	1,609	1,877	2,146
175	1,628	1,900	2,171
180	1,648	1,922	2,197
185	1,667	1,945	2,222
190	1,686	1,967	2,248
195	1,704	1,988	2,272
200	1,723	2,010	2,298
205	1,742	2,033	2,323
210	1,762	2,055	2,349
215	1,781	2,078	2,374
220	1,800	2,100	2,400
225	1,819	2,122	2,426
230	1,838	2,145	2,451
235	1,858	2,167	2,477
240	1,877	2,190	2,502
245	1,896	2,212	2,528
250	1,914	2,233	2,552
255	1,933	2,255	2,578
260	1,952	2,278	2,603
265	1,972	2,300	2,629
270	1,991	2,323	2,654
275	2,010	2,345	2,680
280	2,029	2,367	2,706
285	2,048	2,390	2,731
290	2,068	2,412	2,757
295	2,087	2,435	2,782
300	2,106	2,457	2,803

Choosing a Diet with a Calorie Level That's Right for You

The energy value of one pound of excess weight is equal to 3,500 calories. Therefore, to lose one pound, you need to eat approximately 3,500 fewer calories than your body requires to maintain its present weight. Since relatively few people require as many as 3,500 calories a day, this deficit usually takes several days to achieve. That's why significant weight loss is rarely achieved as quickly as you might wish.

A safe and recommended weight loss—a loss that we believe is more likely to be permanent—is between one-half pound to two pounds per week. The rate at which you lose depends on how much you reduce your daily caloric intake. Use the formula below to estimate in advance the rate of your weight loss. Remember, this is a rough estimate and does not take into account calories expended with physical activity.

To Lose:	Reduce Your Daily Intake by:
½ pound a week	250 calories
1 pound a week	500 calories
1½ pounds a week	750 calories
2 pounds a week	1,000 calories

We recommend that you eat no fewer than 1,000 calories daily, divided into three meals. Contrary to popular opinion, we've found that a 1,200-, 1,300-, 1,400-, or 1,500-calorie plan can be as successful as a lower calorie plan, probably because it is more easily accepted and therefore followed more readily.

Begin by determining your expected weekly rate of weight loss. The formula below will help you to calculate how long it will take to reach your goal weight. Our sample formula is based on a man who weighs 220 pounds, has a low level of physical activity, and thus needs 2280 calories a day to maintain that weight. He has chosen to follow a diet plan of 1,300 calories a day, which would result in a weekly deficit of 6860 calories, or the loss of almost two pounds a week. As he loses weight, the number of calories he must consume to maintain his weight also decreases, and he will lose fewer pounds per week if his calorie intake remains the same. For example, when that man reaches a weight of 200 pounds, his maintenance calories will decrease to 2171, reducing his weekly calorie deficit to 6097 and his weekly weight loss to about one and three quarters pounds per week.

How to Calculate Weekly Weight Loss (for a woman who weighs 220 lbs. and has a low level of physical activity)

1. Maintenance calories	1,800
2. Proposed daily caloric intake	1,300
3. Daily caloric deficit (subtract #2 from #1)	500
4. Weekly caloric deficit (multiply #3 by 7)	3,500
5. Expected weekly weight loss in pound(s) (divide #4 by 3,500)	1 lb.

My Weekly Weight Loss

1. Maintenance calories _____
2. Proposed daily caloric intake _____
3. Daily caloric deficit _____
4. Weekly caloric deficit _____
5. Expected weekly weight loss in pound(s) _____

Be Patient with Your Rate of Weight Loss

In choosing the calorie level of your diet, consider more than just the speed of weight loss. People often make the mistake of choosing a calorie level that is too low to maintain comfortably, thus jeopardizing their chances of success. An excessively low caloric intake will make you feel hungry, lethargic, and deprived, and you may end up thinking constantly about foods you wish you could eat (which then increases the risk of your eating them). If you are a high-energy person, you may feel worn out, even on 1,300 calories a day. Evaluate your own special needs. If your lifestyle makes maintaining a 1,000-calorie-a-day plan extremely difficult, choose a higher level. If, for example, you always eat lunch out, you'll have to plan enough calories to give you variety, adequate portions, and enough flexibility to make each lunch a successful dining experience.

Mark Loomis was one DFC client who chose a 1,000-calorie-a-day plan. Since Mark weighed 220 pounds and was moderately active, he needed 2,660 calories a day to maintain his weight. He calculated that a 1,000-calorie diet would give him a deficit of 1,660 calories a day or 11,620 calories in seven days, a loss of three and a third pounds a week. It sounded good, but after two weeks and the loss of almost seven pounds, Mark was worn out. He was annoyed at feeling limited when he ate at restaurants, and he was so tired at night that he didn't have the energy to use his rowing machine.

Mark found that he felt much better on a higher calorie diet. By increasing his caloric intake to 1,660 calories a day, his caloric deficit was 1,000 calories a day, or 7,000 calories for the week, which meant he could lose two pounds a week. While this meant a slower rate of weight loss, he felt it was worth it to feel more satisfied and less tired. He worked out a plan to use his added energy by rowing thirty minutes each day and thereby improving his physique and rate of weight loss.

Keep in mind that small changes in your diet can have a powerful impact. Seemingly insignificant habits can cost calories, and simply eliminating them from your diet can make a difference in the long run. For instance, you may normally use one or more tablespoons of butter or margarine on bread or in cooking every day. If you stopped using just one tablespoon a day, you would lose approximately one-half pound in two weeks—which means, everything else being equal, a loss of thirteen pounds in one year from this one small change in your diet.

Above all, be patient. There are only so many calories that you can eliminate from your diet each day. Even fasting, which we do not recommend because it leads to excessive loss of lean tissue, does not produce instant weight loss. Let's say that your total daily requirements amounted to 2,000 calories and you decided to fast, giving you a caloric deficit of 2,000 calories a day. Fasting for seven days would create a deficit of 14,000 calories, or the loss of four pounds. Compare fasting and that weight loss with a diet of 1,000 calories a day for a week consisting of fruit and a muffin for breakfast, tuna fish in a pita sandwich with seltzer and a salad for lunch, and crisp chicken, a baked potato, and a salad for dinner, and a resulting loss of two pounds that week. Which diet would you choose?

Use Your Calories Wisely

One key to our nutrition plan is to think of calories as money in a checking account to be spent on three meals a day. At a dollar a calorie, you can "spend" 1,200 calories a day, if that is your caloric budget. Next, how should you budget or distribute your calories throughout the day? You could spend 250 for breakfast, 450 for lunch, and 500 for dinner. The distribution of your calories throughout the day will largely depend on your lifestyle. For instance, if you are physically active in the morning, perhaps you should budget more calories for breakfast.

Spend your calories wisely, and use your best judgment in choosing the foods you eat. Usually, before making a major purchase you think seriously about it and evaluate your priorities. Do the same for your food choices. Be a bargain shopper and consider both quality and quantity. For example, compare the following list of foods in Diet A and Diet B and decide which of the two diets is a better buy.

Diet A

⅛ of a 9-inch apple pie
1 cup rich ice cream (16% milk fat)
TOTAL: 1,000 calories   DAILY TOTAL: 1,000 calories

or

Diet B

Breakfast

1 oz. toasted bagel
1 tsp. margarine
½ large grapefruit
coffee or tea (without milk or sugar)
TOTAL: 185 calories

Lunch

Tuna-tomato melt on whole wheat*:
   2 oz. water-packed tuna
   1 Tb. low-calorie mayonnaise
   1 slice tomato
   1 oz. part-skim milk mozzarella cheese, shredded
   ¼ cup alfalfa sprouts
   1 oz. whole wheat bread
½ large apple
TOTAL: 345 calories

Dinner

3 oz. beef loaf†
½ cup linguine
½ cup steamed cauliflower
1 cup mixed greens
1 Tb. reduced-calorie salad dressing
1 fresh fruit crepe‡
TOTAL: 500 calories   DAILY TOTAL: 1,030 calories

*See recipe on page 229.
†See recipe on page 197.
‡See recipe on page 273.

We hope you selected Diet B. Although both diets have about the same number of calories, Diet B is nutritious and varied and a better long-term investment.

How to Use the DFC Checkbook System

The DFC checkbook system will help you plan meals to suit your food preferences and will provide you with a healthy, calorically controlled and enjoyable way of eating for a lifetime. Learning this system requires some homework, but once mastered you will find it easier to select and maintain your weight loss diet.

Our system is designed to help you budget your calories and nutrients from six basic food groups:

1. Breads and other starches
2. Meat and meat substitutes (lean, medium fat, and high fat)
3. Vegetables
4. Fruits
5. Milk and milk products
6. Fats

Each of the food groups contains foods that are similar in size, calorie, and nutrient value. These are called the exchange lists.* For example, one vegetable exchange equals 25 calories for ½ cup of cooked or 1 cup of raw vegetables.

To use this system, you can then "write a check" for any vegetable exchange. As long as you eat either ½ cup cooked or 1 cup raw vegetables, you are only spending 25 calories from your daily caloric allowance. By using the exchange lists and measuring your food, you will never have to count calories again unless you choose to.

By writing checks for the appropriate number of daily exchanges from each food group, you will develop a system that is easy to remember and

---

*The exchange lists are the basis of a meal-planning system designed by a committee of the American Diabetes Association and the American Dietetic Association. While designed primarily for people with diabetes and others who must follow special diets, the exchange lists are based on principles of good nutrition that apply to everyone. © 1986 American Diabetes Association, the American Dietetic Association

has built-in variety. The number of checks you write will depend on the number of allowed exchanges for the calorie level of the diet you choose. For example, the 1,000-calorie diet calls for two daily bread/starch exchanges, the 1,200-calorie diet calls for three and one half bread/starch exchanges, and the 1,500-calorie diet allows five bread/starch exchanges.

The plans we offer automatically provide a nutrient distribution we have found to be effective in losing weight: high in protein, moderate in carbohydrate, and low in fat. The protein calories we recommend are proportionally higher than you need on a long-term basis, but in our experience higher protein levels will increase your feeling of fullness and may reduce the loss of body protein that normally occurs during the early phase of weight loss. Eventually, you should aim for a distribution of nutrients with a higher proportion of complex carbohydrates.

The following are the 1,000-, 1,200-, and 1,500-calorie weight loss diets we use at the Duke Diet and Fitness Center. We believe you will find that the recommended number of exchanges allocated to each food group will provide a distribution of nutrients that is satisfying and thus will enable you to achieve long-term success.

Table 6.

1,000-Calorie Weight Loss Diet

Food Group	Checks Per Day	Calories Per Check	Total Calories
Bread/Starch	2	80	160
Meat & Meat Substitutes	7	55	385
Vegetables	3	25	75
Fruit	3	60	180
Skim Milk	1½	90	135
Fat	2	45	90

Total Daily Calories 1,025

Table 7.

1,200-Calorie Weight Loss Diet

Food Group	Checks Per Day	Calories Per Check	Total Calories
Bread/Starch	3 1/2	80	280
Meat & Meat Substitutes	7	55	385
Vegetables	4	25	100
Fruit	3	60	180
Skim Milk	2	90	180
Fat	2	45	90

Total Daily Calories 1,215

Table 8.

1,500-Calorie Weight Loss Diet

Food Group	Checks Per Day	Calories Per Check	Total Calories
Bread/Starch	5	80	400
Meat & Meat Substitutes	7	55	385
Vegetables	4	25	100
Fruit	5	60	300
Skim Milk	2	90	180
Fat	3	45	135

Total Daily Calories 1,500

A Calorie and Nutrient Guide to the Six Food Groups

By learning the controlled portion of food corresponding to each exchange, you can easily estimate the number of calories in any food or combination of foods you choose. This system will help you to design a diet with a proper balance of nutrients from the six food groups.

Another advantage of our system is that it will enable you to become more conscious of high-calorie items and of those foods that contain fat, a major dietary cause of weight gain. It will also teach you which nutrients are contained in a wide variety of foods and help you to decide whether you want to spend your calories on any particular food.

For example, many people would place bacon in the meat group; however, we list bacon as a fat because most of its calories are derived from fat. Thus, when you eat bacon, you are really eating fat, not meat.

In planning your diet, remember to start each day with the number of calories in your daily budget. Every time you choose a food item, you will be writing a check against your account. At the end of each day, you should have a zero balance. If you show a minus balance, you have overdrawn your account, and you will either be gaining weight or not losing it as quickly as you want.

Group 1: Breads and Other Starches

One check from this group contains approximately 80 calories, 15 grams of carbohydrate, and 3 grams of protein. One check from this group could be ½ cup cooked pasta or cereal, or ¼ cup baked beans or 1 ounce of a bread product.

Guidelines for Meal Planning from This List

For starchy foods that are not included in this list, the general rule is that ½ cup of cooked cereal, grain, or pasta equals one bread and starch check.

Foods marked with an asterisk (*) contain 3 or more grams of dietary fiber per serving, and we highly recommend that you write at least one check per day from these sources.

Starches with added fat have about 125 calories per serving. We suggest that you do not spend these extra calories because the added fat is usually saturated (lard, butter, palm oil, or coconut oil). Read the labels of products in this category and avoid purchasing them.

A word of warning: As you'll see, the portioned amount of food corresponding to one check varies for many items in this food group. For example, one slice of bread and ½ cup of oatmeal are each worth 80 calories. Start by memorizing only the portioned amounts of food corresponding to one check for items that you often eat or plan to eat on your diet.

Breads and Other Starches • 1 check = 80 calories

Cereals/Grains/Pasta	Portioned Amount per Check
*Bran cereals, concentrated	⅓ cup
*Bran cereals, flaked, such as Bran Buds or All Bran	½ cup
Bulgur, cooked	½ cup
Cooked cereals, such as oatmeal	½ cup
Cornmeal, dry	2½ Tb.
Grits	½ cup
Other ready-to-eat unsweetened cereals	¾ cup
Pasta, cooked	½ cup
Rice, white or brown, cooked	⅓ cup
Shredded wheat	½ cup
*Wheat germ	3 Tb.

Dried Beans/Peas/Lentils	
*Beans and peas, cooked, such as kidney, white, split, and blackeye	⅓ cup
*Lentils, cooked	⅓ cup
*Baked beans	¼ cup

Starchy Vegetables	
*Corn	½ cup
*Corn on the cob, 6 in. long	1

*3 or more grams of fiber per serving

	Portioned Amount per Check
*Lima beans	½ cup
*Peas, green, canned or frozen	½ cup
*Plantain	½ cup
Potato, baked	1 small (3 oz.)
Potato, mashed	½ cup
Squash, winter, acorn, butternut	¾ cup
Yam, sweet potato, plain	⅓ cup

Bread

Bagel	½ (1 oz.)
Bread sticks, crisp 4 in. long by ½ in.	2 (⅔ oz.)
Croutons, low-fat	1 cup
English muffin	½
Frankfurter or hamburger bun	½ (1 oz.)
Pita, 6 in. diameter	½
Plain roll, small	1 (1 oz.)
Raisin bread, unfrosted	1 slice (1 oz.)
*Rye or pumpernickel	1 slice (1 oz.)
Tortilla, 6 in. diameter	1
White, including French and Italian	1 slice (1 oz.)
Whole wheat	1 slice (1 oz.)

Crackers/Snacks

Animal crackers	8
Graham crackers	3
Matzoh	¾ oz.
Melba toast	5 slices
Oyster crackers	24
Popcorn, popped, no fat added	3 cups
Pretzels	¾ oz.
Rye crisp, 2 in. by 3½ in.	4
Saltine-type crackers	6
Whole wheat crackers, no fat added, and crisp breads, such as Finn, Kavli, Wasa	2–4 slices (¾ oz.)

*3 or more grams of fiber per serving

Starches with Added Fat (1 check = 125 calories)	Portioned Amount = 1 starch/bread check and 1 fat check
Biscuit, 2½ in. diameter	1
Chow mein noodles	½ cup
Corn bread, 2 in. cube	1 (2 oz.)
Cracker, butter	6
French fried potatoes 2 in. to 3½ in. long	10 (1½ oz.)
Muffin, plain, small	1
Pancake, 4 in. diameter	2
Stuffing, bread, prepared	¼ cup
Taco shell, 6 in. diameter	2
Waffle, 4½ in. square	1
Whole wheat crackers, fat added, such as Triscuits	4–5 (1 oz.)

Group 2: Meat and Meat Substitutes

Of the three lists in this group, we recommend that you write most of your checks from the lean meat group. Note that lean meat substitutes include eggs and certain cheeses. (Whole egg consumption should be limited to three to four per week. Egg white consumption can be unlimited.)

If you choose food items from the medium- and high-fat groups, be sure to add the correct number of fat calories and remember that these extra calories will be largely spent on saturated fat.

Guidelines for Meal Planning from This List

If you choose to eat red meat, which is not essential for optimal nutrition, limit your consumption to three times per week.

Increase your consumption of fish to at least three times a week. Fish is low in saturated fat and has beneficial Omega-3 fatty acids.

Complement your remaining meals with skinless turkey or chicken, egg whites, or other choices from the lean meat and lean meat substitute items.

Lean Meat and Lean Meat Substitutes

One check from this group contains approximately 55 calories, 7 grams of protein, 3 grams of fat, and corresponds to a one-ounce portioned amount. In preparing meat, trim all visible fat.

Lean Meat and Lean Meat Substitutes • 1 check = 55 calories

		Portioned Amount Per Check
Beef	USDA Good Choice grades of lean beef, such as round, sirloin, flank steak, tenderloin, and chipped beef*	1 oz.
Pork	Lean pork, such as fresh ham, or boiled ham,* tenderloin	1 oz.
Veal	All cuts are lean except for veal cutlets (ground or cubed). Examples of lean veal are chops and roasts	1 oz.
Poultry	Chicken, turkey, and cornish hen (without skin)	1 oz.
Fish	All fresh and frozen fish	1 oz.
	Crab, lobster, scallops, shrimp, and clams (fresh or canned in water)*	2 oz.
	Oysters	6 medium
	Tuna (canned in water)*	¼ cup
	Herring (uncreamed or smoked)	1 oz.
	Sardines (canned)	2 medium
Wild game	Venison, rabbit, and squirrel	1 oz.
	Pheasant, duck, and goose (without skin)	1 oz.
Cheese	Any low-fat cottage cheese	¼ cup
	Grated Parmesan	2 Tb.
	Diet cheeses (with less than 55 calories per ounce)*	1 oz.
Other	Egg whites	3
	Egg substitutes with less than 55 calories per ¼ cup	¼ cup

*Refers to a selection with 400 mg. or more of sodium per check.

Medium-Fat Meat and Medium-Fat Meat Substitutes

One check from this group contains approximately 75 calories, 7 grams of protein, and 5 grams of fat, and also corresponds to a one-ounce portioned amount. Items from this list are simply fattier and can be thought of as one lean meat check (55 calories) with ½ added fat check (20 to 22 calories). Again, as with lean meats, trim all visible fat.

Medium-Fat Meat and Meat Substitutes • 1 check = 75 calories

		Portioned Amount Per Check
Beef	Most cuts: ground beef, roast (rib, chuck, rump), steak (cubed, porterhouse, T-bone), and meat loaf	1 oz.
Pork	Most cuts: chops, loin roast, Boston butt, cutlets	1 oz.
Lamb	Most cuts: chops, leg, and shoulder roast	1 oz.
Veal	Cutlet, ground or cubed (unbreaded)	1 oz.
Poultry	Chicken (with skin), domestic duck and goose (well drained of fat), ground turkey	1 oz.
Fish	Tuna (canned in oil and drained)* and salmon (canned)*	¼ cup ¼ cup
Cheese	Skim or packaged skim milk cheeses, such as ricotta	¼ cup
	Mozzarella	1 oz.
	Diet cheeses (56 to 80 calories per ounce)*	1 oz.
Other	86% fat-free luncheon meat*	1 oz.
	Egg (high in cholesterol, limit to 3 per week)	1 oz.
	Egg substitutes (56 to 80 calories per ¼ cup)	¼ cup
	Tofu	4 oz.
	Liver, heart, kidney, and sweetbreads (high in cholesterol)	1 oz.

*Refers to a selection with 400 mg. or more of sodium per check.

High-Fat Meat and High-Fat Meat Substitutes

One check (1 ounce) from this group contains approximately 100 calories, 7 grams of protein, and 8 grams of fat. Items from this list count as one meat serving and one fat serving. Remember to trim all visible fat before preparing the meats.

High-Fat Meat and High-Fat Meat Substitutes • 1 check = 100 calories

		Portioned Amount Per Check
Beef	Most USDA Prime cuts of beef, such as ribs and corned beef*	1 oz.
Pork	Spareribs, ground pork, and pork sausage* (patty or link)	1 oz.
Lamb	Patties (ground lamb)	1 oz.
Fish	Any fried fish product	1 oz.
Cheese	All regular cheeses,* such as American, blue, cheddar, Monterey Jack, and Swiss	1 oz.
Other	Luncheon meats,* such as bologna, salami, pimento loaf	1 oz.
	Sausage,* such as Polish, Italian	1 oz.
	Knockwurst (smoked), bratwurst*	1 oz.
	Frankfurter (turkey or chicken)*	1 (10/lb.)
	Peanut butter (contains unsaturated fat)	1 Tb.

Group 3: Vegetables

One check from this list contains approximately 25 calories, 5 grams of carbohydrate, and 2 grams of protein. Vegetables average about 2 to 3 grams of dietary fiber per serving.

*Refers to a selection with 400 mg. or more of sodium per check.

Guidelines for Meal Planning from This List

All the vegetables on this list are excellent low-calorie choices. For optimal nutrition, choose a dark green and yellow vegetable each day. For variety in salad preparation, mix greens such as spinach, cabbage, and romaine lettuce. Starchy vegetables, such as corn, peas, and potatoes, are found in the bread/starch group.

Vegetables • 1 check = 25 calories
Portioned Amount per Check: ½ cup of cooked vegetables or vegetable juice, or 1 cup of raw vegetables, or 2 cups of salad greens.

Artichoke (½ medium)
Asparagus
Bamboo shoots
Beans (green, wax, Italian)
Bean sprouts
Beets
Broccoli
Brussels sprouts
Cabbage, cooked
Carrots
Cauliflower
Celery
Chinese cabbage
Cucumber
Greens
   (collard, mustard, and turnip)
Green onion
Hot peppers
Salad greens:
   Endive
   Escarole
   Lettuce
   Romaine

Kohlrabi
Leeks
Mushrooms
Okra
Onions
Peppers (green)
Radishes
Rhubarb
Rutabaga
*Sauerkraut
Spinach, cooked
Snow peas
Summer squash (crookneck)
Tomato (one large)
*Tomato/vegetable juice
Turnips
Water chestnuts
Zucchini, cooked

*Refers to a selection with 400 mg. or more of sodium per check.

Group 4: Fruits

One check from this group contains approximately 60 calories and 15 grams of carbohydrate. The portioned amount per fruit check varies depending on the fruit. Thus, one fruit check could be half a banana, three medium dried prunes, or ½ cup of apple juice. However, the general rule for fruit checks is that ½ cup of fresh fruit, ½ cup fruit juice, and ¼ cup of dried fruit contain approximately 60 calories each.

Guidelines for Meal Planning from This List

The challenge of this group is to learn the 60-calorie portion sizes of your favorite fruits since serving size varies so much.

Try to select fruits that are good sources of Vitamin C, such as strawberries, grapefruit, oranges, or tangerines. All the fruits in this list are also excellent sources of fiber.

Fruits • 1 check = 60 calories

Fresh, Frozen, and Unsweetened Canned Fruit	Portioned Amount per Check
Apple, raw, 2 in. diameter	1
Applesauce, unsweetened	½ cup
Apricots, medium, raw	4
Apricots, canned	½ cup or 4 halves
Banana (9 inches long)	½
*Blackberries, raw	¾ cup
*Blueberries, raw	¾ cup
Cantaloupe, 5 in. diameter (cantaloupe cubes)	⅓ 1 cup
Cherries, large, raw	12
Cherries, canned	½ cup
Cranberries, unsweetened	1½ cups
Figs raw	2
Fruit cocktail, canned	½ cup
Grapefruit, medium	½
Grapefruit, segments	¾ cup
Grapes, small	15

*Refers to a selection with 400 mg. or more of sodium per check.

Fresh, Frozen, and Unsweetened Canned Fruit	Portioned Amount per Check
Honeydew melon, medium (melon cubes)	1/8 · 1 cup
Kiwi, large	1
Mandarin orange	3/4 cup
Mango, small	1/2
*Nectarine, 1 1/2 in. diameter	1
Orange, 1 1/2 in. diameter	1
Papaya	1 cup
Peach, 2 3/4 in. diameter	1
Peaches, canned	1/2 cup or 2 halves
Pear	1/2 large or 1 small
Pears, canned	1/2 cup or 2 halves
Persimmon, medium, native	2
Pineapple, raw	3/4 cup
Pineapple, canned	1/3 cup
Plum, raw, 2-in. diameter	2
*Pomegranate	1/2
*Raspberries, raw	1 cup
*Strawberries, raw, whole	1 1/4 cups
Tangerine, 2 1/2 in. diameter	2
Watermelon, cubes	1 1/4 cup

Dried Fruit	
*Apples	4 rings
*Apricots	7 halves
Dates	2 1/2 medium
*Figs	1 1/2
*Prunes	3 medium
Raisins	2 Tb.

Fruit Juice	
Apple juice/cider	1/2 cup
Cranberry juice cocktail	1/3 cup
Grapefruit juice	1/2 cup

*3 or more grams of fiber per serving.

Fruit Juice	Portioned Amount per Check
Grape juice	1/3 cup
Orange juice	1/2 cup
Pineapple juice	1/2 cup
Prune juice	1/3 cup

Group 5: Milk and Milk Products

Of the three milk groups listed, we feel that selections from the skim milk or very low-fat milk list are your best choices. Low-fat milk and whole milk have more calories, and those calories come from saturated fat—a poor nutritional investment.

Guidelines for Meal Planning from This List

Because the average adult (especially female) usually does not meet the recommended daily allowance for calcium, the milk group assumes special importance. We recommend that you choose milk products that do not contain more than 1 percent milkfat. Think of milk and yogurt as healthy "fast foods." Make a parfait of fresh fruit and yogurt with cinnamon—a nutritious dessert for the whole family.

Skim Milk or Very Low-Fat Milk

One skim milk or very low-fat (1/2 percent or 1 percent) milk check contains approximately 90 calories, 12 grams of carbohydrate, 8 grams of protein, and a trace of fat.

Skim Milk or Very Low-Fat Milk • 1 check = 90 calories

	Portioned Amount per Check
Skim milk	1 cup
1/2% fat milk	1 cup
1% fat milk	1 cup
Low-fat buttermilk	1 cup
Plain, nonfat yogurt	1 cup
Evaporated skim milk	1/2 cup
Dry nonfat milk	1/3 cup
Plain nonfat yogurt	8 oz.

Low-Fat Milk

One low-fat milk check contains approximately 120 calories, 12 grams of carbohydrate, 8 grams of protein, and 5 grams of fat. One low-fat milk check is equivalent to one skim milk check (90 calories) and half a fat check (20 to 22 calories).

Low-Fat Milk • 1 check = 120 calories

	Portioned Amount per Check
2% low-fat milk	1 cup
Plain low-fat yogurt (with added nonfat milk solids)	8 oz.

Whole Milk

One whole milk check contains approximately 150 calories, 12 grams of carbohydrate, 8 grams of protein, and 8 grams of fat. One whole milk check is roughly equivalent to one skim milk check and one fat check.

Whole Milk • 1 check = 150 calories

	Portioned Amount per Check
Whole milk	1 cup
Evaporated whole milk	½ cup
Whole plain yogurt	8 oz.

Group 6: Fats

One fat check contains approximately 45 calories and 5 grams of fat. The portioned amount of food corresponding to one fat check varies with the food item. As with breads, starches, and fruits, start by memorizing those food items you are most likely to include in your diet. Each of the following is a fat check:

  1 Tb. cashews
  5 large olives
  1 tsp. margarine

Guidelines for Meal Planning from This List

Whenever you choose to spend calories on fat, select items from the unsaturated fats list only. These fats may help to reduce the level of cholesterol in your blood. Since most animal products contain saturated fat (even when the fat is carefully trimmed), there is no reason to select items from the saturated fat list.

Unsaturated Fats • 1 Check = 45 Calories

	Portioned Amount per Check
Avocado	⅛ medium
Margarine	1 tsp.
Margarine, diet	1 Tb.
Mayonnaise	1 tsp.
Mayonnaise, reduced-calorie	1 Tb.
Nuts and seeds:	
Almonds, dry roasted	6 whole
Cashews, dry roasted	1 Tb.
Peanuts	20 small or 10 large
Pecans	2 whole
Walnuts	2 whole
Other nuts	1 Tb.
Seeds, pine nuts, sunflower (without shells)	1 Tb.
Pumpkin seeds	2 tsp.
Oil (corn, cottonseed, safflower, soybean, sunflower, peanut, olive)	1 tsp.
Olives	10 small or 5 large
Salad dressing, mayonnaise-type	2 tsp.
Salad dressing, reduced-calorie mayonnaise-type,	1 Tb.
Salad dressing, all varieties	1 Tb.
Salad dressing, reduced calorie	2 Tb.

Saturated Fats

Remember that most saturated fats tend to raise the blood cholesterol level. While you may occasionally want to choose a saturated fat, we recommend that you *severely limit* or entirely exclude any choices from this list.

Saturated Fats • 1 check = 45 calories

	Portioned Amount per Check
Butter	1 tsp.
*Bacon	1 slice
Coconut, shredded	2 Tb.
Coffee whitener, liquid	2 Tb.
Coffee whitener, powder	4 Tb.
Cream (light, coffee, table)	2 Tb.
Cream (heavy, whipping)	1 Tb.
Cream, sour	2 Tb.
Cream cheese	1 Tb.

How to Plan Meals Using the DFC System

You are now ready to develop a meal plan. You first might want to highlight the foods in each food group that you most enjoy. Then review the 1,000-calorie weight loss diet table (page 91). Notice that on this diet, you can write checks for two bread/starch servings, seven meat and meat substitute servings, three vegetable and three fruit servings, one and a half milk servings, and two fat servings. With these numbers in mind, first plan your breakfasts. Then subtract the number of checks you have used and go to the next meal. You might have to change a few foods once you have planned all three meals, but that is to be expected.

*If more than one or two servings are eaten, these foods have 400 mg. or more of sodium.

Two Sample Meal Plans for the 1,000-Calorie DFC Diet

Food Group	Checks	Meal Plan I	Meal Plan II
		BREAKFAST	
BREAD/ STARCH	1	½ cup oatmeal	½ toasted bagel
FRUIT	1	½ medium banana	½ grapefruit
MILK	½	½ cup skim milk	½ cup yogurt
		LUNCH	
MEAT	2	2 oz. water-packed tuna	3-egg white omelet w/¼ cup 1% low-fat cottage cheese
VEGETABLE	1	1 cup raw vegetables	½ cup cooked mushrooms, green peppers, and onions
FRUIT	1	½ large apple	½ cup mixed fruit or 1 cup cubed cantaloupe
FAT	1	1 Tb. low-calorie mayonnaise	1 tsp. oil
		DINNER	
MEAT	5	5 oz. broiled fish	5 oz. stir-fry chicken
BREAD/ STARCH	1	3 oz. baked potato	⅓ cup steamed rice
VEGETABLE	2	1 cup steamed broccoli	1 cup stir-fry vegetables
FAT	1	1 tsp. margarine	1 tsp. oil
FRUIT	1	1 cup cubed cantaloupe	1 cup fruit kabobs
MILK	1	1 cup nonfat yogurt	1 cup skim milk

If you are on a 1,200- or 1,500-calorie diet, check the tables on page 92. On a 1,200-calorie plan, you will have an extra half check to spend in the milk group, and one more check each in the meat, bread/starch, and vegetable groups.

Two Sample Meal Plans for the 1,200-Calorie DFC Diet

Meal Plan I

Food Group	Checks	Foods
BREAKFAST		
BREAD/STARCH	1½	¾ cup oatmeal
FRUIT	1	½ banana
MILK	1	1 cup skim milk
LUNCH		
MEAT	2	2 oz. water-packed tuna
BREAD/STARCH	1	1 slice (1 oz.) whole wheat bread
VEGETABLE	1	½ cup raw vegetables
FAT	1	1 Tb. low-calorie mayonnaise
FRUIT	1	½ large apple
DINNER		
MEAT	5	5 oz. broiled fish
BREAD/STARCH	1	3 oz. baked potato
VEGETABLE	3	2 cups mixed salad greens
		1 cup steamed broccoli
FAT	1	1 tsp. margarine
FRUIT	1	1 cup cubed cantaloupe
MILK	1	1 cup nonfat yogurt
		1 Tb. low-calorie salad dressing

Meal Plan II

Food Group	Checks	Foods
	BREAKFAST	
MEAT	1	1 poached egg
FAT	½	
BREAD/STARCH	1	½ English muffin, toasted
FRUIT	1	½ grapefruit
MILK	1	1 cup skim milk
	LUNCH	
VEGETABLE	2	1 cup chicken-vegetable soup
MEAT	1	
BREAD/STARCH	1	1 1 oz. hard roll
FRUIT	1	1 small orange
	DINNER	
MEAT	5	5 oz. marinated flank steak
BREAD/STARCH	1½	4½ oz. parsleyed new potatoes
FAT	1½	1½ tsp. margarine, optional, on potatoes or green beans
VEGETABLE	2	1 cup steamed green beans
FRUIT	1	1 cup mixed fresh fruit
MILK	1	1 cup skim milk

Two Sample Meal Plans for the 1,500-Calorie DFC Diet

Meal Plan I

Food Group	Checks	Foods
BREAKFAST		
BREAD/STARCH	2	1 cup oatmeal
FRUIT	2	½ medium banana
		2 Tb. raisins
MILK	1	1 cup skim milk
LUNCH		
MEAT	2	2 oz. water-packed tuna
BREAD/STARCH	1	1 slice (1 oz.) whole wheat bread
VEGETABLE	1	1 cup raw vegetables
FRUIT	2	1 large apple
FAT	1	1 Tb. low-calorie mayonnaise
DINNER		
MEAT	5	5 oz. broiled fish
BREAD/STARCH	2	6 oz. baked potato
VEGETABLE	3	1 cup steamed broccoli
		2 cups mixed salad greens
FAT	1	1 tsp. margarine or 1 Tb. oil and vinegar dressing
FRUIT	1	1 cup cubed cantaloupe
MILK	1	1 cup nonfat yogurt

Meal Plan II

Food Group	Checks	Foods
		BREAKFAST
MEAT	2	cheese toast
BREAD	1	1 slice (1 oz.) whole wheat bread
FRUIT	1	½ grapefruit
		black coffee
		LUNCH
MEAT	3	turkey sandwich
		3 oz. turkey
BREAD	2	2 slices (2 oz.) whole wheat bread
VEGETABLE	1	lettuce, tomato, onion
FAT	1	1 Tb. mayonnaise (reduced calories)
MILK	1	1 cup nonfat yogurt
FRUIT	1	15 grapes
		DINNER
MEAT	3	spaghetti and meat sauce
		lean ground beef (3 oz.)
VEGETABLE	2	tomato sauce (1 cup)
BREAD	2	spaghetti (1 cup)
VEGETABLE	1	½ cup yellow squash and onions, cooked
FAT	1	with 1 tsp. margarine
MILK	1	1 cup skim milk
FRUIT	3	banana and pineapple fruit cup
		(1 banana, ⅓ cup pineapple)

How You Can Benefit from the DFC System

1. *Personal choice.* You are the one who decides how to distribute your daily calories. In the sample meal plans, if there is any food you want to change, go right ahead! It's vital to your success that you make choices to fit your individual tastes.

2. *No calorie counting.* Look at the summary of the day's sample menu and you will see that you did not have to count calories. Yet you could be confident that you spent very close to the correct number of calories in your budget for the day because you knew the approximate number of calories from each of the six food groups.

3. *Nutritional balance from a variety of foods.*

Adjusted Spending Patterns

Because many people on weight loss diets must cook for others as well as for themselves, the following guide provides plans for a number of different caloric levels. The "spending" patterns of these higher calorie plans are ideal in terms of balanced nutrition. They supply 50 percent to 60 percent of the calories as carbohydrates, about 20 percent as protein, and less than 30 percent as fat, all in accordance with current recommendations by scientists and physicians.

Table 9.

Caloric Budget Adjustments for the DFC System*

Food Groups	Number of Checks for Different Calorie Levels		
	1,800	2,000	2,200
BREAD/STARCH	10	10	11
MEAT (LEAN)	6	7	7
VEGETABLE	3	4	5
FRUIT	5	5	6
MILK (SKIM)	2	3	3
FAT	7	8	9

*This chart was developed from *Exchange Lists for Meal Planning* (Chicago: American Dietetic Association and American Diabetes Association, 1988).

As you master the basics of our healthy and low-calorie DFC system, you can begin to apply it to your own life. Keep in mind that the sample diets we have outlined are only goals. If occasionally you don't include any items from one of the food groups, don't worry. Our bodies have enough reserve and resilience to survive such shortages. On the other hand, if you want to substitute an occasional "other food" not listed, go ahead and do so. You need to be flexible. For this system to become a permanent part of your life, you must enjoy yourself and your food choices.

7

Making the Right Nutritional Choices

Once you have learned some basic principles of good nutrition and as your eating habits begin to change, you will find it easier to make healthy food choices.

As you begin planning your diet, keep the following nutritional goals in mind:

- Reduce total fat, saturated fat, and cholesterol intake.
- Use salt in moderation.
- Eat more complex carbohydrates.
- Eat fewer simple sugars.
- Eat more dietary fiber.
- Reduce alcohol consumption.

You can meet these dietary goals by developing meal plans based on the six food groups. If your current eating habits are at odds with these goals, don't panic. You have time. Make changes gradually, one at a time, and, as you do, remember that the cumulative effect of these changes may significantly reduce your risk of diseases such as atherosclerosis and coronary artery disease, hypertension, diabetes, arthritis, and possibly, certain cancers.

Reduce Total Fat, Saturated Fat, and Cholesterol Intake

The expression "Too much of a good thing" certainly holds true for fat and cholesterol.

Both fat and cholesterol are necessary for normal body functioning. However, both can be harmful when eaten in excess, a problem for most Americans. Forty percent of our total daily calories are in the form of fat, and about half of these are from saturated fat—the harmful type of fat. Dietary saturated fat and cholesterol have been shown to increase blood cholesterol levels, and studies clearly indicate that high blood cholesterol levels are associated with a greater risk of developing coronary heart disease, America's number one cause of death. Furthermore, since fat contains more than twice as many calories per unit weight as carbohydrate or protein, it is the major contributor to excess calories and weight gain. Fortunately for most people, a reduction in dietary fat and cholesterol consumption can lead to weight loss and improved blood cholesterol levels.

In this book, we refer to fat and cholesterol separately. However, both share the common property of being insoluble in water, and are chemically classified together as lipids. What the layperson refers to as "fat" is really triglyceride and has a different chemical structure than cholesterol.

Fats

Fat is one of the three sources from which we derive energy. Carbohydrates and protein are the other two. Fat has several important functions:

- It is a source of energy and is stored in fat cells as a reserve for future energy needs.
- It provides a physical cushion for vital organs.
- It serves as a thermal insulator.
- It is the source for the essential fatty acids.
- It aids in the intestinal absorption of the fat-soluble vitamins A, D, E, and K.

Dietary fats contain a combination of saturated, monounsaturated, and polyunsaturated fatty acids and are classified accordingly, depending on the predominant type of fatty acid they contain.

Saturated fats raise the blood cholesterol level and contribute to the formation of low-density lipoprotein (LDL) cholesterol, which contributes to the development of plaque inside arteries. Saturated fats can be identified easily because they tend to be firm or solid at room temperature.

Highly saturated fats are mainly of animal origin and can be found in lard and other animal fats contained in meat, and in dairy products such as cheese and butter. Very few vegetable products contain significant amounts of saturated fats; the major ones that do are coconut oil, cocoa butter, and palm oil.

Monounsaturated fats have no known undesirable effects on blood cholesterol, and evidence indicates that, in fact, they may contribute to lowering blood cholesterol if substituted for dietary saturated fat. Foods high in monounsaturates include olive oil, peanuts, peanut butter and peanut oil, avocados, and some nuts, such as pecans and almonds.

Polyunsaturated fats, like monounsaturated fats, have been shown to lower blood cholesterol if substituted for dietary saturated fat. Some oils high in polyunsaturates are corn, cottonseed, sunflower, safflower, sesame, and soybean.

Omega-3 fatty acids are polyunsaturated fats found predominantly in fish oils. Studies have shown that they lower triglyceride levels in the blood. They also reduce the tendency of blood to clot and promote vasodilation, effects which may be of benefit in the prevention of heart attack.

Both monounsaturated and polyunsaturated fats (in contrast to saturated fat) are liquid or extremely soft at room temperature.

The Three Types of Fat—Health Hazard or Helper?

Fat	Physical Nature	Sources	Health Hazard or Helper?
SATURATED	Usually firm or solid at room temperature	Lard and other animal fats, red meat, fish, egg yolks, dairy products. Found in coconut oil, cocoa butter, and palm oil	Hazard— raises blood cholesterol
MONOUNSATURATED	Liquid or extremely soft at room temperature	Olive oil, peanuts, peanut butter, peanut oil, avocados, and some nuts, such as pecans and almonds	Helper— contributes to lowering blood cholesterol
POLYUNSATURATED	Liquid or extremely soft at room temperature	Oils—corn, cottonseed, sunflower, safflower, sesame, soybean, and fish	Helper— contributes to lowering blood cholesterol level

Cholesterol

Cholesterol is a waxy, fatty substance found only in foods of animal origin such as meat, egg yolks, and cheese. Organ meats such as brains, liver, and kidney are particularly high in cholesterol. The two major sources of blood cholesterol are

- The cholesterol contained in the foods we eat.
- The cholesterol that we manufacture in our body.

Cholesterol has several useful functions. It is a component of all cell membranes and is a building block for many hormones such as estrogen, testosterone, progesterone, and the steroid hormones of the adrenal gland.

Concern about dietary cholesterol is based on studies that show that the amount of cholesterol we eat influences our blood cholesterol level. As we've said before, elevated blood cholesterol is associated with an increased buildup of cholesterol plaque within the arteries of the heart, which can lead to coronary heart disease and heart attack.

Research has shown that a one percent reduction in blood cholesterol level produces a two percent drop in the risk of a heart attack. Thus, reducing the amount of saturated fat and cholesterol in our diet is a first step in striving for a lower blood cholesterol and a reduction in the risk of coronary heart disease.

Both saturated fat and cholesterol in the diet can increase blood cholesterol levels. Of the two, however, dietary saturated fat has a greater influence on blood cholesterol levels. Therefore, it is particularly important to reduce the amount of saturated fat in your diet.

Recommended Daily Budget for Fat and Cholesterol

In keeping with current standards advocated by the American Heart Association and the American Dietetic Association, we recommend that you limit your total fat consumption to no more than 30 percent of your total daily calories, and that your fat choices be distributed evenly between saturated monounsaturated and polyunsaturated fats. For cholesterol, the goal is to reduce your consumption from the current American average of 400 to 500 milligrams of cholesterol a day to 300 milligrams a day, with an eventual reduction to 100 to 200 milligrams a day.

Dietary Strategies to Reduce the Total Fat, Saturated Fat, and Cholesterol in Your Diet

Meal Planning and Purchasing

1. Choose low-fat foods from all food groups:
   - Choose low-fat (1 percent) milk or skim milk (½ percent fat), not whole milk (4 percent fat) or 2 percent fat milk.

- Eat vegetables without added butter or margarine.
- Choose whole wheat breads, pita, and other low-fat grains. Avoid biscuits, crackers, stuffing, and grains made with added fat.
- Choose lean meat, fish, poultry, dry beans, and peas for your major sources of protein. Limit your consumption of cheese, sandwich meats, whole eggs, and especially organ meats (such as liver, brain, or kidney), which contain significant amounts of cholesterol.

2. Limit portions of all fats, and restrict intake of all saturated fats: butter, cream, hydrogenated margarines, shortening, lard, palm and coconut oils, cocoa butter, and foods made from these products.

3. Increase the amount of fish you eat every week.

4. Read margarine labels and select those brands that contain liquid oil as their major ingredient.

Food Preparation and Cooking

1. Use plain low-fat yogurt, blender-whipped low-fat cottage cheese, evaporated skim milk, or buttermilk in recipes that call for sour cream or mayonnaise.

2. Season vegetables with herbs and spices, not with sauces, butter, margarine, or oil.

3. For a fruit salad, use low-fat yogurt and cinnamon as a topping instead of sour cream.

4. Read the product instructions that recommend adding butter or margarine in preparation. Usually the fat is suggested for added flavor and is not essential in meal preparation.

5. Trim all visible fats from meats and remove skin from poultry before cooking.

6. If you enjoy beef or pork, eat it, but not more than three times a week, and limit your portions. Instead of an eight-ounce filet mignon, limit your cooked portion to three to five ounces.

7. Use preparation methods that require very little or no added fat, for example, roasting, broiling, baking, steaming, and simmering. Bake or broil your meat or poultry on a rack so the fat will drain off.

8. Use a nonstick pan to keep the use of added fat to a minimum.

9. Chill meat or poultry broth until the fat hardens on the surface. Skim that fat off before using the broth.

10. *Never* use a saturated fat in cooking. Substitute a soft margarine or a polyunsaturated or monounsaturated oil for butter or lard. Limit

any fat used in preparing food. A good rule of thumb to follow in stir-frying is one teaspoon of oil per person.

11. Substitute egg whites in recipes calling for whole eggs. Use two egg whites for one whole egg. For example, if you are making a three-egg omelet, use one whole egg and four egg whites.

12. Plan to have a meatless meal at least one day a week.

13. Measure any added fat used in a recipe or as a topping. Remember that one teaspoon contains approximately 45 calories.

Use Salt in Moderation

One teaspoon of salt, a combination of the essential minerals sodium and chloride, contains about 2,300 milligrams of sodium. The body needs only a fraction of that amount to meet its daily sodium requirements.

The salt we eat is derived from four major sources:

• Table salt
• Salt added in food preparation
• Salt added in the processing of foods
• Sodium naturally occurring in foods

The average American consumes approximately 4,000 to 10,000 milligrams (2 to 5 teaspoons) of sodium a day. Excess salt intake is believed to contribute to the development of hypertension (high blood pressure) in some individuals. By simply reducing the amount of sodium in their diet, some hypertensive people may effectively lower their blood pressure, sometimes enough to enable them to reduce or discontinue antihypertensive medications. If you do not have hypertension or cardiovascular disease, you don't need to be as careful in restricting sodium as we recommend below.

Recommended Daily Budget for Salt

Try to limit your daily salt intake from all sources to 1,000 to 3,000 milligrams.

Dietary Strategies to Reduce Salt in Your Diet

1. Cover an item you normally salt with a piece of wax paper and salt the paper. Then pour the salt from the wax paper into a measuring spoon and estimate how much table salt you use in a day. Think about how much salt you could eliminate from your diet by not adding salt at the table.

2. Read labels carefully and look for the following words: salt, sodium alginate, sodium benzoate, sodium hydroxide, sodium propionate, sodium sulfite, sodium pectinate, sodium caseinate, sodium bicarbonate, disodium phosphate, monosodium glutamate.

3. Learn to enjoy the flavors of unsalted foods. Use herbs, spices, and other flavoring agents.

4. Replace the salt shaker you use at the table with an herb and spice blend or peppermill.

5. Eat only limited amounts of high-sodium foods, such as potato chips, pretzels, salted nuts and popcorn, cheese, pickles, pickled foods, cured meats, and condiments such as soy sauce, steak sauce, and garlic salt.

6. Eat more fresh fruits and vegetables, grains, and cereals.

7. Remember that baking soda, baking powder, and many medications such as antacids contain sodium.

Eat More Complex Carbohydrates and Fewer Simple Sugars

Carbohydrates, one of the three basic nutrients, supply energy to the body in the form of blood sugar (glucose). There are two basic kinds of carbohydrates:

- Simple carbohydrates contained in such foods as table sugar, fruit, and candies
- Complex carbohydrates contained in such foods as bread, pasta, potatoes, and legumes

If you are on a limited caloric budget, the simple sugars are not a good buy because they provide only energy calories. Foods that contain complex carbohydrates give you much more for your calories than just energy since they contain additional nutrients and fiber. For example, compare the value of a can of soda to the value of a potato. One 12-ounce can of soda has 150 calories, or 9 teaspoons of the simple sugar sucrose, but these calories are "empty" because they supply only energy. In contrast, a 5-ounce potato has about 100 calories but also contains protein, iron, phosphorus, thiamine, niacin, vitamin C, vitamin B_6, folacin (folic acid), trace minerals, and fiber.

Complex carbohydrates can also help you to lose weight. They give you the satisfaction of chewing and provide dietary bulk which may help to make you feel full with fewer calories. Since they are naturally low in fat, complex carbohydrates are a good buy because they can help you decrease the amount of fat in your diet. In contrast, many of the simple sugar products Americans eat are also high-fat items since saturated fats are often added in food processing, for example, in candy bars.

Nutritious complex carbohydrates that should be included in your diet are beans, peas, vegetables, whole-grain breads, cereals, and other whole-grain products. Limit the amount of butter and other fats added to bread, potatoes, or pasta, so you can pay more attention to the variety of flavors, textures, and nutrients the complex carbohydrate group provides.

Recommended Daily Budget for Carbohydrates

From 50 percent to 60 percent of your daily calories should consist of carbohydrates, with the majority in the form of complex carbohydrates.

Dietary Strategies to Increase Complex Carbohydrates in Your Diet

1. As a substitute for meats or cheeses, use a combination of legumes, such as split peas, lima or kidney beans, and grains.

2. Eat more legumes, fruits, and vegetables.

3. Eat more whole grains, including pasta and cereals. Use 100 percent whole wheat flour, stone-ground whole wheat flour, oats, corn, rice, and barley.

To Decrease Simple Carbohydrates in Your Diet

1. Use less sugar, including white sugar and brown sugar, and sweeteners such as honey, molasses, and syrup.

2. Choose fresh fruit for dessert instead of foods high in sugar such as candy, fruit-flavored punches, ice cream, pies, cakes, and cookies.

3. Drink fewer soft drinks, punches, and other sugar-filled beverages. Instead, drink water, seltzer with a twist of lime, or lemonade without sugar added.

4. Select fresh fruits or fruits canned in their own juice rather than fruits packed in light or heavy syrup.

Eat More Dietary Fiber

Fiber is important in our diet as a source of roughage or bulk. A naturally occurring component of plants, it includes substances known as cellulose and lignin, which are water insoluble, hemicellulose (some of which is water soluble), and gums and pectin, which are water soluble. Dietary fiber is resistant to human digestive enzymes and for the most part is not absorbed from the digestive tract.

The two types of dietary fiber are

- *Insoluble fiber,* found in foods such as wheat bran and other whole grains
- *Soluble fiber,* found in oat bran, pectins (from fruits and vegetables), and various gums found in nuts, seeds, and legumes such as beans, chickpeas, lentils, and peas

Each type of fiber plays an important but different role in disease prevention.

Fiber and Weight Control

High-fiber foods tend to be low in fat and simple sugars and therefore save calories for dieters. High-fiber foods also bind water, giving the body a feeling of fullness and increased satisfaction. Because high-fiber foods usually require more chewing than other foods, they slow your eating pace and give your stomach a chance to signal your brain that you're full.

Insoluble Fiber, Colon Disease, and Constipation

Wheat bran, an insoluble fiber, functions like a sponge that draws water into the digestive system and softens the stool. Insoluble fiber–containing foods help speed the transit of food through the digestive tract, thus limiting the duration of contact between potential carcinogens and the surfaces of the intestinal wall. This may reduce the risk of colon cancer. Finally, insoluble fiber helps to prevent constipation.

Soluble Fiber and Cardiovascular Disease

Recent studies have shown that oat bran and other water-soluble fiber-containing foods, such as beans and chickpeas, can reduce blood cholesterol levels, thus lessening your risk of coronary heart disease. However, a recent study in the *New England Journal of Medicine* suggests that fiber in itself does not lower blood cholesterol but that people on high-fiber diets tend to eat less dietary fat, which then leads to lower blood cholesterol levels.

Recommended Daily Budget for Fiber

Aim for a daily intake of 25 grams of fiber. Increase your consumption of all fiber-containing foods, but go easy at first. Increase gradually, one food at a time over the course of several days. This will give your intestinal system a chance to get used to this "indigestible" but healthy food. As you increase dietary fiber also increase your fluid consumption.

Dietary Strategies to Increase Fiber in Your Diet

1. Eat more whole grains such as whole wheat and cracked wheat, breads and pasta, cornmeal, bulgur, brown rice, rye, and barley.

2. At breakfast, eat oatmeal or whole-grain cereals with added bran.

3. Eat more legumes such as dry beans and peas, nuts, and seeds. To reduce the flatus-producing effect of dried beans, soak them overnight, change the water, and cook them slowly over a low temperature.

4. Eat whole fruits, especially those with edible seeds or skins, such as apples, pears, raspberries, strawberries, and prunes.

5. Eat more vegetables, especially those with edible skins, stems, and seeds, such as peas, corn, potatoes, and carrots. When cooking vegetables, decrease the cooking time to a minimum. Serve more raw vegetables and salads.

6. Remember that a "crunchy" or "fibrous" food doesn't necessarily make it a good source of fiber. For example, green peas are a good source of fiber, while lettuce and celery are two very low-fiber sources.

Reduce Alcohol Consumption

Alcoholic beverages tend to be high in calories but low in other nutrients. When following a low-calorie diet, you should severely limit your use of alcohol. Replacing nutritious foods with alcohol can lead to malnutrition, particularly certain vitamin deficiencies.

Because alcohol provides 7 calories per gram, it is a potential contributor to weight gain. A major problem with these calories is that they are empty calories with no nutritional value. In fact, alcohol may alter the absorption and use of some of the body's essential nutrients. It contributes to cardiovascular disease by its direct toxic effect on the heart as well as its tendency to increase blood pressure, a risk factor for coronary heart disease. Alcohol also contributes to a variety of serious conditions, such as cirrhosis of the liver and some neurological disorders.

In spite of recent studies which suggest a beneficial effect of moderate alcohol intake on the risk of heart attack and stroke, we believe that alcohol consumption should be carefully controlled, especially for those whose goal is weight loss. When you are limiting your calories, it's extremely difficult to drink alcohol, eat a balanced diet, *and* stay within your caloric budget.

Recommended Daily Budget for Alcohol

We recommend that you limit your intake to no more than 1 ½ to 2 ounces a day, keeping in mind that 1 ½ to 2 ounces of hard liquor such as scotch or bourbon is equal to 12 ounces of beer or 4 ounces of wine.

Dietary Strategies to Reduce Alcohol in Your Diet

1. Plan the calories you want to spend on alcohol. Pick a time when you most enjoy having alcohol, then plan to have it only at that time.
2. Pay attention to the exact amounts of alcohol you drink.
3. Substitute nonalcoholic beverages such as club soda, diet soda, or water for an alcoholic beverage at cocktail hour.

Read Nutrition Labels

To reduce the fat, sugar, and salt in your diet, and to increase complex carbohydrates and fiber, you must be aware of their presence or absence in the foods you eat. The best way to do this is to read food labels.

Understanding and evaluating food labels, however, can be tricky. Labels saying "low-fat," "all-natural," "sugar-free," or "no cholesterol" can fool you into purchasing high-calorie products that you would not buy if you read and understood the fine print. Foods with labels that read "no salt added" can actually be full of sodium!

The U.S. Food and Drug Administration (FDA) regulates the information required on packaged foods. The least amount of information the food manufacturer must provide is the product name, the manufacturer's name and address, and the weight of the net content. The FDA doesn't require an ingredient list on items such as ketchup, peanut butter, margarine, mayonnaise, and some three hundred other staples because they are made according to a standard recipe that contains specific amounts of the various ingredients. For instance, mayonnaise must contain vegetable oil, vinegar or lemon juice, and egg yolk. These ingredients do not have to be listed. However, if optional ingredients such as sweeteners or spices are included, they must be listed.

Most food products do not fall into this category, and the ingredients they contain must be listed in descending order according to their weight or quantity. Thus, the sequence of ingredients gives you an idea of the relative amount of any particular item the product contains. For instance, if sugar is listed first, you'll know that sugar is used more than any other ingredient in the product.

Standard Information for a Nutrition Label

The nutrition label was created to make it easier for shoppers to evaluate the nutritional content of food products. If a product makes a nutritional claim, such as "low sodium" or "high in iron," the label must contain the following information:

Serving size: the amount of food for which the nutritional
    information is given
Servings per container
Calorie content per serving
Protein content in grams

Fat content in grams

Percent of United States recommended daily allowances (USRDAs)
for protein, vitamin A, vitamin C, thiamine, riboflavin, niacin,
calcium, and iron.

The USRDAs (a term distinct from RDA or Recommended Dietary
Allowance) were designated for use on food labels and represent the
most generous amounts of protein, and the vitamins and minerals shown
above, that an adult should eat every day to stay healthy. These amounts
are listed as percentages of the recommended daily amount. If the food
product is a major part of the meal, it's a good rule of thumb that it
should supply one-third of the USRDA at each meal. It isn't necessary
to purchase a product that has 100 percent USRDA because you should
obtain your nutrient needs from fresh fruits, vegetables, grains, meats,
and other foods eaten at all three meals in a day.

Don't Be Fooled by Words

The terms listed here are often misleading. Spend your caloric budget
in the wisest way. Learn the true meaning of these words and don't let
them trick you into unwise investments.

Sugarless and *sugar-free* are a devious pair. By FDA definition, "sugar"
means sucrose (table sugar) but does not cover other forms of sugar
such as honey, fructose, sorbitol, or mannitol, which all contain as many
calories as sugar. Sorbitol and mannitol are often used in products
labeled as suitable for diabetics. They're suitable sugar substitutes that
fit into a diabetic's food plan, but they do contain calories, and the
calories must be taken into account.

Natural should be read as a warning rather than as a reassurance. This
word has not been defined by the FDA, and any manufacturer who
wishes to can put "natural" on his/her products. Many so-called "natural" foods are highly processed, packed with fat and sugar, and loaded
with additives and/or preservatives.

Light or *lite* is an inviting, but often misleading word to someone who
wants to cut calories. Light can mean a pale color, reduced sodium
content, reduced taste, reduced alcohol, or a "fluffier" texture—none of
which mean reduced calories. If the word actually refers to reduced
calories, the label must contain nutritional information, so read carefully.

Fortified foods contain added nutrients that are not naturally found in the food in question. For example, cornflakes may be fortified with vitamin C.

Enriched foods have an added nutrient that has been lost during processing. When choosing refined products such as white bread or white rice, make sure that the food has been enriched because you want the benefit of the nutrients added back into the product.

Low-calorie products must contain no more than 40 calories per serving and no more than 0.4 calories per gram. If the product is low-calorie, it must have a nutrition label.

Reduced-calorie products must be at least one-third lower in calories and similar in taste, smell, and texture to the standard version of the same food. Reduced-calorie foods must also bear nutrition labels.

Low-fat foods contain a reduced amount of fat or oil. Many low-calorie versions of dairy products and salad dressings are made by reducing the amount of fat or oil. Remember: A "low-fat" product isn't necessarily low in calories.

Imitation is a label that must be used when the product is not as nutritious as the product it resembles. If a product is similar to an existing one and just as nutritious, it can be given a new name instead of being called an imitation.

Organic is a word that's used often, but it does not have a standard FDA definition.

Flavored means that the product contains extracts for flavoring.

Lite beer or *lite wine* has fewer calories and less alcohol, grain, or sugar than regular wine or beer.

Watch Out for Saturated Fat and Cholesterol

When choosing a product, read the label carefully and remember to consider both the cholesterol and saturated fat content. Meeting both dietary recommendations simultaneously is fairly simple—if a food contains saturated fat, it will probably raise your blood cholesterol level. Many nutrition labels, unfortunately, list only the total grams of fat in a serving. A breakdown of the kinds of fats (saturated, polyunsaturated or monounsaturated) contained in the product is essential for a proper evaluation.

The terms *100% vegetable oil* or *cholesterol-free* are extremely misleading. Do not purchase a vegetable oil unless it notes the specific type of vegetable or vegetables used. Choose unsaturated oils such as corn, safflower, sunflower, cottonseed, soybean, peanut, or olive.

As for *cholesterol-free,* the fact is that only animal products contain cholesterol. Even if certain foods are cholesterol-free, they could still contain highly saturated fats, such as palm oil or coconut oil, which alone raise the cholesterol level in the blood.

Also watch out for foods that contain *saturated fatty acids.* Other words to avoid are *hydrogenation* or *hydrogenated,* which means that the oil or margarine has been partially saturated and can contain anything from 5 percent to 60 percent saturated fat.

Avoid all of the following ingredients, which are high in saturated fatty acids: beef fat, butter, cream, lard, cocoa butter, palm oil, and coconut oil.

If the label is not specific about the type of oil that is used, don't buy the product. If the label says, "Contains one and/or more of the following: soybean, hydrogenated cottonseed, and/or palm kernel oil," assume the worst. The manufacturer probably used more saturated oils as they tend to be cheaper and have a longer shelf life.

Choose foods that are made with *unsaturated fatty acids.*

Watch Out for Sugar

When reading food labels, remember that the following foods all contain sugar and will provide only empty calories in your diet:

sugar	honey	brown sugar
sucrose	invert sugar	raw sugar
galactose	lactose	maple sugar
glucose	maltose	dextrose
fructose	corn sweetener	molasses
mannitol	sorbitol	sorghum
xylitol	corn syrup	

Watch Out for Sodium

Read food labels to determine how much sodium the product contains. Remember that you want to limit your daily intake of salt to between 1,000 and 3,000 milligrams.

The following items all contain sodium:

salt	monosodium glutamate (MSG)
sodium benzoate	brine
sea salt	garlic salt
"lite" salt	disodium phosphate
onion salt	meat tenderizer
celery salt	sodium caseinate
bouillon	sodium citrate
baking powder	sodium nitrite
baking soda	sodium phosphate
sodium saccharin	sodium propionate

A few condiments to beware of because of their high levels of sodium:

soy sauce	Worcestershire sauce
steak sauce	salad dressings
barbecue sauce	"lite" soy sauce
catsup	chili sauce
mustard	relish

Once you have learned to read the fine print on labels, you will be able to evaluate and wisely choose the processed products you want to purchase. When you feel satisfied that the ingredients of a particular product are healthy, make a note of the brand name and buy that specific product again when you need it. You're taking control of your dietary choices, and ultimately, your health.

8

Meal Plans, Menus, and Recipes

Planning Your Meals

Planning your meals is central to successfully managing your weight for the rest of your life.

Meal planning isn't just cooking. You may be someone who doesn't cook at all. But whether you eat most of your meals out or prepare all of them at home, you still need to plan in order to control your daily food choices.

In order to work on a long-term basis, this food plan has to fit you and your life. If you're in charge of cooking, you should be able to decide what to have for dinner. If you're not in charge of cooking, you still need to plan what *you* are going to eat.

Step 1. Think About You and Your Lifestyle

Before you begin planning, take a few moments to review your lifestyle. Take time to think about the other people and events involved in your daily routines. Look at your schedule for the week and keep it in mind. Think about your moods, your appetite, the foods that are available, and the costs involved before you sit down to write out your plan. Ask yourself:

- How much time do I have to prepare meals?
- How much time do I *want* to spend in meal preparation?
- When is the best time to go shopping?

- Will there be a night at home when I won't feel like cooking at all?
- Will I be eating alone or with other people? How many servings should I plan?
- What foods should I avoid because they tempt me to eat more than I should?
- Does anyone else in the family have special food requirements?

Explore your feelings. Figure out what is and isn't realistic for you. Some of us don't mind being in the kitchen, but others don't like it at all.

"I discovered that if I prepare meals for the week, all day on Saturday, I'm frustrated because I've spent half my weekend working!" says Nina Halloran. "That's why I now prepare meals in thirty minutes or less. I go for the most nutritious meals in the least amount of time."

On the other hand, you may be the kind of person, like Mark Loomis, who finds cooking a way to relax and be creative.

"I work out my problems when I'm cooking," says Mark. "It's a time for me when I get to dream a bit. I suppose you could call it my therapy, but it's also a lot of satisfaction for me. I love to put out meals that look and taste beautiful."

You are important. Your schedule and *your* wishes are *important.* Make decisions according to *your* time restraints and *your* food preferences.

Plan only one meal for the whole family. DO NOT plan to prepare separate meals for your children, your spouse, or your parents. You can give your family members bigger servings—particularly of the bread and milk groups. They can have margarine on their baked potatoes. Instead of the half cup of pasta you're having, they can have one and a half cups or more, depending on their individual dietary requirements.

Don't worry; you can still make favorite family dishes. If you love lasagna, tacos, or fried chicken, plan them into your diet, but eat less of them.

Step 2. Think About Your Meals and Your Minutes

Anticipate the whole week. Look at your calendar to determine the number of meals you'll be eating at home and at work (do you take lunch with you?), and the number of meals you'll be eating out.

Here is how Nina Halloran set up her plan for one week of meals: Nina always eats breakfast at home, so she plans seven breakfast meals. She's decided to take a brown-bag lunch to work three days a week since it's difficult to eat a low-calorie lunch out. Nina, her husband, and their children are going to a noontime cookout on Saturday, so she only needs to plan four lunch meals (three brown-bag meals and one regular) at home. Dinner always seems to be a chore after a long day, and sometimes she doesn't feel like cooking. She decides to compromise by serving one store-bought frozen entree a week and having one meal out, which means she needs to plan five evening meals at home.

One strategy for success is to have the planned meals readily available. You may change the evening that you're going to eat out, but if you have planned five dinners, you will have the ingredients for them in your refrigerator, ready to prepare.

Sometimes, because you just can't anticipate a day when you don't want to be in the kitchen, it's a good idea to have several low-calorie dinners in the freezer. You might want to make meals in advance and freeze them to save time and reduce the opportunity for overeating. Or, you may want to buy several low-calorie, already-prepared frozen dinners. Some of our clients hesitate to purchase commercially prepared frozen dinners because of their high sodium content. But we believe in calorie control first and sodium control second—unless, of course, you are hypertensive or have heart disease, in which case you must follow your doctor's specific instructions regarding sodium intake.

Choose a caloric distribution that works for you (see table 10). Be consistent on a day-to-day basis. If you stick with your planned distribution, you will be less likely to deviate from it.

Table 10.

Distribution of Calories

Total No. of Calories	Breakfast	Lunch	Dinner	Mini-Meal
1,000	150	350	500	
	300	350	350	
	150	500	350	
	250	250	500	
1,200	200	450	550	
	400	400	400	
	250	350	450	150
	250	400	550	
1,500	200	600	700	
	500	500	500	
	300	500	500	200
	350	450	550	150

However, you do need to be flexible. There may be times when your schedule requires a planned mini-meal. For instance, if you know that you're going to eat a late dinner and will be very hungry at 5 P.M., plan a mini-meal as part of your meal distribution and calculate your calories to include it. Usually a mini-meal of oatmeal or some other filling food containing 100 to 200 calories (for example, half a sandwich, plain yogurt, or fruit) will satisfy your hunger, and keep you from feeling deprived and later overeating at your next meal. The important thing is to incorporate it into your early planning.

Step 3. Set Up Your Weekly Meal Plan

When you're ready to write out your weekly meal plan, choose a time when you won't be interrupted or rushed. Try to give yourself at least an hour. Choose a time when you are not hungry—preferably right after you've eaten a meal. Pour yourself a large glass of water or club soda to drink while you're looking at menus and recipes (this will help to relieve feelings of emptiness in your stomach). If possible, sit down to write out your meal plans and shopping list at the same time and place every week.

Sometimes it's easiest to begin by planning your largest meal. Choose the main dish, your portion size according to your allotment of calories, and then plan around it. Complement your entree with dishes from the remaining six food groups. Remember how many checks you have from each of the food groups. Write the calories beside each item and show the total calories for the meal. Consider the ingredients used in the food preparation and include them in your menu plan so that your calorie count is accurate. We recommend using recipes that include a calorie counts and fat and sodium content (see recipes, pages 179–283).

Now add the remaining meals. Try to plan a variety of foods and think about the nutritional balance. Do you have items from the six basic food groups included in your meals every day? Will your breakfasts, lunches, and dinners have attractive contrasts in texture, flavor, color, form, and temperature?

When you're setting up a week-long plan, you can also figure on using leftovers. For instance, you can cook an extra chicken breast for dinner one night and use it in a chicken salad for the following lunch meal, saving yourself time and money. Of course, if you have difficulty resisting leftovers, this may not be a strategy that will work for you.

If you're not quite ready to make your own personalized weekly meal plan, follow our two-week 1,000-calorie meal plan on page 144. Use it as it is, or set up your own alternatives and just refer to our plan as a guideline.

Step 4. Use Your Weekly Meal Planner

Meal planning takes time and will not go away. In order to save time in the long run, however, plan three to four weeks' worth of meals and then rotate them on a regular basis. Keep your corresponding shopping list with each week's menus so that the list can be used again. Minor modifications can be made as needed, but the major work has been done. After you have planned several weeks' worth of meals a few times, you will have built up many sets of menu plans that work for you and minimize your planning time.

Don't make the mistake of being too repetitive. "Diet boredom" leads to trouble. Whenever you see an appealing recipe, write it down and store it in another section of your weekly meal planner. Use it when you are tired of what you've been eating and need a change.

The weekly meal planner is a good tool for organizing your meals on a weekly basis. A copy of our planner is on page 107. Photocopy this planner as often as you need and create a notebook in which you keep your weekly meal plans and shopping lists.

It's a good idea to let your weekly meal planner serve as a food diary as well as a planning booklet (see the sample food diary, page 136). Record what you planned to eat and then what you actually ate. Make minor revisions in your plans when they're needed, and save your corrected copies, along with notes and suggestions.

If you prefer, use a filing system and index cards with your menu plans for breakfasts, lunches, and dinners. You can also keep corresponding shopping lists on index cards. If you do this, however, keep a separate food diary to record what you actually ate.

Whatever record-keeping system works best for you, we recommend that you rotate at least four weekly sets of menus every month. Remember to keep creativity in meal planning a top priority.

Daily Meal Planner

Date _____

Portion	Food	Calories

Breakfast:

Total

Lunch:

Total

Dinner:

Total

Progress, not perfection.

PLANNED EATING TOTAL

Self-Monitoring

Weight _____ Total Weight Loss _____

Behavior   *Mood*   *Positive*   *Neutral*   *Negative*
                Motivation   *High*   *Moderate* *Low*

Exercise (Note activity and duration)

Comments and Reminders

_____

_____

UNPLANNED EATING (Note time, situation, feelings, foods eaten, and calories consumed with each episode)

UNPLANNED EATING TOTAL _____

Daily Food Diary

The diary is an educational tool of the Duke Diet and Fitness Center. Participants in our program report that consistent use of the diary has benefited their lifestyle change efforts in a number of ways: improved self-awareness, increased responsibility for behavior change, and ongoing evaluation of progress. The diary can be used as a learning device to help you do the following:

- Organize and plan your meals and other selected activities in advance.
- Establish short-term goals as a means of evaluating progress toward long-term change.
- Learn the nutritional and caloric values of specific food portions.
- Identify specific problems or patterns of behavior that might hinder your weight control efforts.
- Incorporate a regular exercise program as an integral part of your lifestyle.

Recommendations for Use of the DFC Diary

1. Whenever possible, plan meals a week in advance and write food plans in your weekly meal planner. If weekly planning doesn't work for you, plan your meals at least a day in advance.
2. Record all actual food intake in the food diary.
3. Total your calorie intake for planned eating.
4. Complete Self-Monitoring section of diary. (Evaluate behavioral and exercise progress, and record your activities and goals.)
5. Record any incidents of unplanned eating (UPE), and describe the circumstances. (For example, you "grab" a frozen yogurt at the mall while shopping.) Total your UPE calories for the day.
6. Periodically look for patterns of UPE that may be occurring.
7. Periodically evaluate your goals and overall progress.

Step 5. Write a Lean Shopping List

Successful shopping begins with a list. When you write down your menu in your weekly meal planner, make a list of the specific ingredients you need to make the recipes you will be using.

You may never have thought that a shopping list could be such a big deal, but it is. It is your key to eliminating food cues at the grocery store as well as at home.

Organize your shopping list according to food categories and the layout of the store. For instance, if you walk to the produce section first, "Produce" should top your list. Other headings will include: Canned Goods, Frozen Foods, Meat and Fish, Dairy, Condiments, Miscellaneous, Grains and Cereals, Paper Products, Cleaning Supplies, Deli, and, if you have a pet, Animal Food. Reorganize these headings according to the aisles in your grocery store so that you can proceed quickly through the store. This organization will allow you to pick up all food items in one visit to each aisle, without backtracking because you forgot something. In addition to saving time, this organization will prevent unnecessary temptation and impulse buying.

Write down exact portion sizes determined from the number of servings you need for each item on your list. The list should have "15 ounces Swiss cheese," not simply "Swiss cheese." If you can't purchase the exact amount, purchase the size closest to the one you need. If you live alone or with only one other person, it is easier to predict the quantity of food that you need. If you have young children or teenagers in your house, you'll have to approximate the amounts of food they eat between meals and add those amounts to your list. No matter what your living situation, be as precise as possible with the quantities of the food you need to buy, and think in terms of the amounts you need for the entire week.

Step 6. Tips for Shopping Trips

- Go shopping when you have enough time so you can read labels and choose your purchases with care.
- Don't go shopping until you've made out your shopping list. Trying to figure out what you want for dinner while you're surrounded by food creates unnecessary temptations.
- Shop *after* you've eaten. Never go to the store at mealtime or at key snack times, and never go when you are hungry.
- Try to shop when you are calm. If you tend to buy extra food and go home for a pig-out when you're angry, don't go to the food store right after you've had a fight with your spouse or when you're furious with your boss.
- Check the newspaper for sale items *before* you go shopping. (You might want to check it even before you make your meal plan.)
- Clip coupons to buy those items you use regularly. Don't save coupons for things you don't need.
- Shop by yourself or with someone who will not grab things and throw

them into your basket. Don't go shopping with someone you know is an impulse buyer.

- Purchase only the items on your list. Buy the exact amount that you need. Don't buy a bunch of bananas if your recipe calls for only one.
- If an item on your list is unavailable, don't run to the candy section. Make a substitution from the same food group and make a note of the change in your weekly meal planner when you return home.
- Buy only those foods that have been planned. Don't buy anything on impulse.
- Don't rationalize the purchase of additional foods "just in case company comes" or "because this particular item is on sale."
- Don't buy any food without having a specific plan for its use.
- Avoid the aisles that are tempting. You don't *need* to walk past the cookies or the candies. If there's something you must buy near items that tempt you, don't dawdle.
- Don't buy anything to eat while you're waiting in the checkout line or on your way home. Don't buy a candy bar and don't buy a small bag of chips. They're not on your list, and they're not part of your plan.
- If you hate to shop and you don't have a family member who can shop for you, consider hiring someone to do it. Anyone can follow a list.

Step 7. Take Your Groceries Home

Put the groceries in the trunk or in the backseat where you can't reach them on the way home. You won't need a reward for having shopped well. Your rewards will come in looking and feeling better about yourself.

When you get home, sit down with a large glass of ice water or a diet soda before you begin to deal with your shopping bags. Slowly sip your drink. When you get up to put away your groceries, remember that all of this food will be used during the week. Don't nibble while you're putting it away.

Step 8. Keep Planning!

After a couple of weeks or a few months of planning your meals and shopping lists, you may become bored and want to drop the weekly meal planner. You may be tempted to go shopping without a list. But no matter how tempting it is, *keep planning.* Planning will continue to be crucial to your successful weight management.

You may think that after a month or so you have broken the habits that took a lifetime to develop, but you are wrong. You will need at least a year of planning to establish better habits that replace the old, familiar ones.

Boredom with planning ahead may be a fact of life for you, and if so, accept it. Meal planning is always there. If you're in charge of it every day of the week, you have to do it, even if you don't like it or even if you eat a low-calorie frozen dinner three or four nights a week.

If a week comes along, and for some reason you haven't planned ahead, at least think a day ahead, or at the very least, a few moments ahead. Let's say you haven't planned and you suddenly realize you're ready to eat. Stop and take a deep breath before you pop food in your mouth. Think: "What are my options, what can I do in this situation?" Even that much will help you, because it's a form of planning. It gives you some control.

With every step you take in controlling your interaction with food, you are changing your lifestyle. Your growing sense of finally managing your food habits reinforces your new behaviors, and you begin to feel stronger, more optimistic, and more confident each day.

DFC Menu Plans and Shopping Lists

The following section contains four weeks of menus with corresponding shopping lists and recipes. Each day's menu contains approximately 1,000 calories, less than 30 percent calories from fat, 150 milligrams of cholesterol and 1,100 milligrams of sodium.

The menus have been planned to provide a variety of foods and are based on our DFC participants' favorites. We encourage you to plan your own menus using those listed here as a starting point. These examples emphasize the exact calorie content of each food.

Using the Checkbook System to Plan Menus

If you hate counting calories, our checkbook system will make planning your meals easier. The recipes list the number of exchanges from the six food groups for each serving. Each exchange has a checkbook equivalent.

We took the first three days of Week 1 and converted the foods and recipes into corresponding checks. We then added the total number of checks for the day and compared them against the recommended amounts for 1,000 calories. Note that the total recommended amounts are close but do not exactly match since recipes vary.

While it is acceptable to be only one or two checks over or under the recommendation, it is more important that you include foods from all groups and plan your meals and stick to them. We feel that you should try to spend your checks at close to the recommended amounts. Watch out for adding more of any food group on a regular basis. An extra two fat checks daily will be a significant increase in calories. At 45 calories per check, this increase adds enough calories to equal 9 pounds of weight gain over a year.

Planning for Higher Caloric Amounts

We have included examples to help you plan your menus using 1,200 or 1,500 calories. We recommend that you do this by increasing the portion size or the number of checks of your bread/starch group and the milk group.

In the Week 1 menu we give examples of a 1,200-calorie diet for Monday, Tuesday, and Wednesday. Note that we increased the bread/starch, milk, and fruit groups in the various meals.

An example for a 1,500-calorie diet is shown for Thursday through Sunday of Week 1. A 200-calorie mini-meal has been added for each day. This should be eaten at a time when you might experience hunger between meals. The two most common times are late afternoon and evening. If you are going to use a mini-meal, plan for it. Having a mini-meal without planning may lead to overeating and an unwanted increase in your daily calories.

The DFC Philosophy on Beverages

We use few beverages at DFC. The only caloric beverage used is skim milk. We do not recommend using fruit juices because compared to fruit they are usually lower in fiber and not as satisfying. For example, compare the time it takes to eat one-half fresh grapefruit (one fruit check) to the time it takes to drink one-half cup grapefruit juice (one fruit check).

We recommend drinking 64 ounces of low-calorie beverage, preferably water, each day. At DFC we suggest water, decaffeinated and regular coffee and tea, unsweetened lemonade, unsweetened Kool-Aid, and a variety of artificial sweeteners for DFC participants to use with discretion. Drinking is a useful diet strategy because it helps to create a feeling of fullness. Also, it is important to increase fluid intake when fiber is augmented in the diet.

Shopping List

When possible, the following shopping lists have been tallied using the specific portions of food items needed by one individual. Some food items do not represent exact amounts. Our experience is that these items cannot be purchased in single-serving sizes and are more readily available in larger quantities. Staples such as grains, macaroni, and frozen vegetables fit this category. When the exact amount is not given, the words "small," "container," or "package" without portion size are used for bulk purchase.

Since the recipes that we use have serving yields for more than one person, it will be necessary to adjust your shopping list when cooking for one individual. Depending on the number of people you are serving, the recipes may have to be increased or decreased. For example, if your recipe indicates a yield of six servings and you want to prepare it for three, you can safely reduce the recipe by one-half.

If you find that calculating the exact numbers is a burden, use the shopping list as a guide. Remember that planning is essential. Having a list of just what you need will deter impulse buying.

Week One Menu

<table>
<thead>
<tr><th></th><th colspan="3">BREAKFAST</th><th colspan="3">LUNCH</th><th colspan="3">DINNER</th><th></th></tr>
<tr><th></th><th>Food</th><th>Portion</th><th>Cal.</th><th>Food</th><th>Portion</th><th>Cal.</th><th>Food</th><th>Portion</th><th>Cal.</th><th>Total Cal.</th></tr>
</thead>
<tbody>
<tr><td rowspan="7">M O N D A Y</td><td>Breakfast Cheesecake*</td><td>1 serving</td><td>194</td><td>Italian Stuffed Potato*</td><td>1 serving</td><td>200</td><td>Crispy Chicken*</td><td>3 oz.</td><td>174</td><td></td></tr>
<tr><td></td><td></td><td>194</td><td>Plain Yogurt</td><td>⅓ cup</td><td>48</td><td>Steamed Green Beans</td><td>1 cup</td><td>44</td><td></td></tr>
<tr><td></td><td></td><td></td><td>Cantaloupe, cubed</td><td>1 cup</td><td>57</td><td>Pasta</td><td>½ cup</td><td>78</td><td></td></tr>
<tr><td></td><td></td><td></td><td></td><td></td><td>305</td><td>Margarine</td><td>2 tsp.</td><td>68</td><td></td></tr>
<tr><td></td><td></td><td></td><td></td><td></td><td></td><td>Sugar-Free Jell-O</td><td>1 cup</td><td>16</td><td></td></tr>
<tr><td></td><td></td><td></td><td></td><td></td><td></td><td>Strawberries</td><td>1 cup</td><td>45</td><td></td></tr>
<tr><td></td><td></td><td></td><td></td><td></td><td></td><td>Skim Milk</td><td>1 cup</td><td>86
511</td><td>1,010</td></tr>
<tr><td rowspan="6">T U E S D A Y</td><td>Toasted Bagel</td><td>1 oz.</td><td>84</td><td>Tuna-Tomato Melt*</td><td>1 serving</td><td>264</td><td>Beef Loaf*</td><td>1 serving</td><td>248</td><td></td></tr>
<tr><td>Grapefruit</td><td>½ large</td><td>37</td><td>Apple</td><td>½ large</td><td>41</td><td>Linguine (cooked firm)</td><td>½ cup</td><td>95</td><td></td></tr>
<tr><td>Nonfat, plain Yogurt</td><td>¾ cup</td><td>95</td><td></td><td></td><td>305</td><td>Steamed Cauliflower</td><td>½ cup</td><td>15</td><td></td></tr>
<tr><td>Blueberry Topping*</td><td>1 Tb.</td><td>8
224</td><td></td><td></td><td></td><td>Mixed Greens</td><td>1 cup</td><td>31</td><td></td></tr>
<tr><td></td><td></td><td></td><td></td><td></td><td></td><td>Reduced-Calorie Salad Dressing</td><td>1 Tb.</td><td>16</td><td></td></tr>
<tr><td></td><td></td><td></td><td></td><td></td><td></td><td>Fresh Fruit Crepe*</td><td>1 serving</td><td>114
519</td><td>1,048</td></tr>
</tbody>
</table>

*Recipe included.

Week One Menu

WEDNESDAY

	BREAKFAST			LUNCH			DINNER			Total Cal.
	Food	Portion	Cal.	Food	Portion	Cal.	Food	Portion	Cal.	
	Omelet Florentine*	1 serving	96	DFC Chicken Salad*	½ cup	107	Lemon-Topped Fish*	4 oz.	137	
	Orange Slices	½ large	31	Whole Wheat Pita Bread	½ pita	53	Baked Potato	4 oz.	105	
	Whole Wheat Toast	1 slice	67	Diced Pineapple	½ cup	39	Margarine	1 tsp.	34	
			194	Skim Milk	1 cup	86	Broccoli Soufflé*	½ cup	60	
						285	Mixed Greens	1 cup	31	
							Reduced-Calorie Salad Dressing	1 Tb.	16	
							Mixed Fresh Fruit	1 cup	83	
							w/Fruit dip*	¼ cup	52	
									518	997

THURSDAY

	BREAKFAST			LUNCH			DINNER			Total Cal.
	Food	Portion	Cal.	Food	Portion	Cal.	Food	Portion	Cal.	
	Oatmeal	½ cup	73	Broccoli Soufflé*	1½ cups	180	Tortilla Casserole*	1 serving	344	
	Skim Milk	½ cup	43	Toasted Bagel	1 oz.	84	Sautéed Squash	1 cup	36	
	Pear	½ large	49	Margarine	1 tsp.	34	w/1 tsp. margarine		34	
			165			298	Mixed Greens	1 cup	31	
							Frozen Banana*	1 serving	110	
									555	1,018

*Recipe included.

Week One Menu

		BREAKFAST			LUNCH			DINNER			
		Food	Portion	Cal.	Food	Portion	Cal.	Food	Portion	Cal.	Total Cal.
F		Bran Muffin*	1	102	Sombrero*	1 serving	185	Marinated Flank Steak*	3 oz.	171	
R		Egg White Omelet*	1	69	Sliced Kiwi Fruit	1/2	23	Parsleyed New Potato*	4 oz.	131	
I		Margarine	1 tsp.	34	Skim Milk	1 cup	86	Margarine	1 tsp.	34	
D				205			294	Brussels Sprouts	1/2 cup	33	
A								Whole Wheat Bread	1 slice	69	
Y								Yogurt-Gelatin Whip*	1 serving	27	
								w/sliced apples	1/2 cup	32	
										497	996
S		French Toast*	2 slices	107	1% Low-Fat Cottage Cheese	1/2 cup	82	Blackened Fish*	1 serving	245	
A		Margarine	1 tsp.	34	Sliced Peaches	3/4 cup	44	Steamed Broccoli	1 cup	46	
T		Grapefruit	1/2 large	39	Bran Muffin*	2	204	Brown Rice	1/3 cup	77	
U				180			330	Skim Milk	1 cup	86	
R								Margarine	1 tsp.	34	
D										488	
A											998
Y											

*Recipe included.

	BREAKFAST			LUNCH			DINNER			Total Cal.
	Food	Portion	Cal.	Food	Portion	Cal.	Food	Portion	Cal.	
S	Poached Egg	1	79	Sea Slaw*	1 cup	159	Chicken Breast Florentine*	1 serving	250	
U	Toasted English Muffin	1/2	77	Honeydew Melon	1 cup	60	Cappelini w/Parmesan Cheese	1/2 cup	95	
N				Skim Milk	1 cup	86		1 Tb.	29	
D	Sunrise Spread*	1 Tb.	18			305	Steamed Carrots	1 cup	52	
A	Strawberries	1/2 cup	23				Pineapple	1/2 cup	40	
Y			197				Margarine	1 tsp.	34	
									500	1,002

*Recipe included.

Week One Check System

Food		Meat	Milk	Bread/Starch	Fruit	Veg.	Fat
Monday/Breakfast							
Breakfast							
Cheesecake	1 serv.	0.5	.15	1.0	1.0		0.5
Monday/Lunch							
Italian Stuffed							
Potato	1 serv.	0.75		1.5		0.5	0.5
Plain Yogurt	⅓ cup		0.3				0.2
Cantaloupe, cubed	1 cup				1.0		
Monday/Dinner							
Crispy Chicken	3 oz.	3.0		0.25			
Steamed Green Beans	1 cup					2.0	
Pasta	½ cup			1.0			
Margarine	2 tsp.						1.5
Sugar-Free Jell-O	1 cup	0.3					
Strawberries	1 cup				1.0		
Skim Milk	1 cup		1.0				
TOTAL		4.55	1.45	3.75	3.0	2.5	2.7
Recommended		7.0	1.5	2.0	3.0	3.0	2.0

Food		Meat	Milk	Bread/Starch	Fruit	Veg.	Fat
Tuesday/Breakfast							
Toasted Bagel	1 oz.			1.0			
Grapefruit	½ lg.				1.0		
Yogurt, Nonfat, Plain	¾ cup		0.75				
Blueberry Topping	1 Tb.				0.1		
Tuesday/Lunch							
Tuna-Tomato Melt	1 serv.	2.5		1.0		0.3	1.6
Apple	½ lg.				1.0		
Tuesday/Dinner							
Beef Loaf	1 serv.	3.8		0.3		0.7	0.1
Linguine	½ cup			1.0			
Steamed Cauliflower	½ cup					1.0	
Mixed Greens	1 cup					1.0	
Reduced-Calorie Salad	1 Tb.						0.4
Dressing							
Fresh Fruit Crepe	1 serv.		0.7	0.3	0.4		0.1
TOTAL		6.3	1.45	3.6	2.5	3.0	2.2
Recommended		7.0	1.5	2.0	3.0	3.0	2.0

Week One Check System

Food		Meat	Milk	Bread/ Starch	Fruit	Veg.	Fat
Wednesday/Breakfast							
Omelet Florentine	1 serv.	2.0				1.0	
Orange Slices	½ lg.				0.5		
Whole Wheat Toast	1 sl.			1			
Wednesday/Lunch							
DFC Chicken Salad	½ cup	1.5			0.25		1.0
Whole Wheat Pita	½			0.7			
Diced Pineapple	½ cup				0.7		
Skim Milk	1 cup		1.0				
Wednesday/Dinner							
Lemon-Topped Fish	4 oz.	3.0		0.25		0.5	
Baked Potato	4 oz.			1.5			
Margarine	1 tsp.						0.8
Broccoli Soufflé	½ cup	1.0				0.5	
Mixed Greens	1 cup					1.0	
Reduced-Calorie Salad	1 Tb.						
Dressing							
Mixed Fresh Fruit	1 cup				1.4		
w/Fruit Dip	¼ cup		0.25				
TOTAL		7.5	1.25	3.45	2.85	3.0	1.8
Recommended		7.0	1.5	2.0	3.1	3.0	2.0

Example of Increasing 1,000-Calorie Diet to 1,200-Calorie Diet*
Week One
Monday—Wednesday

	BREAKFAST			LUNCH			DINNER			
	Food	Portion	Cal.	Food	Portion	Cal.	Food	Portion	Cal.	Total Cal.
M O N D A Y	Breakfast Cheesecake	1 serving	194	Italian Stuffed Potato	1 serving	200	SAME			
	Skim Milk	1 cup	90	Plain Yogurt	2/3 cup	96				
			284	Cantaloupe, cubed	2 cups	114			511	1,205
						410				
T U E S D A Y	Toasted Bagel	2 oz.	168	SAME			Beef Loaf	1 serving	248	
	Grapefruit	1/2 lg.	37				Linguine	1 cup	190	
	Nonfat Yogurt	3/4 cup	95				Steamed Cauliflower	1/2 cup	15	
	Blueberry Topping	1 Tb.	8				Mixed Greens	1 cup	31	
			308			305	Reduced-Calorie Salad Dressing	1 Tb.	16	
							Fresh Fruit Crepe	1 serving	114	1,227
									614	

*Items underlined have been added or their portion increased.

	BREAKFAST			LUNCH			DINNER			Total Cal.
	Food	Portion	Cal.	Food	Portion	Cal.	Food	Portion	Cal.	
W				DFC Chicken Salad	½ cup	107	Lemon-Topped Fish	4 oz.	137	
E							Baked Potato	6 oz.	160	
D				W. Wheat Pita	1	105	Margarine	1 tsp.	34	
N							Broccoli Soufflé	½ cup	60	
E		SAME		Diced Pineapple	1 cup	77	Mixed Greens	1 cup	31	
S							Reduced-Calorie Dressing	1 Tb.	31	
D				Skim Milk	1 cup	86	Mixed Fresh Fruit w/Fruit Dip	⅓ cup	83	
A						375			70	
Y			194						606	1,175

*Items underlined have been added or their portion increased.

Example of Increasing 1,000-Calorie Diet to 1,500-Calorie Diet*
Week One
Thursday—Sunday

	BREAKFAST			LUNCH			
	Food	Portion	Cal.	Food	Portion	Cal.	
T H U R S D A Y	Oatmeal	1 cup	146	Broccoli Soufflé	1½ cups	180	
	Skim Milk	1 cup	86				
	Pear	½ lg.	49	Toasted Bagel	2 oz.	168	
	Raisins	2 Tb.	54	Margarine	1 tsp.	34	
			335			382	
F R I D A Y	Bran Muffins	2	204	Sombrero	1	230	
	Egg White Omelet	1	69	Sliced Kiwi Fruit	1	46	
	Margarine	2 tsp.	68	Skim Milk	1 cup	86	
	Vegetables (mixed), cooked	½ cup	25			362	
			366				
S A T U R D A Y	French Toast	2 slices	107	1% Low-Fat Cottage Cheese	¾ cup	123	
	Margarine	1 tsp.	34				
	Grapefruit	½ lg.	39	Sliced Peaches Dressing	¾ cup	44	
	Skim Milk	1 cup	86	Bran Muffin	2	204	
			266			371	
S U N D A Y	Poached Egg	1	79	Sea Slaw	1½ cups	241	
	Toasted English Muffin	½	77	Honeydew Melon	1 cup	60	
	Sunrise Spread	2 Tb.	36	Rye Wafers	4	88	
	Strawberries	½ cup	23			389	
	Skim Milk	1 cup	86				
			301				

*Items underlined have been added or their portion increased.

DINNER			MINI-MEAL			
Food	Portion	Cal.	Food	Portion	Cal.	Total Cal.
Tortilla Casserole	1 serving	344	Rice Cakes	2	70	
Sautéed Squash	1 cup	36				
w/Margarine	1 tsp.	34	Peanut Butter	1 Tb.	95	
Frozen Banana	1 serving	110				
Mixed Greens	1 cup	31			165	
Skim Milk	1 cup	86				
		641				1,523
Marinated Flank Steak	3 oz.	171	Pear	large	98	
Parsleyed New Potato	4 oz.	131	Nonfat Yogurt	1 cup	127	
Margarine	1 tsp.	34				
Brussels Sprouts	½ cup	33			225	
Whole Wheat Bread	2 slices	138				
Yogurt-Gelatin Whip	2 servings	54				
w/Sliced Apples	½ cup	32				
		593				1,546
Blackened Fish	1 serving	245	Raisins	2 Tb.	54	
Steamed Broccoli	1 cup	46	Popcorn	4 cups	100	
Brown Rice	1 cup	232	Margarine	1 tsp.	34	
Skim Milk	1 cup	86			188	
Margarine	1 tsp.	34				
		643				1,468
Chicken Breast Florentine	1 serving	250	Bran Cereal	½ cup	106	
Cappelini	1 cup	188	Skim Milk	1 cup	86	
w/Parmesan Cheese	1 Tb.	29				
Steamed Carrots	1 cup	52			192	
Pineapple	½ cup	40				
Margarine	2 tsp.	68				
		627				1,509

*Items underlined have been added or their portion increased.

Week One Shopping List
(Check your supply of basics while making your list.)

FRUIT

Apples (5 oz. each)-2 small
Banana (9 in.)-1 medium
Blueberries, frozen or fresh-2 oz.
Cantaloupe (5 in. diameter)-½
Grapefruit (4 in. diameter)-1 large
Honeydew (7 in. diameter)-½
Kiwi fruit-1 small
Lemons-2 small

Orange (5 oz.)-1 small
Peaches (in own juice)-8 oz. can
Pear, Bartlett (6 oz.)-1
Pineapple, diced (in own juice)-8 oz. can
Raisins-1 sm. box
Strawberries-1 pint

VEGETABLES

Alfalfa sprouts-1 pkg.
Beans, green or snap-5 oz.
Beans, kidney or pinto-15 oz. can
Broccoli-1 lg. stalk
Brussels sprouts-3 oz.
Cabbage, green, shredded-sm. head
Cabbage, red, shredded-sm. head
Capers-3½ oz. jar
Carrots-½ lb. bag
Cauliflower-2 oz.
Celery-1 sm. stalk
Garlic-1 bunch
Leeks-Sm. bunch
Lettuce, iceberg-1 head

Lettuce, romaine-1 head
Mushrooms-1 oz.
Onions, red-2 small
Onions, Spanish or yellow-4 medium
Parsley-1 bunch
Peppers, green-2 large
Pimientos-4 oz. jar
Potatoes, baking, (5 oz. each)-2
Potatoes, red-5 oz.
Spinach, fresh or frozen-6 oz.
Squash, summer-6 oz.
Tomatoes-3 small
Tomatoes, low-sodium-14½ oz. can
Tomatoes, low-sodium-8 oz. can

MISCELLANEOUS PRODUCE

Chili pepper, fresh or canned-1
Gingerroot-1
Tofu (soybean curd)-1 lb.

CEREALS

Bran cereal-1 small box
Corn flakes-1 small box
Miller's bran-1 small box

Oat bran-1 small box
Oatmeal-1 small box

BREADS

Bagels (made with water) (2 oz. whole)-1 pkg.
Bread crumbs-1 small box
English muffins-1 pkg.
Lite whole wheat bread-1 loaf
Whole wheat pita bread-1 pkg.
Very Thin Wheat Bread (40 calories/slice)-1 loaf

GRAINS

Brown rice-1 pkg.
Cappelini or other pasta-1 pkg.
Linguine or other pasta-1 pkg.
Tortillas, corn-1 pkg.
Wheat flour (enriched)-1 small bag
Whole wheat flour-1 small bag

SPICES AND HERBS

Basil
Caraway seed
Chili powder
Cinnamon
Cumin seed
Dry mustard powder
Garlic powder
Gumbo filé powder
Ginger
Herb blend, low-sodium
Mustard seed
Nutmeg
Onion powder
Oregano
Paprika
Parsley, fresh
Pepper, black
Pepper, red or cayenne
Pepper, white
Safflower
Sage
Tarragon
Thyme, whole leaf

SAUCES AND DIPS

Steak sauce, low-calorie, low-sodium-1 bottle
Mustard, prepared, low-sodium-1 bottle

FATS AND OILS

Mayonnaise, light-1 jar
Margarine, unsalted (corn/soy)-1 container
Margarine (safflower/soy)-1 container
Safflower or other poly-unsaturated vegetable oil-1 bottle
Vegetable oil cooking spray-1 can

DAIRY PRODUCTS AND EGGS

Buttermilk-1 pint
Cottage cheese, 1% milk fat-12 oz.
Eggs-1 dozen
Milk, nonfat-½ gallon
Monterey Jack cheese-1 sm. package
Mozzarella cheese, part–skim milk-1
  sm. package
Parmesan cheese, grated-1 sm.
  package

Ricotta cheese, part–skim milk-15 oz.
  container
Yogurt, plain (low-fat)-16 oz.
  container
Yogurt, vanilla (low-fat)-8 oz.
  container
Yogurt, nonfat-8 oz. container

MEATS AND POULTRY

Chicken breasts-¾ lb.
Flank steak, lean-¼ lb.

Ground beef, lean-¼ lb.

FISH

Grouper-4 oz.
Tuna fish (water-packed)-6½ oz. can
Red snapper-1 lb.

SUGARS AND SWEETS

Honey-1 sm. bottle

Sugar substitute-1 sm. box

MISCELLANEOUS

Baking soda-1 box
Cornstarch-1 box
Salad dressing, reduced-calorie-1
  bottle

Pickle relish, sweet-1 jar
Sugar-Free Jell-O-2 packages
Vinegar, cider-1 bottle

Week Two Menu

	BREAKFAST			LUNCH			DINNER			Total Cal.
	Food	Portion	Cal.	Food	Portion	Cal.	Food	Portion	Cal.	
M O N D A Y	Whole Wheat English Muffin	1/2 muffin	67	Yogurt-Oatmeal Fruit Salad*	2 servings	244	Seafood Gumbo Filé	2 cups	257	
	Egg White Omelet*	1 serving	69	Rye Wafers	2	45	Rice	1/3 cup	75	
	w/Onion, Mushroom, Green Pepper	1/2 cup	7			289	Chocolate Mint Fluff*	1/2 cup	92	
	1% Low-Fat Cottage Cheese	1/4 cup	41				Skim Milk	1 cup	86	
	Margarine	1 tsp.	34						510	
			218							1,017
T U E S D A Y	Rice Cakes	2	70	Turkey-Mushroom Soup*	1½ servings	236	Spaghetti and Meat Sauce*	3/4 cup	143	
	Blueberry Topping*	2 Tb.	15	Cantaloupe	1 cup	57		1 cup	251	
	Nonfat Yogurt	1 cup	127			293	Mixed Greens	1 serving	31	
	Grapefruit	1/2	39				Oil and Vinegar	1 tsp.	40	
			251				Parmesan Cheese	1 Tb.	29	
									494	1,038

*Recipe included.

Week Two Menu

WEDNESDAY

	BREAKFAST			LUNCH			DINNER			Total Cal.
	Food	Portion	Cal.	Food	Portion	Cal.	Food	Portion	Cal.	
	Oatmeal w/Cinnamon	3/4 cup	109	Stuffed Potato*	2 servings or 1 potato	188	Crispy Fish*	4 oz.	155	
	Raisins	2 Tb.	54	Vanilla Yogurt w/Cinnamon	1/4 cup	50	Brown Rice	1 cup	173	
	Skim Milk	1/2 cup	43	Sliced Peaches	3/4 cup	44	Margarine	2 tsp.	68	
			206			282	Orange-Glazed Carrots*	3/4 cup	73	
							Sugar-Free Jell-O	1 cup	16	
							Grapes	1 cup	58	
									543	1,031

THURSDAY

	BREAKFAST			LUNCH			DINNER			Total Cal.
	Food	Portion	Cal.	Food	Portion	Cal.	Food	Portion	Cal.	
	Bran Cereal	1/2 cup	106	Gazpacho*	1 cup	91	Sautéed Chicken Breast*	3 oz.	167	
	Plain Yogurt	1/2 cup	72	Mixed Chef Salad	1 cup	31	Steamed Spinach	1/2 cup	21	
	Banana	1/2 medium	55	Turkey	1 oz.	38	Pasta	1/2 cup	78	
			233	Egg	1/4	20	Margarine	1 tsp.	34	
				Low-Calorie Salad Dressing	1 Tb.	16	Carrot-Pineapple Salad*	1 cup	118	
				Whole Wheat Pita	1/2 pita (2/3 oz.)	53	Skim Milk	1 cup	86	
				Margarine	1 tsp.	34			504	1,009
						283				

*Recipe included.

FRIDAY

	BREAKFAST			LUNCH			DINNER			Total Cal.
	Food	Portion	Cal.	Food	Portion	Cal.	Food	Portion	Cal.	
F	Toasted Bagel	½ (1 oz.)	84	DFC Tuna Salad*	1 serving	76	Stir-Fry Beef w/Snow Peas and Mushrooms*	1½ cups	252	
R	"Light" Cream Cheese	1 oz.	66	Whole Wheat Bread	1 slice	62				
I							Brown Rice	¾ cup	174	
D	Orange Sections	½ cup	43	Banana	½ medium	55	Fresh Strawberries	1 cup	45	
A			193	Skim Milk	1 cup	86	Vanilla Yogurt	¼ cup	50	
Y						279			521	992

SATURDAY

	BREAKFAST			LUNCH			DINNER			Total Cal.
	Food	Portion	Cal.	Food	Portion	Cal.	Food	Portion	Cal.	
S	French Toast*	2 slices	107	Italian Pita Pizza*	1 serving	171	Cold Marinated Chicken*	1 serving	206	
A	Margarine	1 tsp.	34	Garden Salad	1 cup	31	Baked Potato	5 oz.	132	
T	Grapefruit	½ large	39	Oil and Vinegar Dressing	1 tsp.	40	DFC "Sour Cream"*	1 Tb.	13	
U			180							
R				Pear	1 large	98	Fresh Pineapple	1 cup	77	
D						340	Skim Milk	1 cup	86	
A									514	
Y										1,034

SUNDAY

	BREAKFAST			LUNCH			DINNER			Total Cal.
	Food	Portion	Cal.	Food	Portion	Cal.	Food	Portion	Cal.	
S	Poached Egg	1	79	Sliced Marinated Chicken (leftover)	1 oz.	32	Scallops Provençale*	1 cup	177	
U	Toasted English Muffin	½	77				Linguine	½ cup	78	
N				Whole Wheat Bread	1 slice	61	Margarine	1 tsp.	34	
D	Cubed Cantaloupe	1 cup	57	Part-Skim Mozzarella Cheese	1 oz.	73	Fresh Green Beans	½ cup	36	
A			213				Mixed Greens	1 cup	31	
Y				Mustard	1 tsp.	4	Reduced Calorie Salad Dressing	1 Tb.	16	
				Low-Calorie Mayo	1 Tb.	40				
				Lettuce Garnish			Strawberry Sorbet*	½ cup	65	
				Tomato	2 slices	9	Skim Milk	1 cup	86	
				Apple	1 large	81				
						300			523	1,036

*Recipe included.

Week Two Shopping List

FRUIT

Apple juice, frozen concentrate-1 can
Apples (5 oz. each)-2 small
Banana (9 in.)-1 medium
Blueberries, fresh or frozen-1 pint
Cantaloupe (5 in. diameter)-1
Grapefruit, white (4 in. diameter)-1
  small
Grapes-¼ lb. (25–30)
Kiwi-1 small

Lemon-1 small
Lime-1 small
Oranges (5 oz. each)-2 small
Pear, Bartlett (6 oz.)-1
Pineapple, fresh or 8 oz. canned-1
Raisins-1 sm. box
Strawberries-1 pint
Peaches (in own juice)-2 (8 oz. cans)
Peaches (water-packed)-8 oz. can

VEGETABLES

Beans, green or snap-⅜ lb.
Carrots-½ lb. bag
Celery-1 sm. stalk
Cucumber-1 small
Garlic-1 head
Gingerroot-1
Lettuce, iceberg-1 large head
Lettuce, romaine-1 large head
Mushrooms-⅜ lb.
Onions, yellow or Spanish-4 medium
Parsley-1 bunch
Peppers, green-3 large

Pepper, hot dried (red)-1
Pimientos-4 oz.
Potatoes (5 oz. each)-2
Scallions-1 small bunch
Shallot-1
Snow peas-1 oz.
Spinach-¼ lb.
Tomato-1 large
Tomatoes, low-sodium-2 8 oz. cans
Tomato paste, low-sodium-6 oz. can
Tomato sauce, low-sodium-6 oz. can
Zucchini squash-1 small

CEREALS

Bran cereal-1 small box
Corn flakes-1 small box
Oatmeal-1 small box

BREADS

Bagels (made with water), 2 oz. each-
  1 pkg.
English muffins-1 pkg.
Lite whole wheat bread-1 loaf

Whole wheat pita bread-1 pkg.
Very Thin Wheat Bread (40
  calories/slice)-1 loaf

GRAINS

Brown rice-1 pkg.
Linguine-1 pkg.
Rice cakes (low-sodium)-1 pkg.
Rye crackers-1 pkg.

Spaghetti or other pasta-2 pkg.
Wheat flour (enriched)-1 sm. bag
White rice (enriched)-1 pkg.

SPICES AND HERBS

Basil
Bay leaf
Celery seed
Cinnamon
Dill weed, dried
Dry mustard powder
Garlic powder
Gumbo filé powder
Mace
Marjoram, ground

Mint
Oregano
Paprika
Parsley, fresh
Pepper, black
Pepper, red or cayenne
Pepper, white
Salt
Thyme, ground
Vanilla extract

SAUCES AND DIPS

Mustard, prepared (low-sodium)-1
  bottle
Tabasco sauce-1 bottle

FATS AND OILS

Corn oil-1 bottle
Mayonnaise, light-1 jar
Margarine (safflower-soft)-1 container
Margarine (safflower/soy)-1 container

Olive oil-1 bottle
Safflower oil or other
  polyunsaturated oil-1 bottle
Vegetable oil cooking spray-1 can

DAIRY PRODUCTS AND EGGS

Cottage cheese, 1% milk fat-12 oz.
  container
Cream cheese, light-1 sm. pkg.
Eggs-1 dozen
Milk, nonfat-½ gallon
Mozzarella cheese-2 oz.
Parmesan cheese, grated-1 pkg.

Romano cheese-1 pkg.
Yogurt, plain (low-fat)-16 oz.
  container
Yogurt, vanilla (low-fat)-8 oz.
  container
Yogurt, plain (non-fat)-8 oz.
  container

MEATS AND POULTRY

Chicken breast-12 oz.

Flank steak, lean-6 oz.

Ground beef, lean-3 oz.

Turkey breast, roasted-1 oz.

FISH

Crabmeat (raw)-2 oz.

Oysters (raw only)-2 oz.

Red snapper-1/4 lb.

Scallops-4 oz.

Shrimp (uncooked)-3 oz.

Tuna fish (water-packed)-6 1/2 oz. can

SUGARS AND SWEETS

Sugar substitute-1 sm. box

Sugar, white-1 sm. bag

MISCELLANEOUS

Cocoa-1 sm. container

Cornstarch-1 sm. box

Salad dressing, reduced-calorie-1 bottle

Gelatin-1 sm. box

Sugar-Free Jell-O-1 sm. box

Vinegar, cider-1 bottle

Vinegar, distilled-1 bottle

Week Three Menu

	BREAKFAST			LUNCH			DINNER			Total Cal.
	Food	Portion	Cal.	Food	Portion	Cal.	Food	Portion	Cal.	
M	Baked Apple Omelet*	1 serving	150	Whole Wheat Pasta-Vegetable Salad*	1¼ cups	135	Veal Scallopini* w/Mushrooms	¼ serving	240	
O	Skim Milk	½ cup	43	Grapes	1 cup	58	Linguine	1 cup	155	
N			___	Nonfat Yogurt	1 cup	110	Steamed Asparagus	½ cup	22	
D			193			___	Margarine	1 tsp.	34	
A						303	Skim Milk	½ cup	43	
Y									___	
									494	990
T	Puffed Rice	1 cup	56	German Potato Soup*	1½ cups	173	Baked Chicken Parmesan*	4 oz.	245	
U	Skim Milk	1 cup	86	Rye Wafers	2	45	Rice w/Peas and Parsley*	¾ cup	185	
E	Banana	½	55	Margarine	1 tsp.	34	Margarine	1 tsp.	34	
S			___	Skim Milk	½ cup	43	Steamed Summer Squash	1 cup	36	
D			197			___			___	
A						295			500	
Y										992

*Recipe included.

Week Three Menu

Day	Breakfast Food	Portion	Cal.	Lunch Food	Portion	Cal.	Dinner Food	Portion	Cal.	Total Cal.
WEDNESDAY	Yogurt-Oatmeal Fruit Salad*	1 serving	122	Tex-Mex Turkey Chili*	1 cup	190	Salmon Quiche*	1 cup	345	
	Plain Toasted Bagel	½ (1 oz.)	84	Carrot Sticks	1 oz.	12	Mixed Greens	1 serving	31	
			206	Whole Wheat Roll	1 oz.	73	Oil and Vinegar	1 tsp.	40	
				Margarine	1 tsp.	34	Fresh Pineapple	1 cup	77	
						309			493	1,006
THURSDAY	Very Blueberry Muffins*	1	145	Rice Frittata*	1 serving	220	Beef Stew*	2 cups	300	
	Cubed Cantaloupe	1 cup	57	Lettuce Garnish	⅔ cup	5	Low-fat Crackers	2	40	
			202	Mixed Greens	1 serving	31	Fresh Strawberries	1 cup	45	
				Oil and Vinegar	1 tsp.	40	Nonfat Yogurt	1 cup	127	
						296			512	1,010

*Recipe included.

164

BREAKFAST

	Food	Portion	Cal.
F R I D A Y	Breakfast Cheesecake*	1 serving	194
			194
S A T U R D A Y	Fruit Frittata*	1 serving	185
			185
S U N D A Y	Oatmeal	3/4 cup	108
	Skim Milk	1/2 cup	43
	Raisins	2 Tb.	54
			205

LUNCH

Food	Portion	Cal.
Yellow Squash Casserole*	1 cup	200
Fresh Pear	1 lg.	98
		298
Black Bean Tortilla Melt*	1 serving	195
Mixed Greens	1 serving	31
Oil and Vinegar	2 tsp.	80
		306
Moroccan Chicken Salad*	1 cup	230
Low-Fat Crackers	3	60
		290

DINNER

Food	Portion	Cal.	Total Cal.
Country Captain Chicken*	1 serving	290	
Whole Wheat Pasta	1/2 cup	78	
Margarine	1 tsp.	34	
Fresh Green Beans	1/2 cup	22	
Skim Milk	1 cup	86	
		510	1,002
Shrimp and Wild Rice*	1 1/3 servings	310	
Broccoli	1 cup	46	
Margarine	1 tsp.	34	
Skim Milk	1 cup	86	
Orange Sections	1/2 cup	43	
		519	1,010
Foil Baked Fish*	6 oz.	145	
Baked Potato	6 oz.	158	
Margarine	2 tsp.	68	
Mixed Fresh Fruit	1 1/2 cups	83	
Nonfat Yogurt	3/4 cup	95	
		549	1,044

*Recipe included.

Week Three Shopping List

FRUIT

Apple (5 oz.)-1 small
Banana (9 in.)-1 medium
Blueberries (or 1 bag frozen)-1 pint
Cantaloupe (5 in. diameter)-1
Grapes, red or green-5 oz.
Lemon-1
Lime-1

Orange (6 oz.)-1
Peaches (in own juice)-8 oz. can
Pears, Bartlett (6 oz. each)-2
Pineapple, diced (in own juice)-8 oz. can
Raisins-1 lg. box
Strawberries-1 pint

VEGETABLES

Artichokes-14 oz. can
Asparagus, fresh-3 oz.
Beans, green or snap-2 oz.
Beans, kidney, low-sodium-14 oz. can
Broccoli-1 bunch
Carrots-½ lb. bag
Celery-1 stalk
Chilies, green-4 oz. can
Garlic-1 head
Leeks-1 bunch
Lettuce, iceberg-1 head
Mushrooms-3 oz.

Onions, Spanish-3 medium
Parsley-1 bunch
Peas-8 oz. pkg.
Peppers, green-2 large
Potatoes, baking (5 oz. each)-2
Scallions-1 bunch
Shallots-1 bunch
Squash, yellow-12 oz.
Tomato-1 large
Tomatoes, low-sodium-8 oz. can
Tomato sauce, low-sodium-6 oz. can

CEREALS

Bran cereal-1 box
Corn flakes-1 box
Oatmeal-1 box

Puffed Rice-1 box
Wheat germ-1 container

BREADS

Bagels (2 oz. each), fresh or frozen-1 pkg.
Crackers, low-fat-1 pkg.

Whole wheat bread-1 pkg.
Whole wheat rolls (1 oz. each), fresh or frozen-1 pkg.

GRAINS

Brown rice-1 pkg.

Linguine-1 pkg.

Tortillas, corn-1 pkg.

White rice-1 pkg.

Lite whole wheat flour-1 sm. bag

Whole wheat pasta-1 pkg.

SPICES AND HERBS

Basil, ground

Bay leaf, crumbled

Bay leaf, whole

Chili powder

Cinnamon, ground

Coriander leaf, dried

Cumin seed

Curry powder

Dill weed, dried

Garlic powder

Ginger, ground

Mace

Mustard powder

Nutmeg

Onion powder

Oregano, ground

Paprika

Parsley, dried

Parsley, fresh

Pepper, black

Pepper, red or cayenne

Pepper, white

Poppy seeds

Poultry seasoning

Tarragon

Thyme, ground

Thyme, whole

Turmeric, ground

FATS AND OILS

Oil, safflower-1 bottle

Margarine, diet-1 container

Margarine, safflower/soy/corn-1
  container

Mayonnaise, low-calorie-1 bottle

Vegetable oil cooking spray-1 can

DAIRY PRODUCTS AND EGGS

Cheddar cheese, shredded-4 oz. pkg.

Cider vinegar-1 bottle

Cottage cheese, 1% low-fat-8 oz.

Eggs-1 dozen

Mozzarella cheese, low-fat-sm. pkg.

Neufchâtel cheese-4 oz.

Parmesan cheese, grated-sm. pkg

Skim milk-½ gallon

Yogurt, plain (low-fat)-8 oz.

Yogurt, plain (nonfat)-24 oz.

MEATS AND POULTRY

Chicken breast, boneless-12 oz.
Steak tenderloin tips-4 oz.

Turkey breast-2 oz.
Veal scallopini-4 oz.

FISH

Fish fillet (red snapper, sole,
    grouper)-8 oz. lean

Salmon-3 oz.
Shrimp, peeled-6 oz.

SUGARS AND SWEETS

Sugar, brown-1 sm. bag
Sugar, white, granulated-1 sm. bag

Sugar, white, powdered-1 sm. bag
Sugar substitute-1 box

SOUPS

Chicken broth, low-sodium-1 can

NUTS AND SEEDS

Almonds, slivered-1 sm. pkg.
Walnuts, unsalted-1 sm. pkg.

MISCELLANEOUS

Baking powder-1 can
Cornstarch-1 box
Dijon mustard-1 sm. jar
Sherry, cooking-1 bottle
Tabasco sauce-1 bottle

Vanilla flavoring-1 bottle
Vermouth-1 bottle
Vinegar, red wine-1 bottle
Worcestershire sauce-1 bottle

Week Four Menu

	BREAKFAST			LUNCH			DINNER			Total Cal.
	Food	Portion	Cal.	Food	Portion	Cal.	Food	Portion	Cal.	
M O N D A Y	Egg White Omelet*	1 serving	69	Lentil and Bulgur Salad*	1⅛ cups	330	Spinach Veal Rolls*	1 roll	260	
	Sautéed Onion, Mushroom, Green Pepper	⅜ cup	9				Vermicelli	½ cup	78	
							Mixed Greens	1 cup	31	
							Reduced-Calorie Dressing	1 Tb.	5	
	Whole Wheat English Muffin	½ cup	67				Strawberry Sorbet*	½ cup	65	
	Margarine	1 tsp.	34				Skim Milk	1 cup	86	
			179			330			525	1,034
T U E S D A Y	Oat Bran	½ cup	106	Banana Oatmeal Muffin*	1	130	Chili Scampi*	6 oz	280	
	Skim Milk	½ cup	43				Brown Rice	¾ cup	174	
	Fresh Blueberries	½ cup	41	Cubed Cantaloupe	1 cup	57	Steamed Zucchini	1 cup	28	
				Nonfat Plain Yogurt	1 cup	127	Margarine	1 tsp.	34	
			190			314			516	1,020

*Recipe included.

Week Four Menu

Day		BREAKFAST			LUNCH			DINNER			Total Cal.
	Food	Portion	Cal.	Food	Portion	Cal.	Food	Portion	Cal.	
WEDNESDAY	Toasted Bagel	½ (1 oz.)	84	Tangy Tomato Soup w/ Lemongrass*	1¼ cups	30	Turkey Scallopini*	4 oz.	240	
	Sunrise Spread*	2 Tb.	36	Tuna (in water)	2 oz.	74	Sweet Potatoes w/Orange Raisin Sauce*	4 oz.	160	
	Skim Milk	1 cup	86	Whole Wheat Bread	2 slices	122	Green Beans	1 cup	44	
			206	Low-Calorie Mayonnaise	1 Tb.	40	Margarine	2 tsp.	68	
				Chopped Lettuce (garnish)	⅔ cup	5			512	
				Apple	½ lg.	40				1,029
						311				
THURSDAY	Cream of Wheat	¾ cup	101	Rice-Vegetable Pilaf*	1 cup	160	Hamburger*	5 oz.	250	
	Skim Milk	1 cup	86	Mixed Greens	2 servings	62	Whole Wheat Bun	1	114	
	Grapefruit	½ lg.	39	Reduced-Calorie Dressing	2 Tb.	10	Zucchini Potato Salad*	¾ cup	113	
			226	Canned Peaches (in own juice or water packed)	1 cup	58	Tomato Slices	2	9	
						290	Lettuce and Onion Garnish	¼ cup	10	
									496	1,012

*Recipe included.

	BREAKFAST			LUNCH			DINNER			Total Cal.
	Food	Portion	Cal.	Food	Portion	Cal.	Food	Portion	Cal.	
F R I D A Y	Banana Oatmeal Muffin*	1	130	Stuffed Cabbage Rolls*	2	200	Chilled Lemon-Poached Salmon*	1	210	
	Grapes	1 cup	58	Apple	½	40	Broccoli and Cheese Sauce	1 serving	100	
			‾‾ 188	Skim Milk	¾ cup	65 ‾‾ 305	Noodles	½ cup	90	
							Margarine	1 tsp.	34	
							Mixed Fruit	¾ cup	42	
							Fruit Dip*	¼ cup	52 ‾‾ 528	1,021
S A T U R D A Y	Puffed Wheat	¾ cup	44	1% Low-Fat Cottage Cheese	1 cup	164	Mideastern Chicken*	4 oz.	210	
	Puffed Rice	¾ cup	56	Pineapple Tidbits (in water)	1 cup	79	Steamed Carrots w/Parsley	1 cup	52	
	Skim Milk	½ cup	43	Raisins	2 Tb.	54 ‾‾ 293	Margarine	2 tsp.	68	
	Banana	½ med.	55 ‾‾ 198				Baked Potato	4 oz.	105	
							Skim Milk	¾ cup	65 ‾‾ 500	995
S U N D A Y	Baked Apple Omelet*	1 serving	150	Chicken and Wild Rice Salad w/ Red Pepper Vinaigrette*	1½ cups	270	Swordfish w/Hot Sauce*	4 oz.	200	
	Skim Milk	½ cup	43 ‾‾ 193	Rye Wafer	1	22 ‾‾ 292	Lo Mein Noodles	½ cup	100	
							Blanched Snow Peas	2 oz.	30	
							Margarine	1 tsp.	34	
							Cubed Cantaloupe	1 cup	57	
							Nonfat Yogurt	¾ cup	95 ‾‾ 516	1,001

*Recipe included.

Week Four Shopping List

FRUIT

Apple-1 large
Apple juice, concentrate-8 oz.
Banana-1 med.
Blueberries, fresh or frozen-1 pint
Cantaloupe-1
Grapefruit-1
Grapes-3 oz.
Lemons-2

Lime-1
Orange-1
Orange juice, frozen, diluted-8 oz. can
Peaches, in own juice-16 oz. can
Pineapple, in own juice-16 oz. can
Raisins-1 sm. box
Strawberries, whole-1 pint

VEGETABLES

Beans, green, fresh-4 oz.
Broccoli-1 bunch
Cabbage, green-6 oz.
Capers-1 bottle
Carrots, shredded-½ lb. bag
Celery, Pascal-1 stalk
Garlic-2 heads
Lentils-1 bag
Mushrooms-3 oz.
Onion, red-1 medium
Onions, yellow-3 medium
Parsley-1 bunch

Pepper, chili-1
Pepper, green-1
Potato, baking (6 oz.)-1
Potatoes, red or new-3 oz.
Scallions-1 bunch
Spinach, frozen-8 oz.
Sweet potato-4 oz.
Tomato-1 medium
Tomatoes (low sodium)-4 oz. can
Tomato paste (low sodium)-4 oz. can
Zucchini squash-½ lb.

CEREALS

Bran cereal-1 box
Cream of Wheat-1 pkg.
Oatmeal-1 box

Puffed Rice-1 box
Puffed Wheat-1 box

BREADS

Bagels (made with water) (2 oz. each)-1 pkg.
Bread crumbs-1 container

Crackers, low-fat-1 box
Whole wheat English muffins-1 pkg.
Whole wheat hamburger buns-1 pkg.

GRAINS

Bulgur-1 pkg.

Flour, wheat, enriched and unsifted-1 bag

Spaghetti or other pasta-1 box

Rice, brown-1 pkg.

Rice, white-1 pkg.

Rice, wild-1 pkg.

SPICES AND HERBS

Basil, ground

Cinnamon, ground

Cloves, ground

Coriander leaves, fresh

Cumin

Curry powder

Dill, fresh

Dill, dry

Garlic powder

Gingerroot

Lemongrass, dry

Mace, ground

Nutmeg, ground

Oregano, ground

Paprika

Parsley, fresh

Pepper, black

Pepper, white

Poppy seeds

Tarragon, ground

Vanilla extract

SAUCES AND DIPS

Dressing, reduced-calorie-1 bottle

Mustard, brown-1 jar

Mustard, Dijon-1 jar

Steak sauce, low-sodium-1 bottle

Tabasco sauce-1 bottle

Tomato catsup, low-sodium-1 bottle

Worcestershire sauce-1 bottle

FATS AND OILS

Chicken bouillon, low-sodium-1 container

Chili oil-1 bottle

Margarine (corn/soy)-1 container

Olive oil-1 bottle

Safflower oil-1 bottle

Vegetable oil cooking spray-1 can

DAIRY PRODUCTS AND EGGS

Cheddar cheese-2 oz.

Cottage cheese, low-fat-12 oz.

Eggs-1 dozen

Milk, nonfat-1 gallon

Mozzarella, skim milk-2 oz.

Muenster cheese-2 oz.

Provolone cheese-2 oz.

Ricotta, skim milk-8 oz.

Yogurt, plain (low-fat)-16 oz.

MEATS AND POULTRY

Chicken breast, boneless-8 oz.

Ground beef, lean-4 oz.

Turkey breast, boneless-4 oz.

Veal, ground-2 oz.

Veal scallopini-4 oz.

FISH

Salmon-6 oz.

Shrimp, peeled-8 oz.

Swordfish-4 oz.

Tuna fish (in water)-6 oz. can

SUGARS AND SWEETS

Brown sugar substitute-1 pkg.

Sugar, brown-1 box

Sugar, white, granulated-1 box

SOUPS

Chicken stock, no sodium-1 can

NUTS AND SEEDS

Pecans, halved-small pkg.

Walnuts, chopped-small pkg.

Chestnuts-1 oz.

BEVERAGES

Sherry-1 bottle

Vermouth (cooking)-1 bottle

Wine, dry red (cooking)-1 bottle

MISCELLANEOUS

Baking powder-1 box

Cornstarch-1 box

Vinegar, balsamic or red wine-1
  bottle

Vinegar, cider-1 bottle

DFC Recipes

Our recipes have passed the most rigorous tests. They are tasty, easy to make, require no special skills, and are nutritionally balanced for safe and effective weight loss. In addition, our participants like them!

Each recipe includes the following information:

Servings: This number indicates the total servings made from the listed ingredients.

Serving size: Most recipes give the size either in cups or ounces. For those recipes that do not, divide the recipe when served into equal number of servings listed.

Calories per serving: This number is the calories in a single serving.

Per Serving nutrient content: Nutrient content for a single serving is listed for protein, fat, carbohydrate, and sodium.

Each serving provides: Our check system is equivalent to the American Dietetic Association and the American Diabetic Association Exchange Lists. You can use the checks when planning your menus.

Salads, 179

Soups and Stocks, 190

Entrees, 196

Salads

Carrot-Pineapple Salad

SERVINGS: 3 • SERVING SIZE: ½ cup • CALORIES PER SERVING: 59

> 1 cup shredded carrot
> ½ cup canned pineapple pieces packed in juice, drained
> 2 tablespoons raisins
> ¼ cup plain low-fat yogurt
> Sugar substitute to taste (optional)

Thoroughly blend together all ingredients. Refrigerate for 1 hour.

PER SERVING NUTRIENT CONTENT:

2 g. protein
negligible fat
13 g. carbohydrate
27 mg. sodium

EACH SERVING PROVIDES:

0.6 Vegetable check
0.6 Fruit check
0.1 Fat check

Chicken and Wild Rice Salad with Red Pepper Vinaigrette

SERVINGS: 4 • SERVING SIZE: 1½ cups • CALORIES PER SERVING: 270

> ¾ cup wild rice
> 1½ cups low-sodium chicken stock
> 1 cup chicken or turkey, cooked and cubed
> ½ cup celery, sliced diagonally
> ¼ cup parsley, chopped
> 2 tablespoons capers, rinsed
> ¼ cup scallion, including tops, sliced diagonally
> 1 teaspoon tarragon
> ¼ cup red pepper, sliced
> ½ cup chestnuts, roasted, diced, peeled
> ½ cup Red Pepper Vinaigrette (page 258)
> Lettuce leaves
> Lemon or tomato wedges (optional)

Wash the wild rice in hot tap water. Add rice to the stock in a saucepan. Bring to a boil; cover and simmer 40 minutes or until rice is tender and water is absorbed. Pour half of the Red Pepper Vinaigrette over the rice and let cool. In a large bowl, combine rice, chicken or turkey, celery, parsley, capers, scallion, tarragon, pepper, and chestnuts. Add the remaining vinaigrette and stir lightly to mix. Cover the bowl and chill. To serve, line a bowl with a bed of lettuce leaves. Stir the salad and spoon onto lettuce. Garnish with lemon or tomato wedges.

PER SERVING NUTRIENT CONTENT:
   17 g. protein
   3 g. fat
   43 g. carbohydrate
   150 mg. sodium

EACH SERVING PROVIDES:
   0.2 Vegetable check
   2.5 Bread/Starch checks
   1.5 Meat/Meat Sub checks
   0.1 Fat check

Cranberry Salad Mold

SERVINGS: 6 • SERVING SIZE: ½ cup • CALORIES PER SERVING: 36

> 1 package raspberry- or orange-flavored low-calorie gelatin
> 1 cup boiling water
> Sugar substitute to taste
> 1 cup chopped raw cranberries
> ½ cup diced celery
> 1 8-ounce can crushed pineapple with juice
> ½ teaspoon grated orange zest

Mix gelatin with boiling liquid in a bowl and stir until dissolved. Chill until mixture begins to thicken.

In a separate bowl, add sugar substitute to cranberries. Add sweetened cranberries, celery, pineapple, and orange zest to thickened gelatin and stir until well mixed. Pour into a large mold or individual ones and chill until set. Unmold and serve on a bed of lettuce.

PER SERVING NUTRIENT CONTENT:
1 g. protein
negligible fat
8 g. carbohydrate
30 mg. sodium
EACH SERVING PROVIDES:
0.1 Meat/Meat Sub check
0.5 Fruit check

DFC Chicken Salad

SERVINGS: 2 • SERVING SIZE: ½ cup • CALORIES PER SERVING: 107

1 teaspoon mustard
2 tablespoons low-calorie mayonnaise
1 teaspoon dried tarragon or 1 tablespoon fresh
1/8 teaspoon grated lemon zest
Dash freshly ground black pepper
2 ounces cooked boneless, skinless chicken or turkey, chopped
3 tablespoons hard-cooked egg white, chopped
2 tablespoons finely sliced whites of leeks
1 tablespoon diced celery
1/4 apple, cored and chopped

In a bowl, blend together mustard, mayonnaise, tarragon, lemon zest, and pepper. Add remaining ingredients and toss well. Serve cold.

PER SERVING NUTRIENT CONTENT:
11 g. protein
5 g. fat
4 g. carbohydrate
50 mg. sodium

EACH SERVING PROVIDES:
1.2 Meat/Meat Sub checks
0.1 Vegetable check
0.2 Fruit check
1.0 Fat check

DFC Tuna Salad

SERVINGS: 7 • SERVING SIZE: ½ cup • CALORIES PER SERVING: 76

1 8-ounce can albacore tuna, rinsed and crumbled
¾ cup chopped, hard-cooked egg white
5 ounces chopped red onion
3 tablespoons chopped scallion
3 tablespoons finely diced celery
2 teaspoons capers, rinsed twice and chopped
½ cup low-calorie mayonnaise
1 teaspoon white vinegar
1 teaspoon dried oregano
½ teaspoon minced garlic
3 tablespoons minced fresh parsley
Freshly ground black pepper to taste
1 teaspoon grated lemon rind

In a large bowl, combine all ingredients and mix well. Serve on lettuce leaves or with bread of choice.

PER SERVING NUTRIENT CONTENT:
5 g. protein
5 g. fat
3 g. carbohydrate
65 mg. sodium

EACH SERVING PROVIDES:
0.5 Meat/Meat Sub check
0.3 Vegetable check
1.0 Fat check

Howard's Caesar Salad

SERVINGS: 12 • SERVING SIZE: 1 cup • CALORIES PER SERVING: 56

     3 quarts bite-sized pieces romaine lettuce, washed and dried
    12 drained anchovy fillets
     4 cloves garlic, minced
       Juice of 1 1/2 medium lemons
     2 tablespoons Dijon mustard
     3 tablespoons Worcestershire sauce
   1/4 cup freshly grated Parmesan cheese
       Freshly ground pepper to taste
     2 tablespoons olive oil
     3 egg whites, lightly whipped

Wash and dry lettuce thoroughly and set aside. In a salad bowl, mash anchovy fillets; add garlic and mix well. Add lemon juice, mustard, Worcestershire sauce, cheese, pepper, and olive oil to garlic-anchovy mixture. Stir in egg whites. Add lettuce and toss. Serve immediately.

PER SERVING NUTRIENT CONTENT:
   4 g. protein
   4 g. fat
   3 g. carbohydrate
   127 mg. sodium
EACH SERVING PROVIDES:
   0.3 Meat/Meat Sub check
   0.3 Vegetable check
   0.5 Fat check

Lentil and Bulgur Salad

SERVINGS: 5 • SERVING SIZE: 1⅛ cups • CALORIES PER SERVING: 330

SALAD:
1 cup lentils
4 cups low-sodium chicken broth
1 cup bulgur
2 cups boiling water
½ cup red onion, finely chopped
1 cup fresh parsley, minced
½ cup scallion, thinly sliced

DRESSING:
2 cloves garlic, minced
1 tablespoon Dijon mustard
¼ cup low-sodium chicken broth
1 tablespoon olive oil
2 tablespoons balsamic or red wine vinegar
1 tablespoon cider vinegar
⅛ teaspoon Tabasco sauce
½ teaspoon Worcestershire sauce
1 teaspoon oregano
¼ teaspoon ground cumin
Freshly ground black pepper to taste

In a medium saucepan, cook the lentils in the broth for 30 minutes. Let the lentils stand 10 minutes longer, then drain them. While the lentils are cooking, put bulgur in a heat-proof bowl and pour boiling water over it. Let stand for 10 minutes, then drain. Combine bulgur and lentils in large bowl.

In a separate jar, combine all the dressing ingredients. Mix well. Pour the dressing over the lentil and bulgur mixture, and toss the salad. Add scallion, red onion, and parsley at serving time and toss salad again.

PER SERVING NUTRIENT CONTENT:
18 g. protein
5 g. fat
55 g. carbohydrate
65 mg. sodium

EACH SERVING PROVIDES:
0.4 Vegetable check
3.4 Bread/Starch checks
0.6 Fat check

Moroccan Chicken Salad

SERVINGS: 1 • CALORIES PER SERVING: 230

3 ounces chicken, cooked, cubed
1/4 cup scallion, chopped
2 tablespoons fresh parsley, chopped
1 tablespoon raisins
2 teaspoons lemon juice
1 tablespoon low-calorie mayonnaise
1/8 teaspoon turmeric, ground
1/8 teaspoon cinnamon, ground
1/8 teaspoon black pepper, ground
1/8 teaspoon garlic powder
2 teaspoons almonds, sliced

Toss chicken with scallion, parsley, raisins, lemon juice, mayonnaise, and spices. Garnish with sliced almonds.

PER SERVING NUTRIENT CONTENT:
29 g. protein
8 g. fat
14 g. carbohydrate
105 mg. sodium

EACH SERVING PROVIDES:
0.3 Vegetable check
0.6 Fruit check
3.0 Meat/Meat Sub checks
1.3 Fat checks

Sea Slaw

SERVINGS: 4 • SERVING SIZE: 1 cup • CALORIES PER SERVING: 160

> 1 pound cooked firm-fleshed fish
> 1/4 cup low-calorie mayonnaise
> 2 tablespoons chopped onion
> 2 tablespoons sweet pickle relish
> 1 tablespoon mustard seed
> 1/4 teaspoon freshly ground white pepper
> 1 tablespoon fresh lemon juice
> 1 cup shredded green cabbage
> 1 cup shredded red cabbage
> 1/2 cup thinly sliced celery
> 1/4 cup diced carrot
> 4 lettuce cups

Flake the fish and place in a large bowl. Add the low-calorie mayonnaise, onion, relish, mustard seed, pepper, and lemon juice. Combine and chill for at least 1 hour to marry flavors. Before serving add shredded cabbage and sliced celery; toss lightly. Serve in lettuce cups.

PER SERVING NUTRIENT CONTENT:
   23 g. protein
   3 g. fat
   10 g. carbohydrate
   130 mg. sodium

EACH SERVING PROVIDES:
   0.3 Bread/Starch check
   3.3 Meat/Meat Sub checks
   0.8 Vegetable check
   1.3 Fat checks

Whole Wheat Pasta-Vegetable Salad

SERVINGS: 8 • SERVING SIZE: 1¼ cup • CALORIES PER SERVING: 135

> ¾ cup carrot, sliced
> 1½ cups fresh broccoli florets
> 1 14-ounce can artichoke hearts, drained and quartered
> 3 cups cooked whole wheat fusilli (corkscrew pasta), cooked without salt or fat
> 1 cup Parmesan-Garlic Dressing (page 256)
> 1¼ cups cherry tomato halves
> 8 lettuce leaves (garnish)

Place carrot in a vegetable steamer over boiling water. Cover and steam 3 minutes. Add broccoli. Cover and steam until broccoli is tender but crispy. Combine carrots and broccoli, artichoke hearts, fusilli, and dressing in a large bowl; toss gently to coat. Chill at least 1 hour. To serve, add cherry tomatoes; toss gently. Serve on lettuce-lined plates.

NOTE: Substitute vegetables of your choice in place of carrots and/or broccoli. Remember to keep the portion size the same as above.

PER SERVING NUTRIENT CONTENT:
- 6 g. protein
- 3 g. fat
- 23 g. carbohydrate
- 90 mg. sodium

EACH SERVING PROVIDES:
- 1.6 Vegetable checks
- 0.8 Bread/Starch check
- 0.6 Fat check

Yogurt-Oatmeal Fruit Salad*

SERVINGS: 2 • CALORIES PER SERVING: 122

1/2 *cup plain low-fat yogurt*
1/2 *teaspoon ground cinnamon*
1/2 *teaspoon vanilla*
1/2 *package sugar substitute*
  1 *cup cubed melon*
1/2 *large apple, diced (2 ounces)*
1/3 *cup grapes, sliced*
1/4 *cup raw old-fashioned oatmeal*
  4 *thin slices melon and apple*

Mix yogurt, cinnamon, vanilla, and sugar substitute in mixing bowl. Add melon, apple, grapes, and raw oatmeal, and mix together. Transfer to individual serving dishes; garnish with fresh fruit slices and serve.

PER SERVING NUTRIENT CONTENT:
   5 g. protein
   2 g. fat
   23 g. carbohydrate
   47 mg. sodium
EACH SERVING PROVIDES:
   0.4 Bread/Starch check
   1.0 Fruit check
   0.5 Milk check
   0.3 Fat check

*We serve this salad for lunch at DFC, but it also could be a delicious breakfast—it includes all six food groups.

Soups and Stocks

Gazpacho

SERVINGS: 8 • SERVING SIZE: 1 cup • CALORIES PER SERVING: 91

      2 1/2 cups low-sodium tomato juice
        3 cups peeled, coarsely chopped tomatoes
      1 1/2 cups diced green pepper
        2/3 cup chopped red onion
        1/3 cup fresh parsley, minced
          1 clove garlic, minced
          3 tablespoons red wine or cider vinegar
        1/2 cup peeled, seeded, and diced cucumber
          2 teaspoons fresh lime juice
          2 teaspoons chopped shallot
          1 tablespoon snipped fresh dill or 1/2 teaspoon dried dill
        1/8 teaspoon celery seed
        1/4 teaspoon paprika
        1/4 teaspoon freshly ground black pepper
      1 1/2 teaspoons Tabasco sauce
          8 fresh basil leaves

In a large bowl, combine all ingredients. Refrigerate until very cold. Mix well before serving. Garnish with whole basil leaf.

PER SERVING NUTRIENT CONTENT:
    2 g. protein
    0 g. fat
    11 g. carbohydrate
    22 mg. sodium
EACH SERVING PROVIDES:
    3.4 Vegetable checks

German Potato Soup

SERVINGS: 10 • SERVING SIZE: 1 cup • CALORIES PER SERVING: 115

3 cups leeks, thinly sliced, white part only
1 cup carrot, thinly sliced
1 cup celery, thinly sliced
4 tablespoons unsalted margarine
4 cups potatoes, peeled and diced
6 cups low-sodium chicken stock
1/4 teaspoon pepper, freshly ground
1/2 cup fresh parsley, chopped

In a large saucepan, sauté leeks, carrot, and celery in margarine until leeks are soft. Do not brown. Add potatoes, stock, and pepper. Simmer, covered, about 15 to 20 minutes, or until vegetables are tender. When the soup is cool enough to handle, puree in batches in a blender. Return to saucepan and heat. Garnish with parsley before serving.

PER SERVING NUTRIENT CONTENT:
2 g. protein
5 g. fat
17 g. carbohydrate
80 mg. sodium

EACH SERVING PROVIDES:
1.0 Vegetable check
0.7 Bread/Starch check
0.9 Fat check

Low-Sodium Chicken Stock

YIELD: 1½ quarts • CALORIES PER SERVING: negligible

2 quarts cold water
1 chicken (2½ to 3 pounds), or any leftover chicken bones
1 large onion with skin, quartered
2 large carrots, halved
2 stalks celery with leaves, halved
1 tablespoon poultry seasoning
1 tablespoon dried thyme
1 tablespoon black peppercorns

Place all ingredients in a stockpot or large saucepan, adding more cold water, if necessary, to cover the ingredients. Bring to a boil over high heat; then lower heat and simmer 2 to 4 hours, replenishing water as needed to keep ingredients covered. The pot may be uncovered or partially covered.

Strain, cool, and refrigerate the stock. Remove congealed fat and strain stock through cheesecloth. Freeze in ice cube trays or small plastic containers.

If whole chicken is used, use meat for salad, soup, or casserole.

Low-Sodium Seafood Stock

YIELD: 1½ quarts • CALORIES PER SERVING: negligible

2 quarts cold water
1½ to 2 pounds rinsed shrimp heads, crab shells, rinsed fish remains, or any
combination of these
1 large onion with skin, quartered
2 large carrots, halved
2 stalks celery with leaves, halved
1 tablespoon black peppercorns

Place all ingredients in a stockpot or large saucepan, adding more cold water, if necessary, to cover ingredients. Bring to a boil over high heat; then gently simmer 30 to 40 minutes, replenishing water as needed to keep ingredients covered. The pot may be uncovered or partially covered. Strain, cool, and refrigerate the stock. Freeze in ice cube trays or small plastic containers.

Tangy Tomato Soup with Lemongrass

SERVINGS: 5 • SERVING SIZE: 1¼ cups • CALORIES PER SERVING: 30

1 quart Low-Sodium Chicken Stock (page 192) or vegetable stock
1 14½-ounce can low-sodium tomatoes
1 fresh lemongrass stalk or 1 tablespoon dried lemongrass
2 teaspoons sugar
1 tablespoon lemon juice
2 tablespoons scallion, finely chopped
1 tablespoon chili pepper, sliced
1 tablespoon fresh coriander, finely chopped
Coriander leaves (garnish)

Put the stock in a saucepan and bring to a simmer. Chop the tomatoes into small chunks. Peel the lemongrass until you find the tender, whitish center and finely chop it. Add the sugar, lemongrass, lemon juice, scallion, chili pepper, and coriander to the simmering stock and stir to mix well. Add the tomatoes and simmer for 3 minutes. Garnish with coriander.

PER SERVING NUTRIENT CONTENT:
1 g. protein
negligible fat
7 g. carbohydrate
15 mg. sodium
EACH SERVING PROVIDES:
1.2 Vegetable check

Turkey-Mushroom Soup

SERVINGS: 5 • SERVING SIZE: 1 cup • CALORIES PER SERVING: 157

> 2 tablespoons unsalted margarine
> 1 quart sliced mushrooms
> 1/2 cup chopped onion
> 1/2 cup sliced celery
> 1/2 cup sliced carrot
> 2 cloves garlic, minced
> 2 teaspoons all-purpose flour
> 1/4 teaspoon salt
> 1/8 teaspoon dried whole thyme leaves
> 1/8 teaspoon dried whole marjoram
> 1/2 cup skim milk
> 1 tablespoon dry sherry
> 1 egg yolk, lightly beaten
> 1 1/4 cups Low-Sodium Chicken Stock (page 192), or 1 10 1/2-ounce can no-salt-added chicken broth
> 1 cup cooked skinless turkey, cubed
> 1/3 cup cooked rice (cooked without salt or fat)
> 1 tablespoon diced pimiento

In a large, heavy saucepan, melt margarine over moderate heat. Add mushrooms, onion, celery, carrots, and garlic and cook for about 5 minutes, stirring often, until onion is tender. Add flour, salt, thyme, and marjoram and stir well. Add milk, sherry, egg yolk, and broth and stir well. Add remaining ingredients, mix well, and cook gently until mixture is slightly thickened; do not allow to boil. Serve immediately.

PER SERVING NUTRIENT CONTENT:
12 g. protein
6 g. fat
13 g. carbohydrate
198 mg. sodium

EACH SERVING PROVIDES:
0.4 Bread/Starch check
0.9 Meat/Meat Sub check
1.0 Vegetable check
0.1 Milk check
0.7 Fat check

Entrees

Baked Chicken Parmesan

SERVINGS: 6 • SERVING SIZE: 4 ounces • CALORIES PER SERVING: 245

> 6 5-ounce chicken fillets, skinned and pounded
> 2 ounces cornflakes, crushed
> 1/4 cup grated Parmesan cheese
> 2 tablespoons dried parsley, chopped
> 1/2 teaspoon poultry seasoning
> 1/4 teaspoon onion powder
> 1/8 teaspoon garlic powder
> Paprika (optional)

Preheat oven to 350°F.

Combine all ingredients except chicken and mix together in a small bowl. Place chicken, meaty side down, in baking pan. Sprinkle 1 tablespoon mixture on each serving of chicken. Turn chicken over and repeat. Sprinkle with paprika, if desired. Bake at 350°F for 60 minutes or until tender.

PER SERVING NUTRIENT CONTENT:
- 38 g. protein
- 5 g. fat
- 8 g. carbohydrate
- 270 mg. sodium

EACH SERVING PROVIDES:
- 0.6 Bread/Starch check
- 5.3 Meat/Meat Sub checks

Beef Loaf

SERVINGS: 4 • CALORIES PER SERVING: 246

1 *pound lean ground beef round*
1/4 *cup dry oatmeal*
1/4 *cup chopped green pepper*
2 *egg whites*
1/4 *cup chopped onion*
1/4 *cup chopped carrot*
1/2 *cup canned low-sodium tomatoes, chopped*
1 *clove garlic, minced*
1 *teaspoon chopped fresh basil or* 1/4 *teaspoon dried*
1 1/2 *tablespoons steak sauce, low-sodium*
1 *teaspoon salt-free blended herb mix*

Preheat oven to 350°F.

In a bowl, combine all ingredients together, mixing well. Divide into 4 equal portions and press into small loaf pans or make free-form loaves on a baking sheet. Bake for 45 to 60 minutes. Do not drain, as the juices will add moisture and flavor.

PER SERVING NUTRIENT CONTENT:
   27 g. protein
   12 g. fat
   7 g. carbohydrate
   121 mg. sodium
EACH SERVING PROVIDES:
   0.3 Bread/Starch check
   3.7 Meat/Meat Sub checks
   0.5 Vegetable check

Beef Stew

SERVINGS: 4 • SERVING SIZE: 2 cups • CALORIES PER SERVING: 300

1 pound beef tenderloin tips
2 tablespoons flour
1 tablespoon safflower oil
1 15 1/2-ounce can low-sodium whole tomatoes
1 1/2 cups onion, diced
2 cups potatoes, peeled, diced
2 cups carrot, diced
2 cups celery, diced
2 tablespoons shallot, chopped
1 bay leaf
1 tablespoon dried parsley flakes
1/4 teaspoon black pepper
1/2 teaspoon dried thyme
1/2 teaspoon dried basil
1/3 cup red wine
2 cups water

Trim any visible fat from beef tenderloin tips. Cut beef into 3/4-inch cubes. Dust in flour. In a 4-quart saucepan, heat oil and brown the beef. Add remaining ingredients. Bring to a boil. Reduce heat and simmer for 1 hour or until vegetables are cooked.

PER SERVING NUTRIENT CONTENT:

28 g. protein
12 g. fat
21 g. carbohydrate
145 mg. sodium

EACH SERVING PROVIDES:

2.5 Vegetable checks
0.4 Bread/Starch check
3.2 Meat/Meat Sub checks
0.7 Fat check

Black Bean Tortilla Melts

SERVINGS: 6 • CALORIES PER SERVING: 195

  1 *15-ounce can black beans, rinsed and drained*
½ teaspoon chili powder
  6 *6-inch corn tortillas*
¼ cup minced fresh cilantro
  1 *lime, cut into 6 wedges*
  2 *4-ounce cans chopped green chilies, undrained*
¾ cup (3 ounces) shredded Cheddar cheese
    Fresh salsa

Preheat oven to 450°F.

Mash beans; add chili powder, stirring well. Spread about 3 tablespoons bean mixture on each tortilla. Sprinkle with fresh cilantro, and squeeze 1 lime wedge over each. Top each tortilla with 2 tablespoons green chilies and 2 tablespoons cheese. Bake tortillas at 450°F for 3 to 5 minutes or until cheese melts. Serve with fresh salsa.

PER SERVING NUTRIENT CONTENT:
10 g. protein
6 g. fat
26 g. carbohydrate
160 mg. sodium

EACH SERVING PROVIDES:
0.5 Vegetable checks
1.8 Bread checks
0.5 Meat/Meat Sub check
0.5 Fat check

Blackened Fish

SERVINGS: 1 • CALORIES PER SERVING: 250

1/2 pound raw boneless fillet of grouper, red snapper, or black bass
    Blackened Fish Seasoning (see next page)
  1 teaspoon unsalted margarine

Preheat oven to 350°F.

Heat a nonstick skillet and add 1 teaspoon margarine. Wash fish, pat dry, and sprinkle one side lightly with blackened fish seasoning. Put fish on hot skillet, spice side down. Sprinkle top with blackened fish seasoning. Turn after 1 minute. Continue to cook 1 minute longer. Remove from skillet and place on baking pan and continue to bake in a 350°F oven until flaky, approximately 10 minutes per inch of thickness.

NOTE: Calories have been calculated for red snapper.

PER SERVING NUTRIENT CONTENT:
  45 g. protein
  6 g. fat
  negligible carbohydrate
  155 mg. sodium

EACH SERVING PROVIDES:
  6 Meat/Meat Sub checks
  1 Fat check

Blackened Fish Seasoning

SERVINGS: 24 • SERVING SIZE: 1 teaspoon
CALORIES PER SERVING: 5

1 teaspoon white pepper
¾ tablespoon red pepper
1 tablespoon black pepper
4 teaspoons onion powder
2 teaspoons garlic powder
4 teaspoons salt-free blended herb mix
1 teaspoon sage
2 tablespoons dried safflower
4 teaspoons paprika
2 teaspoons gumbo filé
4 tablespoons dried oregano leaves
8 tablespoons whole leaf thyme

Put all ingredients in a blender and blend until fine. Store in an airtight shaker jar.

PER SERVING NUTRIENT CONTENT:
4 g. carbohydrate
1 mg. sodium

Chicken Breasts Florentine

SERVINGS: 4 • CALORIES PER SERVING: 250

1 10-ounce package frozen chopped spinach,
  thawed and drained, or 2 cups fresh spinach,
  chopped, steamed, and drained
2 tablespoons chopped pimiento
4 4-ounce skinless, boneless chicken breast halves
4 ounces part-skim mozzarella cheese, grated
1 cup Basic Tomato Sauce (page 260)

Preheat oven to 350°F.

In a bowl, combine spinach and pimiento. Pound each chicken piece until flat, about ¼- to ½-inch thick. Top each piece with one-quarter of the cheese and ½ cup spinach-pimiento mixture. Bring up ends of chicken pieces and secure with toothpicks.

Place chicken in baking dish and pour tomato sauce over chicken. Cover and bake 20 minutes, then uncover and bake until done, about 10 minutes more.

PER SERVING NUTRIENT CONTENT:
  36 g. protein
  8 g. fat
  8 g. carbohydrate
  262 mg. sodium
EACH SERVING PROVIDES:
  3.9 Meat/Meat Sub checks
  1.5 Vegetable checks

Chili Scampi

SERVINGS: 8 • SERVING SIZE: 3 ounces • CALORIES PER SERVING: 140

8 cloves garlic, coarsely chopped
2 tablespoons olive oil
1 teaspoon seeded red chili pepper, minced
2 pounds large fresh shrimp, peeled and deveined
1 tablespoon lime juice

In a large heavy skillet, sauté garlic in oil over medium-high heat. Cook for 1 minute. Add pepper and shrimp; cook for 1 minute stirring constantly. Add lime juice, and cook an additional 3 minutes or until shrimp are done.

PER SERVING NUTRIENT CONTENT:

20 g. protein
4 g. fat
3 g. carbohydrate
165 mg. sodium

EACH SERVING PROVIDES:

2.8 Meat/Meat Sub checks
0.7 Fat check

Chilled Lemon-Poached Salmon

SERVINGS: 4 • CALORIES PER SERVING: 210

1 1/2 *cups water*
1 1/2 *cups white wine*
1 *lemon, sliced*
1/4 *cup scallion, sliced*
Fresh dill
1/8 *teaspoon pepper*
4 *6-ounce salmon steaks, 1 inch thick each*

In a large skillet, combine water, wine, lemon slices, scallion, fresh dill, and pepper. Heat to boiling. Add salmon steaks and cover. Reduce heat to low. Simmer gently 7 to 10 minutes. Remove fish from liquid. Cover and refrigerate until chilled.

PER SERVING NUTRIENT CONTENT:

34 g. protein
6 g. fat
2 g. carbohydrate
110 mg. sodium

EACH SERVING PROVIDES:

0.1 Vegetable check
0.1 Fruit check
5.0 Meat/Meat Sub checks

Cold Marinated Chicken

SERVINGS: 4 • SERVING SIZE: 4 ounces • CALORIES PER SERVING: 206

> *4 6-ounce chicken breast halves, skin removed*
> *1/2 cup reduced-calorie Italian dressing*
> *1/4 cup water*
> *1 tablespoon fresh lime juice*
> *1 tablespoon grated lime zest*
> *1/8 cup dry white wine*
> *2 tablespoons minced garlic*
> *2 tablespoons fresh ginger, peeled and minced*
> *Vegetable oil cooking spray*

Combine dressing, water, lime juice and zest, wine, garlic, and ginger in a shallow bowl. Wash chicken, place in marinade, and refrigerate, covered, overnight.

Preheat broiler.

Drain chicken and reserve the marinade. Grill chicken to score both sides, then place chicken on tray covered with foil and sprayed lightly with cooking spray. Reduce oven temperature to 350°F and bake chicken for approximately 30 minutes. Baste with marinade and continue to cook until done. Refrigerate until cooled.

PER SERVING NUTRIENT CONTENT:

    36 g. protein
    4 g. fat
    4 g. carbohydrate
    385 mg. sodium

EACH SERVING PROVIDES:

    3.9 Meat/Meat Sub checks

Country Captain Chicken

SERVINGS: 4 • CALORIES PER SERVING: 290

1 1/2 pounds chicken breasts, boned and skinned
1 cup onion, chopped
1/2 cup red pepper, sliced
1/2 cup carrot, diced
1 teaspoon oil
1 clove garlic, minced
1 1/2 tablespoon fresh ginger
1 1/2 cups tomatoes, chopped
2 ounces green chilies
2 tablespoons raisins
1 tablespoon dried parsley
1/4 teaspoon ground cumin
1 teaspoon brown sugar
1 tablespoon curry powder
1/8 teaspoon cinnamon
1/4 teaspoon orange zest
1 cup Low-Sodium Chicken Stock (page 192)

Wash chicken breasts. In a nonstick skillet sauté chicken breasts in oil until browned on both sides. Remove from skillet and keep warm. Add onion, red pepper, carrot, garlic, and ginger. Sauté until onions begin to wilt. Add tomatoes, green chilies, raisins, parsley, cumin, brown sugar, curry powder, cinnamon, and orange zest. Add chicken stock. Add chicken breasts. Bring to a simmer and continue to simmer 40 minutes, stirring occasionally. Serve warm; garnish with an orange slice.

PER SERVING NUTRIENT CONTENT:
    42 g. protein
    6 g. fat
    16 g. carbohydrate
    110 mg. sodium
EACH SERVING PROVIDES:
    1.3 Vegetable checks
    0.2 Fruit check
    4.4 Meat/Meat Sub checks
    0.3 Fat check

Crispy Chicken

SERVINGS: 4 • SERVING SIZE: 3 ounces • CALORIES PER SERVING: 174

1 1/2 pounds skinless chicken breasts or legs
1 ounce crushed corn flakes
1 teaspoon dry mustard
1/8 teaspoon black pepper
1/4 teaspoon paprika
1/2 teaspoon garlic powder
1 teaspoon grated lemon zest
1 egg white
1 teaspoon fresh lemon juice

Preheat oven to 350°F.

Remove skin and any visible fat from chicken and wash thoroughly. Combine corn flakes, mustard, pepper, paprika, garlic powder, and lemon zest. In a shallow bowl, combine egg white and lemon juice; beat slightly. Dip meaty side of chicken in egg mixture; coat with crumb mixture. Place in ungreased baking pan and bake at 350°F for 1 hour.

PER SERVING NUTRIENT CONTENT:
27.9 g. protein
3.0 g. fat
7.0 g. carbohydrate
162 mg. sodium

EACH SERVING PROVIDES:
0.3 Bread/Starch check
3.0 Meat/Meat Sub checks

Crispy Fish

SERVINGS: 4 • SERVING SIZE: 4 ounces • CALORIES PER SERVING: 155

> 1 ounce crushed corn flakes
> 1 teaspoon dry mustard
> 1/8 teaspoon freshly ground black pepper
> 1/4 teaspoon paprika
> 1/2 teaspoon garlic powder
> 1 egg white
> 2 teaspoons fresh lemon juice
> 16 ounces red snapper fillets
> 1/2 teaspoon lemon zest

Preheat oven to 350°F. Lightly grease a baking sheet.

On a piece of wax paper, combine crushed corn flakes, mustard, pepper, paprika, and garlic powder. In a shallow bowl, combine egg white and lemon juice and beat until foamy. Dip fish in egg mixture and coat with crumb mixture. Arrange fillets in single layer on baking sheet and bake until fish flakes, approximately 10 minutes per inch of thickness.

PER SERVING NUTRIENT CONTENT:
    27 g. protein
    1 g. fat
    7 g. carbohydrate
    186 mg. sodium
EACH SERVING PROVIDES:
    0.3 Bread/Starch check
    2.7 Meat/Meat Sub checks

Foil Baked Fish

SERVINGS: 4 • SERVING SIZE: 6 ounces • CALORIES PER SERVING: 145

> 4 6-ounce sole fillets
> 1/2 cup fresh carrot, sliced
> 1 cup fresh mushrooms, sliced
> 1/2 cup green pepper, diced
> 1/2 cup onion, diced
> 1/2 cup celery, chopped
> 1 tablespoon dried parsley
> 1/2 teaspoon dried oregano
> 1/2 teaspoon paprika
> 4 teaspoons lemon juice

Preheat oven to 450°F.

In a medium-size bowl, mix carrot, mushrooms, green pepper, onion, celery, parsley, oregano, paprika, and lemon juice. Set aside. Wash fish fillets and place each fillet on a sheet of foil. Divide vegetable mixture among the fillets. Seal foil tightly. Bake at 450°F for 25 minutes.

PER SERVING NUTRIENT CONTENT:
- 26 g. protein
- 1 g. fat
- 6 g. carbohydrate
- 115 mg. sodium

EACH SERVING PROVIDES:
- 0.3 Vegetable check
- 4.0 Meat/Meat Sub checks

Hamburger

SERVINGS: 4 • CALORIES PER SERVING: 250

1 pound lean ground beef
½ cup rolled oats
2 large egg whites
2 teaspoons salt-free blended herb mix
3 teaspoons steak sauce, low-sodium

In a medium bowl, blend ingredients well. Portion into 4 hamburger patties. Broil on high until cooked to your preference.

PER SERVING NUTRIENT CONTENT:
27 g. protein
12 g. fat
7 g. carbohydrate
115 mg. sodium

EACH SERVING PROVIDES:
0.5 Bread/Starch check
3.7 Meat/Meat Sub checks

Sombrero (Mexican pita)

SERVINGS: 2 • CALORIES PER SERVING: 185

1 pita bread (6" diameter)
1 c. mixed vegetables, steamed
½ c. Basic Tomato Sauce
2 oz. tofu, cubed
1 oz. Monterey Jack cheese, grated
Vegetable cooking spray

Preheat oven to 400°. Spray flat baking sheet with vegetable cooking spray. Cut whole pita bread in half so that there are two large circles. Layer half (one circle) of the pita bread with vegetables, thickened and modified sauce, tofu, and top with Monterey Jack Cheese. Bake in oven until cheese is brown on top and remaining ingredients are warm (about ten minutes).

PER SERVING NUTRIENT CONTENT:
11 g. protein
6 g. fat
23 g. carbohydrate
205 mg. sodium

Italian Pita Pizza

SERVINGS: 2 • CALORIES PER SERVING: 135

Vegetable oil cooking spray
1 *(2.24 ounces) pita bread*
1 *cup steamed diced vegetables*
½ *cup Basic Tomato Sauce (page 260), reduced slowly until thick*
1 *ounce part-skim mozzarella cheese, grated*
1 *tablespoon freshly grated Parmesan cheese*

Preheat oven to 400°F. Spray baking sheet with vegetable cooking spray.

Cut pita bread in half, making two large circles. Layer each circle with half the vegetables, sauce, mozzarella, and Parmesan cheese. Bake until cheese is golden brown and ingredients are heated through, about 10 minutes.

PER SERVING NUTRIENT CONTENT:
   8 g. protein
   4 g. fat
   18 g. carbohydrate
   230 mg. sodium
EACH SERVING PROVIDES:
   1.5 Bread/Starch checks
   1.0 Meat/Meat Sub check
   0.7 Vegetable check
   0.8 Fat check

Variation: For a **sombrero** (Mexican pizza), add ¼ teaspoon each of ground cumin, chili powder, and minced fresh chilies to tomato sauce. Layer pizza as described above, adding 2 ounces cubed tofu between sauce and Monterey Jack cheese. Omit Parmesan and bake as above.

Lemon-Topped Fish

SERVINGS: 4 • SERVING SIZE: 4 ounces • CALORIES PER SERVING: 137

For Microwave

> 1 pound lean fish fillets of your choice (red snapper or grouper are good examples)
> 2 tablespoons dry bread crumbs
> 1/2 cup chopped onion
> 1/2 cup chopped green bell pepper
> 4 ounces fresh mushrooms, chopped
> 1/4 teaspoon freshly ground black pepper
> 1/2 thinly sliced lemon

Place fish in a 12-by-8-inch baking dish. In small bowl, combine bread crumbs, onion, green pepper, mushrooms, and black pepper. Spread topping over fish and cover with lemon slices. Cover dish with wax paper. Microwave on high (100 percent) 5 to 7 minutes, or until fish flakes easily. Let stand 3 to 5 minutes before serving.

PER SERVING NUTRIENT CONTENT:
   24 g. protein
   1 g. fat
   9 g. carbohydrate
   101 mg. sodium
EACH SERVING PROVIDES:
   0.2 Bread/Starch check
   2.3 Meat/Meat Sub checks
   0.8 Vegetable check

Marinated Flank Steak

SERVINGS: 4 • SERVING SIZE: 3 ounces • CALORIES PER SERVING: 171

¼ cup reduced-calorie Italian dressing
2 tablespoons fresh lemon juice
2 tablespoons red wine or cider vinegar
1 clove garlic, minced
1 pound flank steak (or other lean steak)

Preheat broiler or prepare grill.

In a bowl, combine all ingredients except steak and mix well. Arrange steak in a shallow dish. Pour in marinade and refrigerate, covered, for at least 4 hours or, preferably, overnight. Turn steak occasionally.

Broil or grill steak for 3 to 5 minutes on each side. Slice meat thinly against the grain and serve.

PER SERVING NUTRIENT CONTENT:
25 g. protein
6 g. fat
2 g. carbohydrate
236 mg. sodium

EACH SERVING PROVIDES:
3.0 Meat/Meat Sub checks
0.1 Fruit check

Mideastern Chicken

SERVINGS: 4 • SERVING SIZE: 6 ounces • CALORIES PER SERVING: 315

> 3 pounds raw chicken breasts or legs, skinned
> 1 teaspoon garlic powder
> 1/2 teaspoon crushed tarragon
> 2 teaspoons paprika
> 1/4 teaspoon black pepper
> 1/2 teaspoon cumin
> 1/2 teaspoon lemon peel
> 1/2 teaspoon orange peel
> 1/4 cup lemon juice
> 1/2 cup orange juice
> 1 tablespoon cornstarch
> 1/4 cup water

Preheat oven to 375°F.

Combine seasonings and sprinkle over chicken. Arrange chicken, meat side down, in a baking dish. Combine lemon peel, orange peel, and juices and pour over chicken. Bake, uncovered, at 375°F for 45 minutes. Turn chicken and continue baking 30 minutes longer, basting frequently with pan juices.

PER SERVING NUTRIENT CONTENT:
    53 g. protein
    6 g. fat
    8 g. carbohydrate
    125 mg. sodium

EACH SERVING PROVIDES:
    0.3 Fruit check
    0.2 Bread/Starch check
    5.9 Meat/Meat Sub checks

Rice Frittata

SERVINGS: 6 • CALORIES PER SERVING: 220

1 cup onion, finely chopped
2 teaspoons margarine
4 large eggs
8 large egg whites
1/2 cup nonfat milk
1 teaspoon Worcestershire sauce
1 teaspoon Tabasco sauce
1 tablespoon green chilies, chopped
1 1/2 cups cooked brown rice
1/2 cup yellow squash, diced
1 cup tomatoes, chopped
3 ounces Cheddar cheese, shredded
1/2 cup lettuce, shredded

In a 10-inch skillet, melt margarine on low heat. Add onions and sauté until translucent. Beat eggs and egg whites together. Add nonfat milk, Worcestershire sauce, Tabasco sauce, and green chilies. Add brown rice, squash, and tomatoes. Pour all ingredients into skillet over cooked onion. Reduce heat to low. Cover and cook until top is almost set, about 15 to 20 minutes. When top is set, sprinkle with cheese. Cover and remove from heat and let stand for 10 minutes. Cut into wedges, garnish with shredded lettuce, and serve.

PER SERVING NUTRIENT CONTENT:
    15 g. protein
    10 g. fat
    17 g. carbohydrate
    235 g. sodium
EACH SERVING PROVIDES:
    0.1 Milk check
    0.4 Vegetable check
    0.9 Bread/Starch check
    1.6 Meat/Meat Sub checks
    1.3 Fat checks

Salmon Quiche

SERVINGS: 6 • SERVING SIZE: 1 cup • CALORIES PER SERVING: 345

1 pound poached salmon
3 cups 1% low-fat cottage cheese, drained
½ cup plain yogurt
1 tablespoon cornstarch
2 tablespoons Parmesan cheese
4 ounces part-skim mozzarella cheese, shredded
¾ cups scallion
2 tablespoons dried dill
2 teaspoons white pepper
1 tablespoon mustard powder
Dash of cayenne pepper
4 egg whites

Preheat oven to 350°F.

In a large bowl crumble the poached salmon. In a blender place cottage cheese, yogurt, and cornstarch and puree until smooth. Transfer to the bowl with salmon and mix. Fold in Parmesan cheese, mozzarella cheese, scallion, and seasonings. Whip egg whites and fold into mixture. Divide batter into six portions and place in individual baking dishes sprayed with vegetable oil cooking spray. Bake at 350°F for approximately 30 minutes.

PER SERVING NUTRIENT CONTENT:
  40 g. protein
  16 g. fat
  8 g. carbohydrate
  635 mg. sodium

EACH SERVING PROVIDES:
  0.1 Milk check
  0.1 Vegetable check
  0.2 Bread/Starch check
  5 Meat/Meat Sub checks

Sautéed Chicken Breasts*

SERVINGS: 4 • SERVING SIZE: 3 ounces • CALORIES PER SERVING: 167

> 1 pound boneless, skinless chicken breasts
> 1 tablespoon unsalted margarine
> 1/4 cup dry sherry or white wine
> 1/2–1 teaspoon dried basil or tarragon (or mixture of both)
> 1/8 teaspoon freshly ground white pepper
> Paprika
> Chopped fresh parsley

Place chicken breasts, one at a time, between sheets of wax paper and, using a wooden mallet or rolling pin, pound chicken until it is approximately 1/2-inch thick.

Melt margarine over medium heat in a nonstick pan. Add chicken and sauté until brown on both sides, approximately 4 to 5 minutes. Add sherry and bring to a boil. Sprinkle tarragon, pepper, and paprika and simmer, uncovered, 4 to 5 minutes. Do not overcook. Sprinkle chicken with parsley and serve.

PER SERVING NUTRIENT CONTENT:
 26 g. protein
 negligible carbohydrate
 100 mg. sodium
 5 g. fat

EACH SERVING PROVIDES:
 2.9 Meat/Meat Sub checks
 1.0 Fat check

*In this elegant, easy dish, the alcohol and its calories evaporate as the wine cooks, leaving only the flavor. This is a quickly made, protein-rich recipe which also provides some polyunsaturated fat.

Scallops Provençale

SERVINGS: 4 • SERVING SIZE: 1 CUP • CALORIES PER SERVING: 177

   2 tablespoons unsalted margarine
   1 pound sea scallops
   1 clove garlic, minced
   2 cups low-sodium chopped canned tomatoes, drained (reserve 1/2 cup juice)
   1/4 cup chopped fresh basil or 1 tablespoon dried basil
   1/8 teaspoon freshly ground black pepper
   3 scallions, cut into julienne strips

In large skillet, over medium-high heat, melt margarine. Pat scallops dry with paper towel. Place scallops in skillet and sauté until opaque and lightly browned on all sides. The scallops will cook more evenly if you do not crowd the pan; cook in several batches if necessary.

With slotted spoon, transfer scallops to platter and keep warm. Add garlic to skillet and sauté 1 minute. Add tomatoes, reserved tomato juice, basil, and pepper and cook until tomatoes render their juices but still retain their shape, about 3 to 5 minutes. Return scallops to skillet, add scallions, and heat through.

PER SERVING NUTRIENT CONTENT:
   19 g. protein
   6 g. fat
   11 g. carbohydrate
   375 g. sodium
EACH SERVING PROVIDES:
   2.5 Meat/Meat Sub checks
   1.2 Vegetable checks
   1.5 Fat checks

Seafood Gumbo Filé

SERVINGS: 4 • SERVING SIZE: 2¼ cups • CALORIES PER SERVING: 289

8 ounces whole shrimp, peeled

SEASONING MIX

1 teaspoon cayenne pepper
1 ½ teaspoons paprika
½ teaspoon freshly ground white pepper
½ teaspoon freshly ground black pepper
½ teaspoon dried thyme
½ teaspoon dried oregano
1 bay leaf, crumbled

2 tablespoons unsalted margarine
2 cups chopped onion
2 cups chopped celery
2 cups chopped green bell pepper
3 tablespoons gumbo filé (filé powder)
1 teaspoon Tabasco sauce (or to taste)
1 teaspoon minced garlic
1 ½ cups canned low-sodium tomato sauce
5 cups Low-Sodium Seafood Stock (page 193)
1 ½ cups packed, picked-over crabmeat (about 8 ounces)
12 oysters, shucked (optional)

Peel the shrimp, rinse, and drain well. Refrigerate shrimp until ready to use. (Shrimp shells may be used to make the stock.)

Combine the seasoning mix ingredients in a small bowl and set aside.

In a 4-quart heavy soup pot, melt margarine over medium heat. Add onion, celery, and bell pepper. Turn the heat to high, and stir in the gumbo filé, Tabasco sauce, garlic, and seasoning mix. Cook 6 minutes, stirring constantly. Reduce heat to medium and stir in tomato sauce. Continue cooking 5 minutes more, stirring constantly. (During this time the mixture will begin sticking to the pan bottom. As it does so, continually scrape pan bottom well with a spoon. The scrapings not only add to the gumbo's flavor, but also decrease the gumbo filé's ability to thicken.) Add the stock and bring gumbo to a boil; reduce heat and simmer, uncovered, 45 to 60 minutes, stirring occasionally. Add shrimp, crabmeat, and oysters (if desired); cover and turn off the heat. Leave the pot covered just until the seafood is poached, about 6 to 10 minutes. Serve immediately.

PER SERVING NUTRIENT CONTENT:
  29 g. protein
  9 g. fat
  24 g. carbohydrate
  318 mg. sodium
EACH SERVING PROVIDES:
  3.6 Meat/Meat Sub checks
  1.8 Vegetable checks
  1.2 Fat checks

Shrimp and Wild Rice

SERVINGS: 2 • SERVING SIZE: 1 1/3 cups • CALORIES PER SERVING: 310

  1/2 cup wild rice, uncooked
  1 cup water
  1/4 teaspoon chicken flavored bouillon granules
  2 tablespoons white wine vinegar
  1 tablespoon Chablis or other dry white wine
  1 teaspoon vegetable oil
  1/8 teaspoon sugar
  1/4 teaspoon curry powder
  2 cloves garlic, minced
    Vegetable oil cooking spray
  3/4 pound large fresh shrimp, peeled and deveined
  2 tablespoons scallion tops, thinly sliced
  2 tablespoons toasted almonds, sliced

Wash wild rice in 3 changes of hot water; drain. Combine rice, water, and bouillon granules in a small saucepan; bring to a boil. Cover, reduce heat, and simmer 40 minutes or until rice is tender; drain and set aside. Combine vinegar and next 5 ingredients in a small bowl; stir, using a wire whisk, until well blended. Set vinegar mixture aside. Coat a medium

(recipe continues)

nonstick skillet with cooking spray; place over medium heat until hot. Add shrimp; sauté 4 minutes, stirring constantly. Add vinegar mixture; cook an additional minute. Combine rice, shrimp mixture, and scallion tops in a medium bowl; toss well. Spoon onto a serving platter; sprinkle with almonds. Serve warm.

PER SERVING NUTRIENT CONTENT:
    35 g. protein
    8 g. fat
    26 g. carbohydrate
    355 mg. sodium
EACH SERVING PROVIDES:
    0.1 Vegetable check
    1.5 Bread/Starch checks
    4.6 Meat/Meat Sub checks
    1.2 Fat checks

Spinach Veal Rolls

SERVINGS: 12 • CALORIES PER SERVING: 260

    3 pounds veal, round top, divided in 12 4-ounce portions
1 1/2 teaspoon oil
    1 large clove garlic
    1 10-ounce package frozen spinach, cooked, finely chopped, drained
 1/4 teaspoon dried oregano
 1/2 teaspoon dried basil
    1 teaspoon chives
    2 ounces mild Cheddar cheese, shredded
    2 ounces Muenster cheese, shredded
    2 ounces Provolone cheese, shredded
    2 teaspoons flour
    2 cups mushrooms, thinly sliced
 3/4 cup water
    2 tablespoons lemon juice
 3/4 cup red wine

Pound veal to ⅛-inch thickness. Set aside. In nonstick pan, heat ½ teaspoon oil. Add garlic. Cook until garlic starts to brown lightly. Add spinach, oregano, basil, and chives. Mix well. Set aside to cool. Combine spinach mixture and cheeses; cover. Lay veal pieces out on plastic wrap. Divide cheese mixture equally over the veal and spread to within ½ inch of the edge of the veal. Roll the veal starting at the long end, keeping it tight and tucking in the sides as you go. Seal each seam of the veal rolls with a pinch of flour. Heat 1 teaspoon oil in large nonstick pan. When hot, add veal rolls, seam side down. Brown well. Turn carefully and cover. Brown all sides. Remove from heat and keep warm. Add mushrooms to pan, cover, and cook until limp. Add 1 teaspoon flour and cook uncovered for 1 minute. Add water, lemon juice, and wine to mushrooms. Reduce liquid to half. Place veal rolls on top of mushroom mixture and cover. Reduce heat to low. Cook 5 to 8 minutes or until heated. Serve veal rolls with mushroom sauce. May be served on top of noodles.

PER SERVING NUTRIENT CONTENT:
   27 g. protein
   15 g. fat
   3 g. carbohydrate
   200 mg. sodium
EACH SERVING PROVIDES:
   0.4 Vegetable check
   3.7 Meat/Meat Sub checks
   0.8 Fat check

Stir-Fry Beef with Snow Peas and Mushrooms

SERVINGS: 4 • SERVING SIZE: 1½ cups • CALORIES PER SERVING: 252

> ¾ cup Low-Sodium Chicken Stock (page 192)
> 1 teaspoon grated fresh ginger
> 1 clove garlic, crushed
> 8 ounces mushrooms, sliced vertically
> 14–16 snow peas, strings removed
> 1 pound lean beef, thinly sliced
> 1 tablespoon cornstarch mixed with 2 tablespoons water

Heat ¼ cup chicken stock in a wok or nonstick frying pan; add ginger, garlic, and mushrooms and stir-fry 1 to 2 minutes. Push ingredients to side of pan. Add snow peas and stir-fry 1 to 2 minutes, or until snow peas turn bright green. Push aside. Add beef and stir-fry 2 to 3 minutes. Stir vegetables back into the meat. Add remaining ½ cup stock and corn-starch mixture. Stir over high heat until sauce boils and thickens, and the beef and vegetables are heated through. Serve over rice.

PER SERVING NUTRIENT CONTENT:
 38 g. protein
 7 g. fat
 7 g. carbohydrate
 89 g. sodium

EACH SERVING PROVIDES:
 0.3 Bread/Starch check
 4.4 Meat/Meat Sub checks
 0.6 Vegetable check

Variation: Create your own recipes using the same stir-fry technique with chicken or fish. For each pound of meat, use 2 to 4 cups of prepared vegetables. Use 1 tablespoon cornstarch for each ½ cup of liquid used.

Stuffed Cabbage Rolls

SERVINGS: 16 • SERVING SIZE: 2 rolls • CALORIES PER SERVING: 200

> 2 1/2 to 3 *pounds cabbage*
> 1 *cup chopped onion*
> 3/4 *pound ground veal*
> 2 *tablespoons fresh parsley, chopped*
> 1/8 *teaspoon black pepper*
> 2 *teaspoons curry powder, medium hot*
> 1 *teaspoon Dijon mustard*
> 1 *cup cooked rice*
> 1/4 *cup raisins*
> 3 *cups Stuffed Cabbage Sauce (page 224)*

Preheat oven to 325°F. Steam cabbage in boiling water until soft enough to remove leaves. Sauté onion and veal in a pan until veal turns brown. Add parsley and pepper; mix well. Remove from heat and add curry powder, mustard, and 1 cup sauce. Add rice and mix well. Drop raisins in hot water to plump; drain well. Add to veal mixture. Blend well. Remove 16 leaves from cooked cabbage. Chop remaining cabbage and add to veal mixture; blend well. Place about 1/3 cup meat and cabbage mixture in each of the cabbage leaves. Fold ends of each cabbage leaf over; roll up. Place cabbage rolls in oven-proof pan. Pour remaining sauce over top, cover, and bake 1 hour.

NOTE: 1/3 cup dry rice equals 1 cup cooked rice.

PER SERVING NUTRIENT CONTENT:
    13 g. protein
    4 g. fat
    31 g. carbohydrate
    85 mg. sodium

EACH SERVING PROVIDES:
    3.5 Vegetable checks
    0.3 Fruit check
    0.4 Bread/Starch check
    1.2 Meat/Meat Sub checks
    0.1 Fat check

Stuffed Cabbage Sauce

SERVINGS: 3 • SERVING SIZE: 1 cup • CALORIES PER SERVING: 110

1 cup onion, chopped
1/3 cup dry white wine
2 1/2 cup low-sodium whole tomatoes, pureed
1 packet sugar substitute
1/8 teaspoon cinnamon
2 teaspoons lemon juice
2 teaspoons lemon rind
1/4 teaspoon ground cloves
1/8 teaspoon red pepper flakes
3/4 cup water

Sauté onion in wine. Add remaining ingredients and simmer for 20 to 30 minutes. Do not cover.

PER SERVING NUTRIENT CONTENT:
  4 g. protein
  negligible fat
  26 g. carbohydrates
  45 mg. sodium
EACH SERVING PROVIDES:
  4.0 Vegetable checks

Swordfish with Hot Sauce

SERVINGS: 6 • SERVING SIZE: 4 ounces • CALORIES PER SERVING: 200

3 swordfish steaks (1/2 pound each)
1/4 cup lemon juice
1/4 cup orange juice
1 tablespoon red wine vinegar
Black pepper to taste
3 tablespoons low-sodium catsup
2 tablespoons dry sherry
1 teaspoon low-sodium Worcestershire sauce (optional)

1/2 cup boiling water
2 teaspoons low-sodium chicken bouillon
1 tablespoon chili oil
1 tablespoon fresh gingerroot, minced, or 1/16 teaspoon ginger powder
2 scallions, chopped, including greens
2 cloves garlic, minced
1/4 cup unsalted walnuts, crushed
2 tablespoons cold water
2 teaspoons cornstarch

In a 9-by-13-inch casserole, combine first 8 ingredients. Cover and refrigerate at least 2 hours, turning fish occasionally. In a bowl, combine boiling water and bouillon. Set aside. In a wok, heat oil over low heat. Add ginger, scallions, garlic, and walnuts. Stir-fry 1 minute. Spoon around fish, along with half of the marinade. Preheat oven to broil. Broil fish 6 inches from heat for 5 minutes. Turn and broil 5 minutes more, or until fish flakes easily. Transfer fish to platter. In a saucepan, combine remaining fish marinade and bouillon mixture. Bring to a slow boil over medium heat. Reduce heat to low. Mix the cornstarch with the water and add to bouillon mixture. Cook, stirring constantly, until mixture thickens. Pour sauce over fish.

PER SERVING NUTRIENT CONTENT:
23 g. protein
10 g. fat
5 g. carbohydrate
55 mg. sodium

EACH SERVING PROVIDES:
0.1 Fruit check
0.1 Bread check
3.0 Meat/Meat Sub checks
1.2 Fat checks

Tex-Mex Turkey Chili

SERVINGS: 6 • SERVING SIZE: 1 cup • CALORIES PER SERVING: 190

> 1 cup onion, chopped
> 2 cloves garlic, minced
> 1 tablespoon vegetable oil
> 1 tablespoon chili powder
> 1 teaspoon cumin
> 1 teaspoon sugar
> 1 8-ounce can no-salt-added tomato sauce
> 1 10-ounce can tomatoes and green chilies, undrained
> 1 15-ounce can red kidney beans, drained
> 2 cups shredded cooked turkey breast
> 1 1/2 cups water

In a 2-quart saucepan combine the onion, garlic and oil; cook for one minute or until the onion is tender. Add chili powder, cumin, sugar, and tomato sauce, and stir until blended. Add remaining ingredients; cover and simmer for approximately 30 minutes until thoroughly heated.

PER SERVING NUTRIENT CONTENT:
  20 g. protein
  3 g. fat
  20 g. carbohydrate
  470 mg. sodium

EACH SERVING PROVIDES:
  1.0 Vegetable checks
  0.9 Bread/Starch check
  1.4 Meat/Meat Sub checks
  0.5 Fat check

Tortilla Casserole

SERVINGS: 4 • CALORIES PER SERVING: 344

> 1 1/2 teaspoons vegetable oil
> 3/4 cup chopped Spanish onion
> 2 teaspoons minced garlic
> 1 4-ounce can low-sodium tomatoes, coarsely chopped, with juice

   1 *tablespoon chili powder*
  3/4 *teaspoon ground cumin*
  3/4 *teaspoon dried oregano*
  1/4 *teaspoon caraway seeds*
  1/8 *teaspoon cayenne pepper*
   2 *cups cooked small red beans or pinto beans*
     (rinsed and drained, if canned), or 1 cup pintos and
     1 cup black beans, partially mashed
   1 *2-ounce can green chilies, finely chopped, or*
     small seraño pepper, chopped
   8 *ounces firm tofu, crumbled or grated*
   6 *corn tortillas, toasted in a preheated 350°F oven 10 minutes until*
     crisp, and broken into large pieces
   2 *ounces Monterey Jack cheese, coarsely shredded*
     Shredded lettuce
     Tomato wedges

Preheat oven to 375°F.

In a large nonstick skillet, heat oil, add onion and garlic, and sauté 4 minutes. Add tomatoes and juice, chili powder, cumin, oregano, caraway seeds, and cayenne pepper. Bring mixture to a boil and simmer 10 to 15 minutes, stirring often. Remove pan from heat. Add beans, chilies (or seraño pepper), and tofu and stir ingredients well.

Spread a thin layer of sauce on the bottom of each of two pie pans or one large shallow pan. In each pan, make a layer of broken tortillas, another layer of sauce, one of tortillas, and top with remaining sauce. Sprinkle cheese on top. Cover with foil and bake at 375°F for 20 minutes. Garnish with shredded lettuce and tomatoes.

The casserole may be frozen, before baking, until ready to use. Bake in a preheated 375°F oven for 30 to 40 minutes.

PER SERVING NUTRIENT CONTENT:
   20 g. protein
   11 g. fat
   46 g. carbohydrate
   200 mg. sodium

EACH SERVING PROVIDES:
   3.0 Bread/Starch checks
   0.8 Meat/Meat Sub checks
   0.8 Vegetable check
   1.0 Fat check

Tuna Casserole

SERVINGS: 4 • CALORIES PER SERVING: 179

1/4 *cup chopped onion*
1/4 *cup chopped green bell pepper*
2 *cups 1% low-fat cottage cheese*
8 *ounces tuna packed in water, rinsed and drained*
1/4 *cup chopped and drained pimiento*
1 *teaspoon mixed dried Italian herbs*
4 *egg whites, stiffly beaten*

Preheat oven to 350°F.

Steam onion and pepper until crisply tender and drain well. In a mixing bowl, combine thoroughly cottage cheese, tuna, onion, pepper, pimiento, and herbs. Fold in beaten egg whites. Divide among 4 small individual loaf pans and bake, uncovered for 20 minutes. Drain before serving if liquid has accumulated during cooking.

PER SERVING NUTRIENT CONTENT:
  33 g. protein
  2 g. fat
  6 g. carbohydrate
  532 mg. sodium

EACH SERVING PROVIDES:
  0.1 Bread/Starch check
  3.8 Meat/Meat Sub checks
  0.2 Vegetable check
  0.3 Milk check

Variation: Serve 1/4 cup Mushroom Sauce (page 262) over each casserole.

Tuna-Tomato Melt

SERVINGS: 1 • CALORIES PER SERVING: 264

2 ounces tuna packed in water, rinsed
1 tablespoon low-calorie mayonnaise
Freshly ground black pepper
1 slice whole wheat bread
¼ cup alfalfa sprouts
2 slices tomato
1 ounce shredded part-skim mozzarella cheese

Preheat broiler.

In bowl, mix tuna, 1½ teaspoons mayonnaise, and pepper. Spread remaining 1½ teaspoons mayonnaise on bread. Layer tuna mixture, alfalfa sprouts, and tomato slices on bread and top with mozzarella. Place under broiler until cheese is lightly browned, 2 to 5 minutes.

PER SERVING NUTRIENT CONTENT:
   26.3 g. protein
   11 g. fat
   16.3 g. carbohydrate
   520 mg. sodium

EACH SERVING PROVIDES:
   0.9 Bread/Starch check
   2.6 Meat/Meat Sub checks
   0.3 Vegetable check
   1.6 Fat checks

Turkey Scallopini

SERVINGS: 3 • SERVING SIZE: 4 ounces • CALORIES PER SERVING: 240

> 1 pound boneless turkey cutlets
> 2 tablespoons flour
> 1 tablespoon margarine
> 1 cup sliced mushrooms
> 2 cloves garlic, minced
> 1/4 cup dry sherry or white wine
> 1/2 teaspoon dried basil
> 1/2 teaspoon dried tarragon
> 1/8 teaspoon white pepper
> 1 teaspoon paprika
> 2 tablespoons fresh parsley, minced

Pound turkey to 1/8-inch thickness. Coat turkey cutlets with flour. Melt half of the margarine over medium to medium-high heat in a nonstick pan. Add mushrooms and garlic and sauté 2 to 3 minutes. Remove from pan. Melt remaining margarine and sauté turkey cutlets, turning once. Add sherry and mushrooms. Bring to a boil. Sprinkle spices over turkey cutlets. Cook another 2 to 3 minutes. Sprinkle with fresh minced parsley before serving.

PER SERVING NUTRIENT CONTENT:
   35 g. protein
   8 g. fat
   6 g. carbohydrate
   120 mg. sodium

EACH SERVING PROVIDES:
   0.2 Vegetable check
   0.3 Bread/Starch check
   3.0 Meat/Meat Sub checks
   0.8 Fat check

Veal Scallopini with Mushrooms

SERVINGS: 4 • CALORIES PER SERVING: 240

1 pound boneless veal cutlets, pounded 1/8-inch to 1/4-inch thick
1 tablespoon unsalted margarine
8 ounces fresh mushrooms, sliced
1 large green pepper, cut into 1/2-inch strips
1/2 cup dry white wine
1/4 cup low-sodium chicken broth
1 tablespoon lemon juice
1 tablespoon cornstarch
2 tablespoons water
2 tablespoons fresh parsley, minced
Freshly ground pepper
Vegetable oil cooking spray
1/4 teaspoon thyme leaves
2 cloves garlic, minced

Trim excess fat from veal and cut into large strips. Pound veal and sprinkle lightly with fresh pepper. Coat a large nonstick skillet with cooking spray; add margarine and melt over medium heat. Add veal, and cook 2 to 3 minutes on each side or until veal is lightly browned. Remove from skillet, and keep warm. Add garlic, mushrooms, and green pepper to skillet; sauté 2 to 3 minutes until pepper is tender but crispy. Stir in wine, broth, lemon juice, and thyme, bring to a boil, and boil 1 minute. In a separate bowl combine cornstarch and water. Add to mushroom mixture and stir constantly until thickened. Add veal and warm. Garnish with parsley.

PER SERVING NUTRIENT CONTENT:
  25 g. protein
  11 g. fat
  8 g. carbohydrate
  105 mg. sodium
EACH SERVING PROVIDES:
  1.1 Vegetable checks
  0.1 Bread/Starch check
  3.1 Meat/Meat Sub checks
  0.8 Fat check

Yellow Squash Casserole

SERVINGS: 6 • SERVING SIZE: ½ cup • CALORIES PER SERVING: 100

½ cup plain low-fat yogurt
½ cup 1% low-fat cottage cheese
¼ cup Parmesan cheese, grated
¼ teaspoon whole thyme, dried
2 eggs, beaten
Vegetable oil cooking spray
1 cup onion, sliced
3 cups yellow squash, sliced
¼ cup soft whole wheat bread crumbs, divided

Preheat oven to 350°F.

Combine first 5 ingredients in a bowl; set aside. Coat a skillet with cooking spray; place over medium heat until hot. Add onion, and sauté until tender; drain and set aside. Place 1 cup squash in a 2-quart casserole coated with cooking spray. Top with ⅓ of onion and ⅓ of yogurt mixture. Repeat procedure with remaining squash, onion, and yogurt mixture. Sprinkle with bread crumbs; cover and bake at 350°F for 25 minutes. Uncover and bake until top is browned.

PER SERVING NUTRIENT CONTENT:

8 g. protein
4 g. fat
8 g. carbohydrate
200 mg. sodium

EACH SERVING PROVIDES:

0.2 Milk check
0.4 Vegetable check
0.4 Bread/Starch check
0.3 Fat check
0.8 Meat/Meat Sub check

Breakfast Entrees

Baked Apple Omelet

SERVINGS: 6 • CALORIES PER SERVING: 100

1/4 cup + 1 tablespoon all-purpose flour
1/2 teaspoon baking powder
3 eggs, separated
2 tablespoons sugar, divided
1/4 cup nonfat milk
1 tablespoon + 1 1/2 teaspoons lemon juice
Vegetable oil cooking spray
1 medium cooking apple, cored and cut into thin wedges
1/4 teaspoon ground cinnamon

Preheat oven to 375°F.

Combine flour and baking powder in a large bowl; set aside. Beat egg whites (at room temperature) until soft peaks form; gradually add 1 tablespoon sugar, beating until stiff peaks form. Set aside. Combine egg yolks and milk; mix well. Add egg yolk mixture to reserved flour mixture, stirring just until dry ingredients are moistened. Fold reserved egg white mixture into flour mixture. Add lemon juice. Coat a 9 1/2-by-9 1/2-inch glass baking dish with cooking spray. Pour mixture into baking dish. Arrange apple wedges in a circle on top of egg mixture. Combine remaining 1 tablespoon sugar and cinnamon; sprinkle over apple slices. Bake at 375°F or until set.

PER SERVING NUTRIENT CONTENT:
    4 g. protein
    3 g. fat
    14 g. carbohydrate
    70 mg. sodium
EACH SERVING PROVIDES:
    0.3 Fruit check
    0.5 Bread/Starch check
    0.5 Meat/Meat Sub check
    0.3 Fat check

Breakfast Cheesecake

SERVINGS: 2 • CALORIES PER SERVING: 194

1/3 cup plain low-fat yogurt
1 package sugar substitute
3/4 cup bran cereal
1/2 cup 1% low-fat cottage cheese
1/4 cup canned peaches, drained
1/2 cup sliced bananas
1 tablespoon raisins

Combine yogurt, sugar substitute, and cereal in a bowl. Reserve 1/4 of mixture for topping and divide remaining mixture equally between 2 small, shallow serving dishes. Form into crust by pressing evenly into dishes. Place 1/4 cup cottage cheese on top of each crust and distribute peaches, bananas, and raisins over cheese. Top with remaining bran mixture and serve at once.

PER SERVING NUTRIENT CONTENT:

14 g. protein
2 g. fat
41 g. carbohydrate
618 mg. sodium

EACH SERVING PROVIDES:

1.5 Bread/Starch checks
0.3 Meat/Meat Sub check
0.9 Fruit check
0.2 Milk check

Egg White Omelet

SERVINGS: 1 • CALORIES PER SERVING: 69

Vegetable oil cooking spray
3 egg whites
¼ cup onion, sautéed with vegetable oil cooking spray
¼ teaspoon white pepper (optional)

Heat nonstick omelet pan on medium heat, then spray surface with vegetable oil cooking spray. In a small bowl, whisk egg whites until foamy. Drop egg whites onto heated pan and cook, without stirring, until the top begins to whiten. Place onion in middle, fold omelet in half, and let cook 30 seconds more. Remove to warm plate and serve at once.

PER SERVING NUTRIENT CONTENT:
  11 g. protein
  1 g. fat
  4 g. carbohydrate
  154 mg. sodium
EACH SERVING PROVIDES:
  1.2 Meat/Meat Sub checks
  0.3 Vegetable check

Variation: Fill this omelet with other cooked vegetables or low-fat cheese. A spoonful or two of Basic Tomato Sauce (page 260) would add an attractive touch of color.

French Toast

SERVINGS: 1 • CALORIES PER SERVING: 107

> *1 egg white*
> *1 tablespoon skim milk*
> *2 slices lite whole wheat bread*
> *Vegetable oil cooking spray*

In a shallow bowl, combine egg white and skim milk and beat to break up whites. Soak bread in egg white mixture. Lightly cover a nonstick skillet with cooking spray. Transfer bread to skillet and brown on both sides. Serve at once with Blueberry Topping (page 251).

PER SERVING NUTRIENT CONTENT:

8 g. protein
3 g. fat
13 g. carbohydrate
190 mg. sodium

EACH SERVING PROVIDES:

1.0 Bread/Starch check
0.4 Meat/Meat Sub check
0.1 Milk check

Fruit Frittata

SERVINGS: 6 • CALORIES PER SERVING: 185

   6 *eggs*
   4 *egg whites*
  ½ *cup nonfat milk*
   1 *teaspoon powdered sugar*
   1 *cup fresh blueberries*
   1 *8-ounce can unsweetened crushed pineapple, drained*
  ½ *cup (4 ounces) Neufchâtel cheese, diced*
    Vegetable oil cooking spray
   2 *tablespoons wheat germ*
    Fresh mint sprig

Preheat oven to 350°F.

Combine eggs, egg whites, nonfat milk, and powdered sugar in a large bowl; beat well. Stir in blueberries, pineapple, and cheese. Coat a 9½-by-9½-inch glass dish with cooking spray. Pour egg mixture into the dish and sprinkle with wheat germ. Bake at 350°F degrees for 20 minutes or until the egg is set. Cut into 6 equal portions. Garnish with mint sprig.

PER SERVING NUTRIENT CONTENT:
   12 g. protein
   1 g. fat
   11 g. carbohydrate
   190 mg. sodium

EACH SERVING PROVIDES:
   0.1 Milk check
   0.5 Fruit check
   0.1 Bread/Starch check
   1.5 Meat/Meat Sub checks
   1.4 Fat checks

Omelet Florentine

SERVINGS: 1 • CALORIES PER SERVING: 96

Vegetable oil cooking spray
3 egg whites
1 cup fresh raw spinach, chopped and steamed
1/2 ounce part-skim mozzarella cheese
1 red bell pepper ring (optional)
1/4 teaspoon freshly grated nutmeg (optional)

Place nonstick omelet pan over medium heat. Lightly coat the surface with vegetable cooking spray. In a small bowl, whisk egg whites until foamy. Drop whites into omelet pan and cook without stirring, until the top begins to whiten and bubble. Add spinach, nutmeg, and cheese to middle. Fold omelet in half and cook 30 seconds more. Turn omelet and cook on other side for 30 seconds. Transfer to warm plate, garnish with red pepper ring, and serve immediately.

PER SERVING NUTRIENT CONTENT:
   15 g. protein
   3 g. fat
   4 g. carbohydrate
   260 mg. sodium
EACH SERVING PROVIDES:
   1.6 Meat/Meat Sub checks
   0.5 Vegetable check

Sunrise Spread

SERVINGS: 16 • SERVING SIZE: 1 tablespoon • CALORIES PER SERVING: 18

½ cup part-skim ricotta cheese
½ cup 1% low-fat cottage cheese
2 tablespoons plain low-fat yogurt
1 teaspoon fresh grated ginger
1 teaspoon grated orange rind
1 package sugar substitute

In a bowl or food processor, combine all ingredients and blend well, using a fork if you are mixing by hand. Cover well with plastic wrap and chill 1 hour before serving. Spread will keep well in the refrigerator, tightly covered, for up to 3 days.

PER SERVING NUTRIENT CONTENT:
- 2 g. protein
- 1 g. fat
- 1 g. carbohydrate
- 40 mg. sodium

EACH SERVING PROVIDES:
- 0.3 Meat/Meat Sub check
- 0.1 Fat check

Vegetables and Side Dishes

Broccoli Soufflé

SERVINGS: 5 • SERVING SIZE: ½ cup • CALORIES PER SERVING: 60

> 2 cups chopped broccoli florets
> ½ cup chopped onion
> 1½ ounces shredded part-skim mozzarella cheese
> ½ cup 1% low-fat cottage cheese
> 1 teaspoon freshly ground white pepper (optional)
> 2 egg whites, stiffly beaten
> Paprika

Preheat oven to 350°F.

Steam broccoli and onion over boiling water until just tender. Drain well and place in 1-quart soufflé dish. Stir mozzarella into hot broccoli, then blend in cottage cheese and pepper with a fork. Fold in egg whites and sprinkle with paprika. Bake 30 minutes, or until soufflé is firm and lightly brown on top.

PER SERVING NUTRIENT CONTENT:
   8 g. protein
   2 g. fat
   4 g. carbohydrate
   162 mg. sodium

EACH SERVING PROVIDES:
   0.8 Meat/Meat Sub check
   0.7 Vegetable check

Broccoli with Cheese Sauce

SERVINGS: 6 • CALORIES PER SERVING: 75

1 medium head fresh broccoli, cut into florets
2 teaspoons unsalted margarine
¼ cup minced onion
2 cloves minced garlic
3 tablespoons all-purpose flour
1 cup skim milk
2 ounces part-skim shredded mozzarella cheese
⅛ teaspoon nutmeg
Freshly ground black pepper, to taste
Vegetable oil cooking spray
1 tablespoon fresh grated Parmesan cheese
1 tablespoon fresh minced parsley
Dash of paprika

Preheat oven to 400°F.

Steam broccoli until tender but crispy; drain. Melt margarine in nonstick skillet, sauté onion and garlic until translucent. In small bowl, mix flour and skim milk. Add mixture to skillet and stir constantly over medium heat until thickened. Stir in mozzarella cheese, nutmeg and pepper. Remove from heat. Place broccoli in casserole dish which has been coated with vegetable spray. Pour cheese and onion evenly over broccoli. Mix Parmesan cheese with parsley and sprinkle over casserole. Top with paprika for color and bake 20 to 25 minutes at 400°F.

PER SERVING NUTRIENT CONTENT:
7 gm. protein
3 gm. fat
9 gm. carbohydrate
90 mg. sodium

EACH SERVING PROVIDES:
0.5 Meat/Meat Sub check
0.5 Fat check
1.0 Vegetable check
0.2 Milk check

Crispy Corn Tortilla Chips

SERVINGS: 32 chips • CALORIES PER CHIP: 8

4 6-inch corn tortillas, each cut into 8 wedges

Preheat oven to 400°F.

Arrange tortilla wedges on cookie sheet and bake 6 to 7 minutes, or until crisp. Cool on cookie sheet. Serve with dips.

PER SERVING NUTRIENT CONTENT:
   negligible protein
   negligible fat
   2 g. carbohydrate
   7 mg. sodium
EACH SERVING PROVIDES:
   0.1 Bread/Starch check

"Fried" Potato Skins

SERVINGS: 24 • CALORIES PER SERVING: 37

6 *5-ounce baking potatoes*
1 *tablespoon melted unsalted margarine*
1/3 *cup plain low-fat yogurt*
1/4 *teaspoon dried thyme*
2 *cloves garlic, minced*
1 1/2 *tablespoons toasted sesame seeds*
Paprika

Preheat oven to 375°F.

Cut the potatoes in half lengthwise. Scoop out the potato flesh from each piece, leaving a layer of potato about 1/8-inch thick on each skin. Reserve pulp for another use. In a bowl, mix margarine, yogurt, thyme, and garlic and brush generously on potato skins. Sprinkle with sesame seeds and paprika. Place the skins on a baking sheet and bake 25 minutes, or until they are crunchy and brown. Cut in half lengthwise and serve hot.

PER SERVING NUTRIENT CONTENT:

1 g. protein
1 g. fat
7 g. carbohydrate
5 mg. sodium

EACH SERVING PROVIDES:

0.4 Bread/Starch check
0.2 Fat check

Variation: Omit the thyme and add chili powder and curry to taste.

Italian Stuffed Potatoes

SERVINGS: 2 • CALORIES PER SERVING: 200

> 2 5-ounce potatoes
> Vegetable oil cooking spray
> 3/4 to 1 cup diced raw vegetables
> 1 clove garlic, crushed
> 1 teaspoon chopped fresh basil or 1/4 teaspoon dried
> 1/8 teaspoon dried oregano
> Dash red pepper flakes
> 1 1/2 ounces part-skim mozzarella cheese, grated

Preheat oven to 350°F.

Bake potatoes until tender, about 1 hour, and remove from oven, leaving heat on.

Place a nonstick skillet over moderate heat and spray with cooking spray. Add diced vegetables and garlic and sauté until tender, 3 to 5 minutes. Add basil, oregano, and red pepper flakes and mix well. Cut baked potatoes in half lengthwise and fluff up flesh with a fork. Divide vegetable mixture between potatoes and mix lightly with potato flesh. Sprinkle mozzarella on top, and bake until cheese melts, about 10 minutes.

(recipe continues)

PER SERVING NUTRIENT CONTENT:

9 g. protein
4 g. fat
34 g. carbohydrate
109 mg. sodium

EACH SERVING PROVIDES:

1.7 Bread/Starch checks
0.7 Meat/Meat Sub check
0.5 Vegetable check
0.3 Fat check

Orange-Glazed Carrots

SERVINGS: 2 • SERVING SIZE: ¾ cup • CALORIES PER SERVING: 73

For Microwave

3 medium carrots, cut into ¼-inch slices
6 tablespoons fresh orange juice
1 teaspoon cornstarch
¼ teaspoon grated orange rind
⅛ teaspoon ground mace

Combine carrots and 3 tablespoons orange juice in a 1-quart casserole. Cover and microwave on high (100 percent) for 5 to 6 minutes, or until carrots are tender but crispy, stirring at 2-minute intervals. In a cup, combine cornstarch, remaining 3 tablespoons orange juice, orange rind, and mace, stirring until blended. Stir into carrot mixture, mixing well. Cover and microwave on high for 1 minute, or until thickened, stirring after 30 seconds.

PER SERVING NUTRIENT CONTENT:

1 g. protein
negligible fat
17 g. carbohydrate
38 mg. sodium

EACH SERVING PROVIDES:

0.1 Bread/Starch check
1.7 Vegetable checks
0.4 Fruit check

Parsleyed New Potatoes

SERVINGS: 4 • CALORIES PER SERVING: 131

1 1/4 *pounds new potatoes, washed and quartered*
1 *tablespoon melted unsalted margarine*
5 *tablespoons minced fresh parsley*
Pepper to taste

Arrange potatoes in a steamer rack. Bring water to a boil and steam until potatoes are tender. Transfer potatoes to a bowl. Add margarine and parsley, then toss.

PER SERVING NUTRIENT CONTENT:
    2 g. protein
    3 g. fat
    24 g. carbohydrate
    7 mg. sodium
EACH SERVING PROVIDES:
    1.5 Bread/Starch checks
    0.6 Fat check

Variation: Substitute butter buds for margarine; this yields 105 calories per serving.

For decorative effect, before steaming, use a vegetable peeler to remove a ½-inch strip around center of each potato.

Pickled Carrots

SERVINGS: 24 • CALORIES PER SERVING: 6

> 3 medium carrots
> 1/2 medium onion, sliced thinly
> 1 teaspoon dill seed or pickling spice
> 2 cloves garlic, crushed
> 1/2 cup water
> 1/2 cup white vinegar
> 3 packets of sugar substitute

Scrape carrots, cut into even sticks, and steam for about 2 minutes. Plunge carrots into cold water to stop cooking. Drain and place with onions in 1-pint jar. Add dill seed and garlic. In a small saucepan, place water, vinegar, and sugar substitute. Bring to a boil. Pour over carrots, seal tightly, and cool. Refrigerate for at least 6 hours.

PER SERVING NUTRIENT CONTENT:
negligible protein
negligible fat
2 g. carbohydrate
3 mg. sodium
EACH SERVING PROVIDES:
0.2 Vegetable check

Variation: Try this recipe with other vegetables (broccoli, cauliflower, green beans). If you use mushrooms, do not cook first.

Rice with Peas and Parsley

SERVINGS: 4 • SERVING SIZE: ¾ cup • CALORIES PER SERVING: 185

> 1 cup long-grain rice
> 1/2 cup fresh peas, cooked, or frozen peas, thawed
> 1/2 cup fresh parsley, minced

Cook rice according to package directions, omitting the salt. When done, stir in peas and parsley; heat through.

PER SERVING NUTRIENT CONTENT:
  4 g. protein
  negligible fat
  40 g. carbohydrate
  25 mg. sodium
EACH SERVING PROVIDES:
  2.5 Bread/Starch checks

Rice-Vegetable Pilaf

SERVINGS: 8 • SERVING SIZE: ½ cup • CALORIES PER SERVING: 80

1 1/3 cups water
1 teaspoon chicken-flavored bouillon granules
1/2 cup long-grain rice, uncooked
1 1/2 cups carrot, coarsely shredded
1/2 cup fresh parsley, chopped
1/3 cup scallion, thinly sliced
1/4 teaspoon pepper
1/4 cup toasted pecans, chopped

Combine water and bouillon granules in a saucepan; bring to a boil. Add rice; cover, reduce heat, and simmer 20 minutes. Remove from heat, and let stand, covered, 5 minutes. Add next 4 ingredients, stir well. Place over low heat; cover and cook 5 minutes. Sprinkle with pecans.

PER SERVING NUTRIENT CONTENT:
  2 g. protein
  3 g. fat
  13 g. carbohydrate
  125 mg. sodium
EACH SERVING PROVIDES:
  0.5 Vegetable check
  0.6 Bread/Starch check
  0.6 Fat check

Stuffed Baked Potato

SERVINGS: 2 • CALORIES PER SERVING: 94

    1 5-ounce potato
    ½ cup 1% low-fat cottage cheese
    1 teaspoon snipped chives or scallion greens
    Dash paprika

Preheat oven to 375°F.

Pierce scrubbed potato repeatedly with fork, then bake until tender. Cut baked potato in half and scoop out inside. Return potato shells to oven. Mash cottage cheese with potato. Mix in chives and paprika. Return potato mixture to potato shells and heat until hot.

PER SERVING NUTRIENT CONTENT:
    8 g. protein
    1 g. fat
    14 g. carbohydrate
    233 mg. sodium
EACH SERVING PROVIDES:
    0.8 Bread/Starch check
    0.5 Meat/Meat Sub check

Stuffed Cherry Tomatoes

SERVINGS: 36 • CALORIES PER SERVING: 13

    36 cherry tomatoes (about 1 pint)
    ⅔ cup 1% low-fat cottage cheese
    2 ounces crumbled blue cheese
    2 tablespoons chopped scallion
    ¼ cup plain low-fat yogurt
       Freshly ground black pepper to taste
    3 tablespoons snipped fresh chives

Cut a thin slice off the top of each tomato. Using a melon ball cutter or grapefruit spoon, scoop out pulp and seeds. Drain tomatoes upside down on paper towels for 15 minutes. Combine cottage cheese, blue cheese, scallion, yogurt, and pepper in blender. Fill tomatoes with mixture and sprinkle with chives.

PER SERVING NUTRIENT CONTENT:
- 1 g. protein
- 1 g. fat
- 1 g. carbohydrate
- 41 mg. sodium

EACH SERVING PROVIDES:
- 0.1 Meat/Meat Sub check
- 0.2 Vegetable check

Sweet Potatoes with Orange Raisin Sauce

SERVINGS: 4 • SERVING SIZE: 4 ounces • CALORIES PER SERVING: 60

1 pound sweet potatoes
1/3 cup orange juice
2 tablespoons raisins
2 tablespoons sherry
1 tablespoon brown sugar substitute

Peel and slice sweet potatoes uniformly. Mix orange juice, raisins, sherry, and brown sugar substitute together. Pour mixture over the sweet potatoes. Cover. Bake at 350°F for 20 to 30 minutes or until done.

PER SERVING NUTRIENT CONTENT:
- 2 g. protein
- 1 g. fat
- 36 g. carbohydrate
- 15 mg. sodium

EACH SERVING PROVIDES:
- 0.4 Fruit check
- 1.5 Bread/Starch checks

Zucchini Potato Salad

SERVINGS: 4 • SERVING SIZE: 1 cup • CALORIES PER SERVING: 150

8 ounces red potatoes, cut into 1/4-inch strips
2 cups zucchini, cut into 1 1/2-inch chunks
3 tablespoons olive oil
1 teaspoon dry vermouth
1 scallion, sliced diagonally
2 tablespoons fresh tarragon
1/2 teaspoon sugar
Dash pepper

In small saucepan, over medium-high heat, bring 1 inch of water to a boil. Add potatoes and cook 7 to 10 minutes until fork-tender. In another pan, in 1 inch of boiling water, cook zucchini 5 minutes until tender but crispy. Drain potatoes and zucchini. In small jar with tight-fitting lid combine oil with remaining ingredients. Shake to combine. Pour over still-hot potatoes and zucchini. Toss to coat. Cover and refrigerate.

PER SERVING NUTRIENT CONTENT:
   2 g. protein
   10 g. fat
   13 g. carbohydrate
   5 mg. sodium
EACH SERVING PROVIDES:
   0.4 Vegetable check
   0.7 Bread/Starch check
   2.1 Fat checks

Toppings, Dips, and Dressings

Blueberry Topping

SERVINGS: 24 • SERVING SIZE: 1 tablespoon • CALORIES PER SERVING: 8

  2 cups fresh or frozen unsweetened blueberries, thawed
  2 packages sugar substitute
  1 teaspoon cornstarch
  1/4 teaspoon ground cinnamon

Combine all ingredients in blender and puree. Transfer mixture to small saucepan and cook over low heat until thickened. Serve warm or cold.

PER SERVING NUTRIENT CONTENT:
  0.2 g. carbohydrate
  negligible sodium
EACH SERVING PROVIDES:
  0.1 Fruit check

Creamy Clam Dip

SERVINGS: 1½ cups • SERVING SIZE: 1 tablespoon
CALORIES PER SERVING: 30

  1 7½-ounce can minced clams
  1 8-ounce package Neufchâtel cheese, cut into cubes and softened
  1 scallion with top, sliced, plus snipped scallion tops for garnish
    Assorted raw and blanched vegetables for dipping

Drain clams, reserving 1 to 2 tablespoons liquid. Set both aside. In blender, place cheese and scallion. Cover and blend until smooth, adding reserved clam liquid until mixture is of dipping consistency. Stir in drained clams. Turn dip into serving dish and garnish with snipped scallion tops. Serve with raw vegetables.

(recipe continues)

PER SERVING NUTRIENT CONTENT:
2 g. protein
2 g. fat
negligible carbohydrate
43 mg. sodium

EACH SERVING PROVIDES:
0.5 Meat/Meat Sub check
0.1 Fat check

Creamy Carrot Dressing

SERVINGS: 8 • SERVING SIZE: 2 tablespoons • CALORIES PER SERVING: 15

½ cup 1% low-fat cottage cheese
½ teaspoon fresh lemon juice
½ cup plain low-fat yogurt
⅓ cup shredded carrot
1 tablespoon grated onion
1 teaspoon grated lemon peel
⅛ teaspoon each thyme, basil, oregano, marjoram, and black pepper

Combine cheese, lemon juice, and yogurt in a blender or food processor and mix until smooth. Transfer to a bowl and stir in remaining ingredients. Chill before serving.

PER SERVING NUTRIENT CONTENT:
2 g. protein
negligible fat
2 g. carbohydrate
35 mg. sodium

EACH SERVING PROVIDES:
0.1 Meat/Meat Sub check
0.1 Vegetable check
0.1 Milk check

Cucumber Lemon Dip

SERVINGS: 8 • SERVING SIZE: 2 tablespoons • CALORIES PER SERVING: 23

1 medium cucumber, peeled, seeded, shredded, and well drained
2/3 cup DFC Sour Cream (below)
Juice and grated rind of 1/2 lemon
2 tablespoons chopped scallion
2 tablespoons chopped fresh parsley
1/2 teaspoon crushed dried rosemary
1 small clove garlic, crushed

In a bowl, combine all ingredients, then chill.
NOTE: Use as a dip for raw vegetables such as zucchini, yellow squash, broccoli, and cauliflower.

PER SERVING NUTRIENT CONTENT:
3 g. protein
negligible fat
2 g. carbohydrate
93 mg. sodium
EACH SERVING PROVIDES:
0.3 Meat/Meat Sub check
0.2 Vegetable check

DFC "Sour Cream"

SERVINGS: 8 • SERVING SIZE: 2 tablespoons • CALORIES PER SERVING: 25

12 ounces 1% low-fat cottage cheese
1 tablespoon fresh lemon juice

Combine ingredients in blender or food processor until smooth. (For easier mixing, leave cottage cheese at room temperature for 30 minutes before placing in blender.)

(recipe continues)

PER SERVING NUTRIENT CONTENT:
 4 g. protein
 negligible fat
 1 g. carbohydrate
 138 mg. sodium
EACH SERVING PROVIDES:
 0.5 Meat/Meat Sub check
 0.1 Milk check

Fruit Dip

SERVINGS: 16 • SERVING SIZE: 1 tablespoon • CALORIES PER SERVING: 13

1 cup low-fat vanilla yogurt
1/2 teaspoon cinnamon (or to taste)

In a bowl, combine ingredients. Let flavors marry 1 to 2 hours, then serve with fruit chunks.

PER SERVING NUTRIENT CONTENT:
 1 g. protein
 negligible fat
 2 g. carbohydrate
 9 mg. sodium
EACH SERVING PROVIDES:
 0.1 Milk check

Fruit Topping

SERVINGS: 12 • SERVING SIZE: 1 tablespoon • CALORIES PER SERVING: 5

2 cups apple, peeled, cored, and thinly sliced
2 tablespoons sugar substitute
1 teaspoon cornstarch
1/4 teaspoon ground cinnamon

Combine all ingredients in a small saucepan. Cook over low heat, stirring, until apples are tender and mixture is thick. Refrigerate until ready to use. Serve warm or chilled.

NOTE: Use this on a muffin, bagel, or toast, or as a topping for French Toast (page 236).

PER SERVING NUTRIENT CONTENT:
   1 g. carbohydrate
   negligible sodium
EACH SERVING PROVIDES:
   0.1 Fruit check

Green Goddess Dressing

SERVINGS: 16 • SERVING SIZE: 2 tablespoons • CALORIES PER SERVING: 5

   2 cups loosely packed fresh mixed greens (spinach, beet, Swiss chard)
   1/4 cup fresh parsley leaves
   1 tablespoon fresh dill
   2 tablespoons fresh lemon juice
   1 cup water or low-sodium vegetable stock
   1/2 cup sliced zucchini, steamed until soft
   1/2 cup coarsely chopped onion, steamed until soft
   1/2 teaspoon dried thyme
   1/4 teaspoon freshly ground black pepper
   1 clove garlic

Place all ingredients in food processor or blender and combine until smooth. Serve on sprout salads.

PER SERVING NUTRIENT CONTENT:
   negligible protein
   negligible fat
   1 g. carbohydrate
   9 mg. sodium
EACH SERVING PROVIDES:
   0.2 Vegetable check

Herbed "Sour Cream"

SERVINGS: 12 • SERVING SIZE: 2 tablespoons • CALORIES PER SERVING: 21

> 12 ounces 1% low-fat cottage cheese
> 1 teaspoon fresh lemon juice
> 1 clove garlic, minced
> 1 tablespoon snipped fresh chives
> 1 tablespoon minced fresh parsley

Place cottage cheese, lemon juice, and garlic in blender or food processor and blend until smooth. Transfer mixture to a bowl, stir in chives and parsley, and refrigerate.

PER SERVING NUTRIENT CONTENT:
    4 g. protein
    negligible fat
    1 g. carbohydrate
    115 mg. sodium
EACH SERVING PROVIDES:
    0.4 Meat/Meat Sub check

Parmesan-Garlic Dressing

SERVINGS: 16 • SERVING SIZE: 1 tablespoon • CALORIES PER SERVING: 14

> 1/2 cup plain low-fat yogurt
> 1/4 cup red wine vinegar
> 2 tablespoons Parmesan cheese, freshly grated
> 2 tablespoons low-calorie mayonnaise
> 1 teaspoon garlic, minced
> 1/4 teaspoon pepper
> 2 tablespoons scallion, chopped

Combine all ingredients in blender. Cover and process at low speed until smooth.

PER SERVING NUTRITIONAL CONTENT:

1 g. protein
1 g. fat
1 g. carbohydrate
20 mg. sodium

EACH SERVING PROVIDES:

0.1 Fat check
0.1 Meat/Meat Sub check

Pesto Dip

SERVINGS: 24 • SERVING SIZE: 1 tablespoon • CALORIES PER SERVING: 16

8 ounces 1% low-fat cottage cheese or part-skim ricotta cheese
1 cup loosely packed fresh basil
2 tablespoons freshly grated Parmesan cheese
1/2 cup skim milk
1 tablespoon olive oil
1 large clove garlic, crushed
1/4 teaspoon freshly ground black pepper

In a food processor or blender, combine all ingredients. Blend until smooth. Transfer to bowl and chill 1 hour. Serve with Crispy Corn Tortilla Chips (page 242), or zucchini and yellow squash slices.

PER SERVING NUTRIENT CONTENT:

2 g. protein
1 g. fat
1 g. carbohydrate
50 mg. sodium

EACH SERVING PROVIDES:

0.1 Fat check
0.1 Meat check

Variation: Instead of basil, use 1 cup shredded fresh spinach leaves, tightly packed, and 2 tablespoons dried basil leaves.

Red Pepper Vinaigrette

SERVINGS: 4 • SERVING SIZE: 2 tablespoons • CALORIES PER SERVING: 10

> 1 tablespoon Dijon mustard, unsalted
> 2 tablespoons white wine
> 1/4 teaspoon Tabasco sauce
> 1/4 teaspoon red pepper flakes, crushed
> 6 tablespoons low-sodium chicken stock
> 1 teaspoon cornstarch

In a bowl, combine the first 4 ingredients. Mix the cornstarch with the cold chicken stock in a small saucepan and heat until clear and slightly thickened. Add the other ingredients and blend well. Remove from heat and cool.

PER SERVING NUTRITIONAL CONTENT:
    1 g. protein
    1 g. carbohydrate
    55 mg. sodium

Shrimp-Cucumber Dip

SERVINGS: 32 • SERVING SIZE: 1 tablespoon • CALORIES PER SERVING: 11

1 medium cucumber, skin on
1 cup cream-style 1% low-fat cottage cheese
2 tablespoons finely chopped onion
2 teaspoons tarragon vinegar
1/2 teaspoon prepared white horseradish
4 ounces shrimp, steamed, shelled, and coarsely chopped, or 1 4 1/2-ounce can shrimp
Assorted raw and blanched vegetables for dipping

Halve cucumber lengthwise and scoop out the seeds with a spoon. Shred enough cucumber to make 1 cup; drain. In a bowl, combine the shredded cucumber, cottage cheese, onion, vinegar, and horseradish. Beat with electric mixer until smooth. Stir in shrimp. Serve with vegetable dippers.

PER SERVING NUTRIENT CONTENT:
2 g. protein
negligible fat
1 g. carbohydrate
37 mg. sodium

EACH SERVING PROVIDES:
0.2 Meat/Meat Sub check

Sauces and Spreads

Basic Tomato Sauce

SERVINGS: 8 • SERVING SIZE: ½ cup • CALORIES PER SERVING: 30

> 1 16-ounce can low-sodium tomatoes or 2 cups fresh, chopped
> ½ cup diced onion
> 1 large green pepper, diced
> ½ teaspoon dried basil or 2 teaspoons fresh, chopped
> ½ teaspoon freshly ground black pepper
> 1 teaspoon minced garlic
> 1 teaspoon dried oregano

Combine all ingredients in medium saucepan, and simmer for 15 minutes, or until thickened.

PER SERVING NUTRIENT CONTENT:
> 1 g. protein
> negligible fat
> 6 g. carbohydrate
> 6 mg. sodium

EACH SERVING PROVIDES:
> 1.0 Vegetable check

Creole Seafood Sauce

SERVINGS: 8 • SERVING SIZE: ¼ cup • CALORIES PER SERVING: 28

> Vegetable oil cooking spray
> 2 cups sliced fresh mushrooms
> 1½ cups undrained, chopped, low-sodium canned tomatoes
> 1 medium green bell pepper, thinly sliced
> ½ cup thinly sliced onion
> 1 tablespoon flour
> 1 cup Low-Sodium Chicken Stock (page 192), defatted
> 1 teaspoon fresh lemon juice
> 1 teaspoon prepared white horseradish
> Dash Tabasco sauce (optional)

Place a large nonstick saucepan over medium heat, coat with vegetable oil cooking spray. Add mushrooms and sauté until lightly browned. Add tomatoes, green pepper, and onion and simmer 10 minutes. In a cup, mix flour, stock, and lemon juice, then stir into saucepan. Cook and stir until thickened. Add horseradish and season with Tabasco sauce.

PER SERVING NUTRIENT CONTENT:
    2 g. protein
    negligible fat
    5 g. carbohydrate
    14 mg. sodium
EACH SERVING PROVIDES:
    0.1 Meat/Meat Sub check
    0.7 Vegetable check

Fresh Salsa

SERVINGS: 14 • SERVING SIZE: 2 tablespoons • CALORIES PER SERVING: 8

    1/2 cup onion, chopped
    1/2 teaspoon low-sodium chicken-flavored bouillon granules
    2 medium tomatoes, chopped
    1 clove garlic, minced
    1 4-ounce can chopped green chilies, undrained
    1/2 cup water

Combine all ingredients in a non-aluminum saucepan; bring to a boil over high heat. Reduce heat and simmer, uncovered, 10 minutes or until liquid has evaporated. Remove from heat. Place in a small bowl; cover and chill. Store in refrigerator in an airtight container.

PER SERVING NUTRITIONAL CONTENT:
    2 g. carbohydrate
    5 mg. sodium
EACH SERVING PROVIDES:
    0.3 Vegetable check

Mushroom Sauce

SERVINGS: 4 • SERVING SIZE: ¼ cup • CALORIES PER SERVING: 72

> 2 teaspoons oil or melted unsalted margarine
> ½ cup fresh mushroom pieces
> ¾ cup skim milk
> 2 teaspoons cornstarch
> 1½ ounces shredded part-skim mozzarella cheese
> Freshly ground pepper to taste

Heat oil or margarine in a saucepan; add mushrooms, and sauté over moderate heat for 3 minutes. In a cup, stir cold milk into cornstarch, then add mixture to mushrooms and stir over low heat until thickened. Add cheese. Stir until melted and smooth. Add pepper. Serve ¼ cup over each individual Tuna Casserole (page 228).

PER SERVING NUTRIENT CONTENT:
   4 g. protein
   4 g. fat
   4 g. carbohydrate
   74 mg. sodium

EACH SERVING PROVIDES:
   0.1 Bread/Starch check
   0.4 Meat/Meat Sub check
   0.1 Vegetable check
   0.2 Milk check
   0.5 Fat check

Spaghetti Meat Sauce

SERVINGS: 11 • SERVING SIZE: ½ cup • CALORIES PER SERVING: 125

> 1 pound lean ground beef round
> 1 teaspoon extra virgin olive oil
> 2 teaspoons fresh minced garlic
> ¾ cup chopped onion
> ½ cup diced green bell pepper
> 2 14½-ounce cans low-sodium tomatoes
> 1 6-ounce can low-sodium tomato paste
> ¾ cup water
> 1 8-ounce can low-sodium tomato sauce
> ½ teaspoon dried oregano
> ½ teaspoon dried basil
> ½ teaspoon red pepper flakes
> 1 tablespoon romano cheese, freshly grated

In a nonstick skillet, brown ground beef and drain off any fat. In separate skillet, heat oil. Add garlic, onion, and green pepper and sauté until tender. Add beef, tomatoes, tomato paste, water, tomato sauce, oregano, basil, Romano cheese, and red pepper flakes. Let simmer, uncovered, 1 hour. Serve with spaghetti.

PER SERVING NUTRIENT CONTENT:
  15 g. protein
  3 g. fat
  9 g. carbohydrate
  62 mg. sodium

EACH SERVING PROVIDES:
  1.2 Meat/Meat Sub checks
  2.0 Vegetable check
  0.1 Fat check

Spicy Creole Sauce

SERVINGS: 10 • SERVING SIZE: ¼ cup • CALORIES PER SERVING: 50

SEASONING MIX:
    2 bay leaves
    3/4 teaspoon dried oregano
    1/2 teaspoon freshly ground white pepper
    1/2 teaspoon freshly ground black pepper
    1/2 teaspoon cayenne pepper
    1/2 teaspoon paprika
    1/2 teaspoon dried thyme
    1/2 teaspoon dried basil

    2 tablespoons unsalted margarine
    1 cup peeled and chopped tomatoes
    3/4 cup chopped onion
    3/4 cup chopped celery
    3/4 cup chopped green bell pepper
    1 1/2 teaspoons minced garlic
    1 1/4 cup Low-Sodium Chicken Stock (page 192)
    1 cup low-sodium canned tomato sauce
    1 teaspoon sugar
    1/2 teaspoon Tabasco sauce

Thoroughly combine the seasoning mix ingredients in a small bowl and set aside. Melt margarine in a large skillet over medium heat. Stir in tomatoes, onions, celery, and bell pepper. Add garlic and seasoning mixture, stir until well blended. Stir in stock, tomato sauce, sugar, and Tabasco sauce and bring to a boil. Reduce heat to maintain a simmer. Cook until vegetables are tender and flavors are married, about 20 minutes, stirring occasionally. Remove bay leaves before serving.

PER SERVING NUTRIENT CONTENT:
    1 g. protein
    3 g. fat
    6 g. carbohydrate
    50 mg. sodium

EACH SERVING PROVIDES:
    0.2 Bread/Starch check
    0.1 Meat/Meat Sub check
    1.0 Vegetable check
    0.5 Fat check

Spinach Spread

SERVINGS: 36 • SERVING SIZE: 1 tablespoon • CALORIES PER SERVING: 15

> 1 10-ounce package frozen chopped spinach, thawed
> 1 cup DFC Sour Cream (page 253)
> ½ cup low-calorie mayonnaise
> ½ cup chopped scallion
> ½ cup minced fresh herbs
> 1 tablespoon fresh lime juice

Squeeze spinach dry and place in a bowl. Add the remaining ingredients and mix well. Refrigerate for several hours. Serve on cucumber slices or in mushroom caps.

PER SERVING NUTRIENT CONTENT:
   1 g. protein
   1 g. fat
   1 g. carbohydrate
   40 mg. sodium

EACH SERVING PROVIDES:
   0.1 Meat/Meat Sub check
   0.1 Vegetable check
   0.1 Fat check

Vegetable-Cheese Spread

SERVINGS: 20 • SERVING SIZE: 1 tablespoon • CALORIES PER SERVING: 9

> 1 cup 1% low-fat cottage cheese
> 1 tablespoon fresh minced chives
> 2 tablespoons minced radish
> 2 tablespoons minced, peeled cucumber
> 1 teaspoon Dijon mustard
> 1 teaspoon fresh lemon juice
> 1/4 teaspoon Worcestershire sauce
> Dash of cayenne pepper

Combine all ingredients in a bowl and stir gently until well blended. Chill and serve with Melba toast or as a sandwich spread.

PER SERVING NUTRIENT CONTENT:

   1 g. protein
   negligible fat
   negligible carbohydrate
   50 mg. sodium

EACH SERVING PROVIDES:

   0.1 Meat/Meat Sub check

Breads

Banana Oatmeal Muffins

SERVINGS: 16 • CALORIES PER SERVING: 130

1 1/2 cups unbleached flour
1/4 cup brown sugar
1 tablespoon baking powder
1/2 teaspoon mace
1 cup rolled oats
1 tablespoon poppy seeds
1/2 cup skim milk
1 egg
1 egg white
1 teaspoon vanilla
3 medium, ripe bananas, mashed
3 tablespoons unsalted margarine
1 tablespoon orange zest
Vegetable oil cooking spray

Preheat oven to 350°F.

In a large bowl blend flour, sugar, baking powder, mace, oats, and poppy seeds. In another bowl blend milk, egg, egg white, vanilla, bananas, margarine, and orange zest. Add wet ingredients to dry ingredients. Stir well until moist. Spray large muffin tins with cooking spray. Use a 1/4-cup measure to portion batter into muffin tins. Bake 20 minutes at 350°F or until toothpick inserted in the middle of a muffin comes out clean.

PER SERVING NUTRIENT CONTENT:
   3 g. protein
   3 g. fat
   22 g. carbohydrate
   75 mg. sodium
EACH SERVING PROVIDES:
   0.4 Fruit check
   1.0 Bread/Starch check
   0.1 Meat/Meat Sub check
   0.6 Fat check

Bran Muffins

SERVINGS: 16 • CALORIES PER SERVING: 102

Vegetable oil cooking spray
1 1/2 cups whole wheat flour
1 cup miller's bran
1/3 cup oat bran
1 teaspoon baking soda
2 teaspoons cinnamon
1 teaspoon freshly grated nutmeg
1/2 cup honey
3 egg whites
1/2 cup buttermilk
1/2 cup water
1/2 cup mashed banana
1 teaspoon vanilla extract
1/2 teaspoon banana extract

Preheat oven to 400°F. Coat 16 muffin cups with vegetable cooking spray.

In a large mixing bowl, combine flour, miller's and oat brans, baking soda, cinnamon, and nutmeg. In another bowl, place the honey, egg whites, buttermilk, water, mashed banana, banana and vanilla extracts, and beat until well mixed. Add the honey mixture to the flour mixture and stir well.

Pour batter into muffin tins and bake at 400°F for 15 minutes, or until a toothpick inserted in the center of a muffin comes out clean.

PER SERVING NUTRIENT CONTENT:
  3 g. protein
  1 g. fat
  24 g. carbohydrate
  122 mg. sodium

EACH SERVING PROVIDES:
  1.0 Bread/Starch checks
  0.1 Meat/Meat Sub check
  0.1 Fruit check

Corn Muffins

SERVINGS: 40 • CALORIES PER SERVING: 42

Vegetable oil cooking spray
1 *cup cornmeal*
1 *cup whole wheat flour*
1 *tablespoon baking powder*
2 *teaspoons baking soda*
1/2 *cup oat bran*
1/2 *teaspoon cinnamon*
1 *cup grated carrot*
3/4 *cup frozen apple juice concentrate*
3/4 *cup skim milk*
3/4 *cup evaporated skim milk*
1 *egg*

Preheat oven to 375°F. Coat miniature muffin tins with vegetable cooking spray.

In a bowl, mix together cornmeal, flour, baking powder, baking soda, bran, and cinnamon. In another bowl, beat together carrot, apple juice concentrate, skim milk, evaporated skim milk, and egg. Add to dry ingredients and mix with swift, quick strokes. Use a 1/8-cup measure to drop batter into muffin tins. Bake 20 minutes at 375°F, or until a toothpick inserted into the center of a muffin comes out clean.

PER SERVING NUTRIENT CONTENT:
2 g. protein
1 g. fat
8 g. carbohydrate
77 mg. sodium

EACH SERVING PROVIDES:
0.4 Bread/Starch check
0.1 Milk check
0.1 Vegetable check
0.1 Fruit check

Very Blueberry Muffins

SERVINGS: 12 • CALORIES PER SERVING: 145

1 1/3 cup all-purpose flour
1 cup rolled oats (quick or old-fashioned, uncooked)
1/4 cup brown sugar
1 tablespoon baking powder
1/2 teaspoon cinnamon
1 cup skim milk
1/4 cup egg whites
3 tablespoons safflower oil
1 cup fresh or frozen blueberries
Vegetable oil cooking spray

Preheat oven to 425°F.

In a bowl combine dry ingredients. Add milk, egg whites, and oil; stir just until dry ingredients are moistened. Fold in blueberries. Spray 12 medium muffin cups with cooking spray or line with paper baking cups. Fill muffin cups 2/3 full. Bake at 425°F for 25 to 30 minutes or until light golden brown.

PER SERVING NUTRIENT CONTENT:

4 g. protein
4 g. fat
23 g. carbohydrate
105 mg. sodium

EACH SERVING PROVIDES:

0.1 Milk check
0.1 Fruit check
1.3 Bread/Starch checks
0.1 Meat/Meat Sub check
0.8 Fat check

Desserts

Bublanina

SERVINGS: 8 • CALORIES PER SERVING: 160

From Czechoslovakia, a cherry cake that's a delicious conclusion to any dinner.

Vegetable oil cooking spray
1/3 cup unsalted margarine
3 tablespoons sugar
1 teaspoon grated lemon peel
1/2 teaspoon vanilla
4 eggs, separated
3/4 cup sifted flour
40 large pitted cherries*

Preheat oven to 350°F. Coat a 9-inch springform pan with nonstick cooking spray; set aside.

In large mixing bowl, using electric mixer, beat together margarine, sugar, lemon peel, and vanilla until fluffy; add egg yolks, one at a time, beating until thick and lemon-colored, about 5 minutes. While beating, gradually add flour.

In separate bowl, using clean beaters, beat egg whites until stiff peaks form; gently fold whites into yolk mixture. Pour batter into prepared pan; using a spatula, smooth top. Arrange cherries on top of batter, spacing them evenly. Bake 25 to 30 minutes, or until lightly browned and a cake tester, inserted in center, comes out clean. Transfer pan to wire rack and let cool 10 minutes; remove cake from pan and let cool completely on wire rack.

PER SERVING NUTRIENT CONTENT:
4 g. protein
7 g. fat
20 g. carbohydrate
125 mg. sodium
137 mg. cholesterol

EACH SERVING PROVIDES:
0.5 Protein check
1.0 Fat check
0.5 Fruit check
0.5 Bread/Starch check

*If fresh cherries are not available, 2 cups drained canned cherries (no sugar added) or frozen cherries (no sugar added), thawed and drained, may be substituted.

Chocolate Mint Fluff

SERVINGS: 6 • SERVING SIZE: ½ cup • CALORIES PER SERVING: 92

> 1 envelope unflavored gelatin
> 2 cups skim milk
> ⅓ cup plus 2 tablespoons sugar
> ⅓ cup unsweetened cocoa
> ½ teaspoon mint extract

Soften gelatin in milk in a small saucepan and let stand 1 minute. Add sugar and cocoa. Place over low heat and cook, stirring constantly, 5 minutes, or until gelatin dissolves. Do not allow to boil. Transfer mixture to shallow pan and stir in mint extract. Cover and chill until dessert is consistency of unbeaten egg white (about 20 minutes in freezer).

Transfer to a bowl; beat with an electric mixer at high speed until chocolate mixture is light and fluffy (about 5 minutes). Spoon evenly into dessert dishes; chill thoroughly.

NOTE: Any flavored extract works well.

PER SERVING NUTRIENT CONTENT:
   5 g. protein
   1 g. fat
   18 mg. carbohydrate
   44 mg. sodium
EACH SERVING PROVIDES:
   0.3 Milk check

Crepes

SERVINGS: 16 • CALORIES PER SERVING: 42

> 1 cup all-purpose flour
> 1½ cups skim milk
> 1 whole egg, slightly beaten
> Vegetable oil cooking spray

In mixing bowl, blend flour, milk, and egg until smooth. Let stand at room temperature for 45 to 60 minutes. Lightly coat a 6-inch nonstick skillet with vegetable oil cooking spray and heat to medium-high temperature. Pour 2 tablespoons batter in skillet; cook until golden brown on bottom. Repeat with remaining batter, lightly coating skillet with vegetable oil cooking spray for each crepe.

NOTE: Leftover crepes may be frozen between 2 layers of wax paper.

PER SERVING NUTRIENT CONTENT:
> 2 g. protein
> negligible fat
> 8 g. carbohydrate
> 16 mg. sodium

EACH SERVING PROVIDES:
> 0.4 Bread/Starch check
> 0.1 Meat/Meat Sub check
> 0.1 Milk check

Fresh Fruit Crepes

SERVINGS: 2 • CALORIES PER SERVING: 113

1/2 cup low-fat vanilla yogurt
1/2 cup sliced or diced fresh fruit or whole berries
1/2 teaspoon cinnamon (optional)
2 crepes (page 272)

Measure 2 tablespoons of vanilla yogurt and set aside. In a small bowl, place remaining yogurt, fruit (reserving 2 pieces for garnish), and cinnamon (if desired), mix together. Place half the yogurt-fruit mixture in each crepe and top with 1 tablespoon yogurt. Garnish with fruit.

PER SERVING NUTRIENT CONTENT:
> 5 g. protein
> 1.0 g. fat
> 21 g. carbohydrate
> 55 mg. sodium

EACH SERVING PROVIDES:
> 0.4 Bread/Starch check
> 0.1 Meat/Meat Sub check
> 0.4 Fruit check
> 0.4 Milk check

Frozen Banana

SERVINGS: 2 • CALORIES PER SERVING: 110

2 medium bananas
1 teaspoon fresh lemon juice
½ cup water

Peel bananas and cut in half. In a shallow dish, mix lemon juice and water. Dip bananas in lemon mixture. Place on wax paper and freeze. When frozen, remove from wax paper, place in plastic bag, seal, and return to freezer until ready to serve.

PER SERVING NUTRIENT CONTENT:
   1 g. protein
   negligible fat
   28 g. carbohydrate
   negligible sodium
EACH SERVING PROVIDES:
   2.0 Fruit checks

Strawberry Sorbet

SERVINGS: 2 • SERVING SIZE: ½ cup • CALORIES PER SERVING: 65

> 1 pint strawberries
> 3 tablespoons plain low-fat yogurt
> 1 tablespoon grated lemon rind
> 2 teaspoons frozen apple juice concentrate
> ¼ cup minced fresh mint
> 2 thin slices kiwi fruit or 2 sprigs fresh mint (garnish)

Wash, core, and cut strawberries into 1-inch pieces. Line a plate with plastic wrap; spread strawberries on plate in a single layer and freeze.

Place frozen pieces in blender or food processor. Add yogurt, lemon rind, apple juice concentrate, and fresh mint and blend until smooth. Turn into serving bowls and freeze until ready to serve. Garnish with kiwi fruit or mint sprigs.

PER SERVING NUTRIENT CONTENT:
  1 g. fat
  2 g. protein
  14 g. carbohydrate
  17 mg. sodium
EACH SERVING PROVIDES:
  1.0 Fruit check
  0.1 Milk check

Yogurt-Gelatin Whip

SERVINGS: 6 • SERVING SIZE: ½ cup • CALORIES PER SERVING: 30

1 box low-calorie fruit-flavored gelatin
1 cup boiling water
2 cups ice cubes
1 cup plain low-fat yogurt
½ teaspoon vanilla

In a mixing bowl, dissolve gelatin in boiling water. Add ice cubes and stir until gelatin starts to thicken, 3 to 5 minutes. Remove any unmelted ice. Add yogurt and vanilla. Beat until light and fluffy (mixture may be thin). Pour into serving dishes and chill until set.

PER SERVING NUTRIENT CONTENT:
    3 g. protein
    1 g. fat
    3 g. carbohydrate
    70 mg. sodium
EACH SERVING PROVIDES:
    0.2 Milk check

Strategies for Modifying Your Favorite Recipes

Changes in lifestyle and eating habits don't mean you have to throw away your favorite recipes or make them just for other family members. Once you learn the three basic principles of recipe modification, you can prepare many of your own favorite recipes and incorporate them into your new, healthy, low-calorie menu plan. Everyone will benefit from reduced fat, sodium, and sugar. Take time to experiment with these new cooking techniques; you'll find that they're well worth the effort.

Three Basic Principles of Recipe Modification

1. Substitution. Substitute low-calorie ingredients and/or cooking methods for high-calorie ones. Low-fat yogurt or blender-whipped low-fat cottage cheese easily replaces sour cream or mayonnaise in a recipe, saving calories and reducing saturated fats. Broil or steam your foods; don't fry them.

2. Reduction. Less is often better. Cut down the amounts of fat, sugar, and salt called for in recipes. Fat can usually be reduced by half.

3. Elimination. If an ingredient isn't essential, leave it out. Dispense with sugar in salad dressings. Butter on broiled fish can be eliminated. Omit salt and oil from the water when boiling pasta. By omitting these nonessential ingredients, you'll not only save calories, but you'll be better able to experience the delicious tastes of your major ingredients.

With these principles in mind, evaluate your recipes and menu choices for fats, sugar, cholesterol, and sodium. Remember that reducing the fat and sugar in recipes automatically reduces the caloric content.

Strategies for Reducing Fats

- Reduce oils, shortening, margarine, and butter by one-third to one-half.
- Choose skim or 1 percent low-fat dairy products instead of those made from whole milk.
- Select the leanest cuts of meat. One ounce of lean beef is only 60 calories compared to its high-fat counterpart at 100 calories.

- Always measure fat so you'll know exactly how many calories you're using. One teaspoon of margarine or butter equals approximately 40–45 calories, and 1 tablespoon equals about 120–135 calories.
- Trim all visible fat from meat. Remove the skin from poultry before cooking. Chances are that if you leave it on, you will eat it.
- Use nonstick cookware to eliminate or reduce the amount of oil used in preparation.
- Instead of oil or margarine, use small amounts of liquid or broth to sauté food.
- Chill soups, stews, broths, and sauces until the fat rises to the top and becomes solid. Then spoon off and discard the fat.
- For sauces and dressings, use low-calorie, low-fat bases such as vinegar, yogurt, mustard, tomato juice, and fat-free broth instead of high-calorie bases such as oil, mayonnaise, and creams.
- Reduce fat and cholesterol by substituting two egg whites for each whole egg. For example, use two egg whites in place of each whole egg in muffin or meatloaf recipes.
- Puree vegetables and combine them with skim milk for "cream" sauces or soups.
- For flavoring vegetables and starches such as rice and potatoes, consider using butter substitutes or butter extract. Also experiment with various herbs, either dried or fresh.
- Add more fish to your diet. It is a very good source of nutrients and is low in fat.
- Roast, broil, bake, or simmer meat, poultry, and fish.

Strategies for Reducing Sodium

- Reduce or eliminate salt when cooking. Begin by decreasing the requested amount by one-half to one-fourth.
- Reduce or eliminate high-salt ingredients such as some canned broths and soups, soy sauce, or condiments, and substitute reduced-sodium products such as salt-free broth and reduced-sodium soy sauce.
- Use fresh vegetables whose flavor can stand alone without added salt.
- Limit purchases of processed foods.
- Use lemon juice, vinegar, wine, or other acidic agents to enhance food flavor.

- Use a salt substitute. (Because salt substitutes contain potassium, it is important to make sure that you have no medical problems, specifically kidney disease, which could be aggravated by additional potassium.)
- Experiment with herbs and spices for added flavor. Record the mixtures that please you so that you can use them again.
- Keep a peppermill on the table instead of a saltshaker.
- Use fresh herbs, vegetables, and fruits. They are more flavorful and generally deliver greater amounts of vitamins and minerals.

Strategies for Reducing Sugar

- Reduce the amount of sugar called for by one-half to one-fourth.
- Use natural sweeteners such as fruits or fruit juices. Blend ripe fruits for a sweet sauce, or use as a replacement for sugar called for in a recipe.
- Use sugar substitutes to replace half of the sugar in baked goods or all of the sugar in other recipes.
- Use extracts and spices to enhance the flavor of baked goods. For example, vanilla extract and cinnamon added to a muffin or french toast batter really spark the flavor.

Recipe Modification

The DFC technique for modifying high-calorie recipes is illustrated in the following two recipes, Rice Frittata and Broccoli with Cheese Sauce. Both were modified to reduce their fat, sodium, and sugar content.

Rice Frittata

(Original Version)

SERVINGS: 6 • CALORIES PER SERVING: 315

> 1 medium onion, finely chopped
> 1 tablespoon unsalted butter
> 8 eggs, beaten
> 1/2 cup heavy cream
> 1 teaspoon salt
> 1 teaspoon Worcestershire sauce
> Dash Tabasco sauce
> 2 cups cooked rice
> 1 medium tomato, chopped
> 4 ounces Cheddar cheese, shredded

In a 10-inch skillet, melt butter over low heat. Add onions and sauté until translucent. To the beaten eggs, add the cream, salt, Worcestershire sauce, Tabasco sauce, cooked white rice, and tomato. Stir well. Pour all ingredients into skillet over cooked onion. Reduce heat to low. Cover and cook until top is almost set, about 15 to 20 minutes. Sprinkle with cheese, cover again, and remove from heat. Let stand for 10 minutes, then cut into 6 wedges and serve.

PER SERVING NUTRIENT CONTENT:
    16 g. protein
    18 g. fat
    22 g. carbohydrate
    640 mgs. sodium

Rice Frittata

(Modified Version)

SERVINGS: 6 • CALORIES PER SERVING: 220

1 cup onion, finely chopped
2 teaspoons unsalted margarine
4 large eggs
8 large egg whites
1/2 cup nonfat milk
1 teaspoon Worcestershire sauce
1 teaspoon Tabasco sauce
1 tablespoon green chilies, chopped
1 1/2 cups cooked brown rice
1/2 cup yellow squash, diced
1 cup tomatoes, chopped
3 ounces Cheddar cheese, shredded
1/2 cup lettuce, shredded

In a 10-inch skillet, melt margarine on low heat. Add onions and sauté until translucent. Beat eggs and egg whites together. Add nonfat milk, Worcestershire sauce, Tabasco sauce, and green chilies. Add brown rice, squash, and tomatoes. Pour all ingredients into skillet over cooked onion. Reduce heat to low. Cover and cook until top is almost set, about 15 to 20 minutes. When top is set, sprinkle with cheese. Cover and remove from heat and let stand for 10 minutes. Cut into wedges, garnish with shredded lettuce, and serve.

PER SERVING NUTRIENT CONTENT:
    15 g. protein
    10 g. fat
    17 g. carbohydrate
    235 g. sodium
EACH SERVING PROVIDES:
    0.1 Milk check
    0.4 Vegetable check
    0.9 Bread/Starch check
    1.6 Meat/Meat Sub checks
    1.3 Fat checks

Broccoli with Cheese Sauce

(Original Version)

SERVINGS: 6 • CALORIES PER SERVING: 370

2 10-ounce packages frozen broccoli, chopped
5 tablespoons salted butter
2 tablespoons minced onion
3 tablespoons all-purpose flour
1/2 cup heavy cream
1/4 teaspoon garlic salt
1/4 teaspoon salt
1 cup shredded Swiss cheese
2 eggs, beaten
4 tablespoons butter
1/2 cup bread crumbs

Preheat oven to 400°F.

Boil broccoli until soft; drain. Melt 5 tablespoons butter in saucepan and sauté onion until transparent. Add flour and cook 2 minutes, stirring constantly. Stir in cream and cook until thickened. Add garlic salt, salt, and cheese. Place broccoli in greased casserole dish. Pour on cheese sauce. Melt 4 tablespoons butter in saucepan. Stir in bread crumbs until crumbs are well coated; sprinkle over top. Bake 20 to 25 minutes at 400°F.

PER SERVING NUTRIENT CONTENT:

11 g. protein
32 g. fat
10 g. carbohydrate
585 mg. sodium

Broccoli with Cheese Sauce

(Modified Version)

SERVINGS: 6 • CALORIES PER SERVING: 75

1 medium head fresh broccoli, cut into florets
2 teaspoons unsalted margarine
1/4 cup minced onion
2 cloves garlic, minced
3 tablespoons all-purpose flour
1 cup skim milk
2 ounces part-skim mozzarella cheese, shredded
1/8 teaspoon nutmeg
   Freshly ground black pepper, to taste
   Vegetable oil cooking spray
1 tablespoon freshly grated Parmesan cheese
1 tablespoon minced fresh parsley
   Dash of paprika

Preheat oven to 400°F.

Steam broccoli until tender but crispy; drain. Melt margarine in nonstick skillet, and sauté onion and garlic until translucent. In small bowl, mix flour and skim milk. Add mixture to skillet and stir constantly over medium heat until thickened. Stir in mozzarella, nutmeg, and pepper. Remove from heat. Place broccoli in casserole dish coated with vegetable spray. Pour cheese sauce evenly over broccoli. Mix Parmesan cheese with parsley and sprinkle over casserole. Top with paprika for color and bake 20 to 25 minutes at 400° F.

PER SERVING NUTRIENT CONTENT:
   7 g. protein
   3 g. fat
   9 g. carbohydrate
   75 mg. sodium

The DFC Fitness Program

9

Getting into Shape

Our Bodies Are Made to Be Used

Exercise is not a luxury; it's one of the most important investments in your health and well-being that you will ever make. It's key to achieving physical fitness, by which we mean a combination of muscular strength, endurance, flexibility, and cardiovascular conditioning. The dividends are tremendous.

Some of the profits that can be earned from regular exercise include
- Lower blood pressure
- A reduced risk of coronary artery disease (heart attack and angina)
- An increase in lung efficiency
- Improved blood sugar control in Type II diabetes
- Strengthened bones, ligaments, and tendons
- A lower risk of osteoporosis
- Greater physical endurance
- Better body tone
- A reduction in body fat and loss of inches
- A more attractive body
- A better self-image
- More self-confidence
- More restful sleep
- More energy
- Improved mood and mental alertness
- Increased ability to concentrate
- Greater productivity
- Greater ease in coping with stress
- Greater sense of well-being
- Possibly, a delay in the aging process

The Risks of Inactivity

Almost every one of our overweight clients has been leading an inactive life. In fact, inactivity is often a major contributor to their excess weight. For many, fatigue has been a major problem, sometimes even debilitating, but once these clients begin to follow our exercise program they feel better, and gain energy and a sense of vitality.

Inactivity is supported by late twentieth-century American culture. Most of our work is sedentary. Jobs involving vigorous labor are fewer than ever before. We drive instead of walking, and we ride elevators and escalators instead of climbing up or down stairs.

The price we may pay for inactivity is a reduction in energy and health, as well as an increased risk of cardiovascular disease, the number one killer in the United States today. There are some risk factors for this disease over which we have no control: age, gender, race, and family history. However, there are many avoidable or modifiable risk factors: inactivity, elevated cholesterol levels, cigarette smoking, diabetes melitus, hypertension, obesity, and possibly Type A behavior.

Physical activity can help to modify five of these factors—inactivity, abnormal cholesterol levels, diabetes, hypertension, and obesity—and has been shown to ameliorate some of the negative effects of Type A behavior. It's been well established that combining aerobic exercise and physical activity with a healthier diet increases HDL, the "healthy" type of cholesterol levels in the blood, and reduces LDL, the harmful type of cholesterol. Exercise can also reduce high blood pressure and diminish free-floating hostility, anxiety, and an excessive competitive drive—all of which characterize people with Type A personalities.

Even if you don't have high blood pressure problems, or a Type A personality, exercise can help you manage stress better. It gives you time to relax your mind and emotions, time to daydream and to think about things.

Start Now

As you begin to build activity into your daily life, think in terms of small adjustments. Anything you can do to move will help you. See how many of the following activities you can incorporate into your everyday life.

• Instead of taking the bus all the way to work, get off one stop earlier and walk the rest of the way. After a week of doing this, get off two stops earlier.

- Walk up a flight of stairs instead of using the elevator.
- Instead of picking up the phone and calling your colleague in the next office, get up and walk over to see her.
- Replace coffee breaks with exercise breaks, such as a short walk or some stretches.
- Walk from store to store instead of driving and reparking.
- Park at the far edge of the lot instead of circling for the space closest to the entrance to the store.
- Walk to work. If it's too far, walk part of the way.
- Do your own yardwork and housework.
- Walk two or three extra blocks when you go out to lunch.
- Walk whenever you can.

Make small adjustments in physical activities such as these, and begin to incorporate regular aerobic exercise in your daily life.

Metabolic Rate, Exercise, and Weight Loss

Before beginning this section, you may want to review the description of metabolic rate on page 82.

People have different metabolic rates primarily because they have different amounts of lean body tissue. The greater the amount of lean body tissue you have, the higher your resting metabolic rate (RMR). This is because lean body tissues such as muscle and organ tissues such as those of the lungs, kidneys, and liver, are more metabolically active and thus require more energy (calories) to function. In contrast, fat is less metabolically active and requires less energy because its primary function is to serve as a warehouse for the storage of excess energy.

This may explain why men, who generally have more lean tissue and less fat than women, have a higher metabolic rate than women—and, thus, generally lose weight more rapidly. This also explains why older people seem to lose weight more slowly—because aging is associated with a gradual loss of lean tissue. The loss of lean tissue in older people is probably related to the fact that they are generally less physically active than young people, a situation that doesn't necessarily have to be. Because physical activity helps to preserve and possibly increase lean body tissue (primarily muscle tissue), it is an important component of any effective weight management program.

An important benefit of aerobic exercise is that metabolic rate rises during exercise and may remain elevated for a short time after an exercise session. Exercise, of course, also burns calories. For these reasons, and because exercise has numerous other health benefits, it's very important to increase your energy output by increasing the amount of time that you devote to aerobic exercise, and by increasing other physical activities associated with daily living, such as climbing stairs or walking.

How to Begin Your Fitness Program

Step 1. Start in Your Doctor's Office

The exercise program you choose should be determined by your health and physical condition, and whether or not you have been exercising regularly. We firmly believe that for most people, the starting line for a fitness program should be in the physician's office.

Each client who comes to the DFC receives a complete assessment, which includes a family and personal health history focusing on current health status, risk factors, and exercise habits. In addition to a complete physical examination, each person takes a graded exercise test, a common diagnostic tool that helps screen for the presence of coronary heart disease and also estimates the body's fitness level. Most often, the exercise test is given on a treadmill. As you walk on the treadmill, your blood pressure and heart rate are monitored and an electrocardiogram (EKG) records the electrical activity of your heart. Because of its value in helping to develop an individually appropriate exercise prescription, we recommend that you take an exercise test before beginning any fitness program, especially if you haven't been active in recent years, are older, or have cardiovascular risk factors as described in chapter 3.

If you have no known health problems or risk factors as described in chapter 3 and decide not to see your physician before beginning this program, start slowly and work steadily. It is probably a lesser risk to work your way gradually into movement and exercise than it is for you to remain inactive.

Step 2. Understand the Components of Your Exercise Prescription

While it's important to incorporate physical activity into all aspects of your daily life, it's also important to engage in a regular program of exercise.

In terms of health and weight management, one of the most important components of a fitness program is aerobic exercise. The word *aerobic* means "in the presence of oxygen," and the term *aerobic fitness* (which is achieved by aerobic exercise) describes a condition in which the body is able to take in, transport, and efficiently utilize oxygen during exercise. Aerobic exercise leads to improvements in cardiorespiratory function, or the capacity of the cardiorespiratory system (heart, blood vessels, and lungs) to function during sustained physical activity.

Other components of physical fitness are muscular strength (the ability to exert force against resistance), muscular endurance (the ability to repeat an activity over a period of time), and flexibility (the ability to move joints and muscles through a range of motions, or to bend, twist, and stretch).

The effectiveness of an aerobic fitness program depends on several factors, including the following:

The type of activity. Aerobic exercise consists of moderate, rhythmic, and continuous movements of large muscle groups. This can be achieved by brisk walking, running or jogging, aerobic dancing, swimming, bicycling, rowing, or any activity of this nature.

The duration of the activity. Aerobic exercise should be performed continuously for twenty to sixty minutes. Duration depends on intensity level and frequency of the exercise. Anyone beginning a program should start with short sessions performed at a low intensity.

The frequency of the activity. Aerobic fitness is best accomplished by aerobic exercise sessions three to six days a week. The American College of Sports Medicine recommends working up to and performing aerobic exercise five to six days each week if you are using exercise as an aid in weight reduction.

The intensity of the activity. The amount of stress sustained by the circulatory and respiratory systems during exercise is also important in developing aerobic fitness. Although a certain intensity level is needed to reap the maximum benefits of aerobic exercise, intensity is sometimes overemphasized—particularly for new exercisers who have a tendency to overdo when they first begin.

Step 3. Monitor the Intensity of Your Workout

At the Duke University Diet and Fitness Center, we teach people to monitor their intensity level in two ways: by heart rate and by perceived exertion.

Heart rate or pulse monitoring is a popular way to measure the intensity of exercise. To determine your heart rate, put your fingers (not your thumb) on the radial artery of your wrist or on the carotid artery in your neck for ten seconds. Count the number of times your pulse beats in this ten-second period. Multiply this ten-second count by six to get the number of beats per minute. For example, twelve beats in ten seconds equals seventy-two beats per minute ($12 \times 6 = 72$).

When you exercise at your target heart rate, your cardiorespiratory system is being effectively but safely stressed to produce aerobic fitness. As mentioned, aerobic fitness is associated with improvements in cardiorespiratory function and health. The following simple calculations can be used to estimate your target heart rate, the rate you should try to achieve during the main aerobic (sometimes called conditioning) phase of your exercise workout.

First, estimate your maximal heart rate for your age. Your maximal heart rate is just what it says—the highest heart rate you can theoretically achieve. Maximal heart rate decreases with age and is estimated as follows:

$220 -$ your age $=$ your maximal heart rate

Estimate your heart rate reserve (the difference in your heart rate from rest to maximal heart rate):

1. Your maximal heart rate: _____
2. Your resting heart rate (your heart rate while at rest): _____
3. Your heart rate reserve (subtract #2 from #1): _____

Next, estimate your target heart rate. If you are at a low fitness level (you are sedentary and never exercise, and wish to exercise at a low intensity level), use the following formula to determine your target heart rate:

1. Your heart rate reserve multiplied by .6: _____
2. Your resting heart rate: _____
3. Your target heart rate (add #1 and #2): _____

If you are at a moderate fitness level, (you are moderately active, and wish to exercise at a moderate intensity level), use the following formula:

1. Your heart rate reserve multiplied by .7: _____
2. Your resting heart rate: _____
3. Your target heart rate (add #1 and #2): _____

If you are at a high fitness level (and you enjoy intense exercise), you may choose to exercise at a higher intensity level. Use the following formula:

1. Your heart rate reserve multiplied by .8: _____
2. Your resting heart rate: _____
3. Your target heart rate (add #1 and #2): _____

Remember that it is possible to improve your aerobic fitness at intensity levels less than your target heart rate. Then, as you gradually improve your aerobic fitness level, you can increase the intensity of your exercise sessions, if you so desire. Don't let the intensity of the exercise limit you!

Perceived exertion is another practical way to monitor exercise intensity. The method is simple: listen to your body. During exercise, your lungs, heart, and muscles send messages to your brain signaling the intensity level of your exercise effort. Studies show that these subjective signals are good estimates of the physiologic changes occurring in response to exercise, for example, increases in heart rate and oxygen consumption. The key is to be aware of your body's response to exercise in terms of perceived exertion, physical stress, effort, and fatigue. Don't concentrate on any single factor such as muscle soreness or breathlessness. Instead, focus on your total sense of exertion. Try to be as objective and honest as you can about the degree of exertion you feel.

Perceived exertion is the way most people monitor their exercise intensity, whether they realize it or not. It's easy, practical, and you can trust it. If you feel that you're exercising comfortably and productively, you are probably receiving a healthy workout.

The following scale, originally devised by a Swedish scientist, Dr. Gunnar Borg, will help you to rate the intensity of your effort during exercise. Your exercise intensity should fall between levels 11 and 15. Be sure, however, to always exercise at a *comfortable* level.

Borg Scale for Rating Perceived Exertion

6 No exertion at all	11 Light	16
7	12	17 Very hard
8 Extremely light	13 Somewhat hard	18
9 Very light	14	19 Extremely hard
10	15 Hard	20 Maximal exertion

Step 4. Follow an Exercise Sequence

The *warm-up phase* warms your muscles and tendons and prepares them for the main conditioning phase of the workout. A slow and steady warm-up will stimulate your heart and lungs, elevate your heart rate slightly, and prepare your muscles and cardiovascular system to handle more rapid and sustained activity. An effective warm-up is to perform your exercise routine at a slower, more controlled pace. Warm-up time will vary, but when you begin to perspire, you are ready for the main conditioning phase.

The *main conditioning phase* challenges your cardiovascular system and trains your body to take in, transport, and use oxygen efficiently. The period, lasting from twenty to thirty minutes, or even longer, depending on your intensity and fitness level, involves performing continuous rhythmic exercise. As muscles contract rhythmically, you experience increases in heart rate, blood pressure, breathing, and the need for oxygen. Monitor the intensity of your workouts (see page 291), and be careful not to overdo it. Work within your limits. Your body will respond over time to the physical challenge and will change as a result.

The *cool-down phase*—from five to ten minutes of exercise at a lower level of intensity—slowly returns your body's physical parameters to the preworkout levels. During exercise, blood has been shunted to working muscle groups and away from nonworking tissues. Therefore, it's important not to stop suddenly but to allow time for blood to return to its normal distribution pattern. The cool-down helps to remove metabolic waste products produced during the conditioning phase. This third stage of your workout should never be omitted. This is an excellent time to stretch as well, since the muscles are warm and stretching will help preserve range of motion and flexibility.

Step 5. Choose an Aerobic Exercise that Suits You

Creating a personal exercise program is something of an art since it involves individual sensibilities, aesthetics, and choices that must satisfy you mentally as well as physically.

Check to see what's available in your area, and always consider your individual tastes. Exercise involves commitment and time, and you should enjoy it. At the minimum, look for an effective workout that you're able to do and that you don't mind doing. If you hate your exercise program, you probably won't continue it and thus you won't receive any benefits from it. For instance, if you loathe the kind of music played in a dance exercise class, you won't continue exercising. If you can't stand getting wet, you won't do well in swimming.

Consider your temperament and how you like to spend your time. If you are a solitary exercise person and enjoy doing things on your own, take up solo walking or bicycling. If you don't like jogging, try fast walking. If you like company, find an exercise partner or join a class.

Recreational pursuits such as golf, tennis, bowling, or volleyball are great fun but are of limited benefit because they involve a great deal of starting and stopping. Muscle-building exercises with weight-training machines may help strengthen and tone your muscles, but may benefit your cardiovascular system in only limited ways.

Don't let medical barriers defeat you before you begin. If you have chronic knee pain or other joint problems, you may have to forego jogging and aerobic dance. Instead, try walking, stationary cycling, and/ or swimming. If you have a heart condition and you need medical supervision, join a cardiovascular conditioning program that is run by a local hospital or YMCA.

Exercise programs that are aerobically beneficial include
- Walking
- Jogging
- Low-impact aerobic dance
- Cycling and stationary cycling
- Swimming
- Pool aerobics

Walking is excellent for your general health and is probably the best choice for anyone who has been inactive for a number of years. Studies have shown that walkers in their sixties, seventies, and eighties have more energy and mental alertness than their nonwalking counterparts.

Besides being convenient, inexpensive, and easy, walking gives you many of the advantages of more vigorous forms of exercise with a lower risk of injury. Walking on level ground may not allow you to reach your target heart rate, but it will still stress your cardiovascular system sufficiently to produce a training effect and enable you to burn a good number of calories. Walking requires no equipment other than a good pair of walking or jogging shoes and can be done in regular clothes. Most people find walking pleasurable, which is probably why studies show that among exercisers, walkers have the lowest dropout rate.

Tips
- Walk comfortably and naturally, maintaining good posture. Follow your natural gait.
- Measure your walk by time, not by mileage. The mileage will come as you put in the time.
- Challenge yourself, but don't overdo it.

Jogging is excellent for weight control and cardiovascular conditioning. Many people love to jog, and some depend on it as a way of relieving tension. Others get a "high" from it, and say they couldn't do without it. However, joggers must guard against injuries as well as aches and pains. Jogging stresses both knees and ankles, and can exacerbate a number of orthopedic problems.

Tips
- Begin slowly.
- Monitor your exercise intensity carefully. Don't push and *never* "run through the pain."
- Buy running shoes that give good support and shock absorption.
- Wear loose and comfortable clothing. Start with walking, then move gradually into jogging.
- Measure your progress by the time you run instead of the distance you cover.
- Stretch your muscles—particularly the leg muscles after you jog.
- Take advantage of the many good books to help the beginning runner.

Low-impact aerobic dance incorporates the benefits of higher impact exercise with a greatly reduced risk of injuries.

Aerobic dance is usually performed to upbeat music, and exercises a variety of muscle groups. There are many good classes available for low-impact aerobics. The exercise requires coordination, but don't be afraid to try it if you feel clumsy or insecure. People in these classes work at various levels of skill. Sometimes the success of the workout depends on the quality of the instructor.

Tips
- Check out the instructor's credentials before beginning a class. You need someone who knows something about the body—not just someone who looks good in a leotard.

- Buy good, supportive exercise shoes to reduce your chances of injury.
- Before you enroll, take a trial class to make sure that you enjoy it.
- Always exercise at *your* pace, not the instructor's.

Cycling works your lower body by pedaling and your upper body by positioning and providing leverage. Variety is built into the bike ride with the rapid change of scenery. It can be a very smooth activity and one that you can perform for extended periods of time. (See page 298 on stationary cycling.)

Tips
- Wear a helmet.
- Have the bike sized to your body.
- Ride defensively and obey traffic laws.
- Pedal smoothly and in a continuous motion.
- Investigate local bike clubs or shops for instruction and planned day trips.
- Consider buying cycling clothing. Padded gloves and bicycling shorts can be particularly helpful for safety and comfort.
- Start slowly and gradually build up your speed and endurance.

Water exercise is a mainstay of the DFC program. As a rule, people enjoy the water and find it an easy place to begin a conditioning program.

Water walking is a good aerobic activity, especially if you have limitations and need to start slowly. Water walking can be tremendously rehabilitating. The buoyancy of the water allows you to move your arms and legs in a controlled fashion, thus reducing orthopedic concerns.

Pool aerobics gives a good cardiovascular workout by using water as the medium of resistance during twenty or thirty minutes of continuous and rhythmic exercises of the upper and lower body.

Swimming is also a good choice for aerobic conditioning. You don't have to be a great swimmer in order to get a good cardiovascular workout. It's never too late to learn to swim. Private and group lessons are available for beginners in many communities. The strengthening and toning benefits of lap swimming are well documented. Vary your strokes to work all the major muscle groups of the body.

If you choose an outdoor exercise as your mainstay, remember that an indoor pool is an excellent all-weather alternative. The water is both warming and cooling; it warms the joints, while the swirling water helps to dissipate body heat built up by vigorous exercise. You don't need to be an accomplished swimmer to do water exercises.

Tips
- Invest in quality eye goggles for comfort and relief from chlorine.
- Consider using earplugs, particularly if you are prone to ear infections or if water in your ears bothers you.
- Start slowly and build up your intensity over time, remembering that your heart rate may be ten to fifteen beats or more per minute slower in the water than it is during a comparable aerobic workout on land (perceived exertion may be a better indicator of exercise intensity in the water).
- Vary your strokes to use a number of muscle groups, so that you can swim longer. Soon you will be able to concentrate less on your strokes and more on your thoughts.

At-Home Aerobic Exercise Options

There are a number of affordable and effective at-home exercise options, but remember that many gadgets will make you thinner only in the wallet. If an exercise machine can't provide continuous and rhythmic motion for at least twenty to thirty minutes, don't buy it. Here are some of the better choices for exercising at home.

A *treadmill* may be of interest to you if you enjoy walking or jogging. The more expensive motorized treadmills give you a smooth walk or jog at a regulated speed and inclination. Also, being off the road and out of the inclement weather can be added to the benefits of walking and jogging. Manual treadmills are noisier, less expensive, and less well controlled.

Stationary bicycles are easy to use and are a readily available option for many people. They provide an aerobic workout and also tone your legs. Some have arm components that allow for an upper body workout. A stationary bicycle is a good option for someone with orthopedic problems because it enables one to exercise without bearing weight.

Look for a bike that is sturdy and has a comfortable and adjustable seat. Adjust the seat height so that there is a slight bend in your knees at extension. As with cycling in general, adjust the tension (resistance) so that you can pedal comfortably (about 70 to 90 rpm). Avoid bargain-basement brands. Invest in a quality machine that works well and that will give you good dividends for the time you spend exercising.

Rowing machines have become popular for working out at home, perhaps because the hydraulic types are relatively inexpensive. Rowing correctly involves good technique, so consult the manufacturer's owner's manual and follow instructions. The rowing motion involves a lot of upper body work and thus may take some getting used to. Make sure that the machine is sized correctly for you, and set the tension so that you can maintain a steady pace at an appropriate heart rate or at appropriate perceived exertion.

Records, cassettes, videos, and books offer a wide variety of exercise classes and routines. Many television channels also regularly broadcast exercise programs. These options allow you the privacy of your own home for exercising. The variety of these offerings may avoid the potential staleness in an exercise program.

Tips
- At home, as in a supervised class, always follow safe and proper techniques.
- Work within your limits.
- Do not let the instructor dictate your level of intensity.

Strategies for Setting Up Your Personal Exercise Plan

Step 1. Identify Your Needs, Interests, and Objectives

Write down why you need to exercise, what kinds of aerobic fitness activities interest you, and what you think exercise will do for you. Also note which lifestyle activities you could change to include more movement, and which aerobic exercises you want to implement.

Step 2. Record Your Short- and Long-Term Goals

Be specific. Write down target times for exercise, and list goals that include health, appearance, body tone, shape, measurements, stamina, and overall physical capacity. Long-term goals may include improved health and a smaller clothing size. Your short-term goal, then, may be to lose five pounds for your sister's wedding in four weeks. This short-term goal will help you realize your long-term goals.

Set reasonable and realistic short-term goals. When you have accomplished one short-term goal, set another one. Once you have gotten into shape for your high school reunion, what is your next short-term motivator? Make something up, and then reward yourself when you have achieved it. Just as you may have experienced a downward, negative spiral in the past, so can you experience an upward, positive spiral. If you like clothes, buy yourself a good-looking running suit or a special outfit as a gift for adhering to your program.

Your long-term goals should be equally realistic. One such goal might be to decrease your amount of body fat or to stay at a particular weight or size. Remember to make your goals personal. You know what will motivate you; use that knowledge to your advantage.

Step 3. Prescribe Your Proper Attire, the Time of Day, and the Location

Make exercise a regular part of your day at a time that works best for you. If you're a morning person—or if you tend to put things off—the best time might be first thing in the morning. Or, depending on your routine, the best time might be the end of the work day to help reduce stress.

Make sure that your exercise is convenient and realistic. Consider where it will take place, and how you will incorporate it into your day. If you have to drive a half hour to get to a health spa, will you be able to maintain a commitment to it?

Wear comfortable clothing. Do you have a gym suit, a leotard, or a bathing suit? Do you have proper supportive athletic shoes? Set realistic goals for yourself in terms of the convenience and the clothing or equipment you need.

Step 4. Set the Amount of Exercise You Need Each Week

We recommend that you begin your exercise training with short but regular sessions, then follow a slow to moderate progression that builds up to exercising three to six times a week depending on the type, intensity, and duration of your activity. If you are at a very low fitness level, start with no more than five to fifteen minutes per exercise session at a safe and enjoyable intensity, using the following guidelines.

Table 11.

Exercise Progression Chart

Fitness Level	Walking	Stationary Cycling	Swimming
Low	Start with 15 min. increase 5 min. per week	Start with 5 min. increase 2–3 min. per week	Start with 10 min. increase 5 min. per week
Moderate	Start with 30 min. increase 5 min. per week	Start with 10 min. increase 2–3 min. per week	Start with 20 min. increase 5 min. per week
High	Start with 45 min. increase 5 min. per week	Start with 15–30 min. increase 2–3 min. per week	Start with 30 min. increase 5 min. per week
Goal	45–60 min.	30 min.	30–45 min.

It's tempting to dive into a dance class or to overdo it on your first day out walking. This overenthusiastic approach can result in sore muscles, an aching back, and little motivation to go out and try again. Always be careful to follow a systematic program, and gradually increase the duration of each session. Don't fall into the temptation of doing too much too soon.

When Rita Caparelli started her walking program, she began with fifteen-minute walks. Now she walks thirty to forty minutes six days a week and maintains a moderate program that makes her feel healthy. Similarly, when Nathan Bennett started his swimming program, he swam for a short period just about every day. Eventually, as he increased the duration of his workout, he began swimming every other day. On the days he doesn't swim, Nathan does the DFC stretch and strengthen routines, which you'll find in chapter 10.

Look at some of the following sample exercise programs that DFC clients have set up for themselves at various points in their own development. This format can be applied to any aerobic activities that you choose. Notice that when clients are doing smaller amounts of exercise, they may do them five or six days a week, whereas at a higher fitness and intensity level, they may do the activity every other day. These time charts are suited to the people who designed them, and thus may not suit you at all. Use them only as a model to help you construct a program that fits you, your temperament, and your life situation.

Sample Walking Programs

Rita's Low Fitness Level Walking Prescription

	Mon.	Tues.	Wed.	Thurs.	Fri.	Sat.	Sun.	Times per Week
			Minutes Per Day					
Week 1	15	15	15	15	15	0	0	5
Week 2	20	20	20	0	20	20	0	5
Week 3	25	25	25	25	0	0	25	5
Week 4	30	30	30	30	30	30	0	6

Rita's Moderate Fitness Level Walking Prescription

	Mon.	Tues.	Wed.	Thurs.	Fri.	Sat.	Sun.	Times per Week
			Minutes per Day					
Week 1	30	30	30	30	30	0	0	5
Week 2	35	35	35	35	0	35	35	6
Week 3	40	40	40	40	40	0	40	6
Week 4	45	45	45	45	0	45	45	6

Rita's High Fitness Level Prescription

	Mon.	Tues.	Wed.	Thurs.	Fri.	Sat.	Sun.	Times per Week
			Minutes per Day					
Week 1	45	45	45	45	45	0	0	5
Week 2	50	50	50	50	50	0	50	6
Week 3	55	55	55	55	55	0	55	6
Week 4	60	60	60	60	60	60	0	6

Sample Stationary Cycling Programs

Marlene's Low Fitness Level Stationary Cycling Prescription

	Mon.	Tues.	Wed.	Thurs.	Fri.	Sat.	Sun.	Times per Week
			Minutes per Day					
Week 1	5	5	5	5	5	0	0	5
Week 2	8	8	8	8	0	5	0	5
Week 3	10	10	10	0	10	10	0	5
Week 4	13	13	13	13	13	0	0	5

Daniel's Moderate Fitness Level Stationary Cycling Prescription

	Minutes per Day							Times per Week
	Mon.	Tues.	Wed.	Thurs.	Fri.	Sat.	Sun.	
Week 1	10	10	10	10	10	0	0	5
Week 2	12	12	12	12	0	12	0	5
Week 3	15	15	15	15	0	15	0	5
Week 4	18	18	18	18	0	18	0	5

Sarah's High Fitness Level Stationary Cycling Prescription

	Minutes per Day							Times per Week
	Mon.	Tues.	Wed.	Thurs.	Fri.	Sat.	Sun.	
Week 1	15	0	15	0	15	0	15	4
Week 2	18	0	18	0	18	0	18	4
Week 3	21	0	21	0	21	0	21	4
Week 4	24	0	24	0	24	0	24	4

Sample Swimming Programs

Nathan's Low Fitness Level Swimming Prescription

	Minutes per Day							Times per Week
	Mon.	Tues.	Wed.	Thurs.	Fri.	Sat.	Sun.	
Week 1	10	10	0	10	10	0	10	5
Week 2	15	15	0	15	15	0	15	5
Week 3	20	20	0	20	20	0	20	5
Week 4	25	25	0	25	25	0	25	5

Nathan's Moderate Fitness Level Swimming Prescription

	Minutes per Day							Times per Week
	Mon.	Tues.	Wed.	Thurs.	Fri.	Sat.	Sun.	
Week 1	20	20	0	20	20	0	20	5
Week 2	20	20	0	20	20	0	20	5
Week 3	25	25	25	0	25	25	0	5
Week 4	30	30	30	0	30	30	0	5

Nathan's High Fitness Level Swimming Prescription

	Minutes per Day							Times per Week
	Mon.	Tues.	Wed.	Thurs.	Fri.	Sat.	Sun.	
Week 1	30	30	0	30	30	0	30	5
Week 2	35	35	0	35	35	0	35	5
Week 3	40	40	0	40	40	0	40	5
Week 4	45	0	45	0	45	0	45	4

Step 5. Start Slowly

Your initial experiences with exercising should be enjoyable, refreshing, and not too demanding either in terms of time or physical exertion. We recommend consistency and moderation. When you're starting out, remember that slow and steady wins the race. This gradual approach will help you to cultivate a positive attitude and enhance the likelihood of your maintaining it. As your fitness level improves, you can safely increase the duration and intensity of your workout, always maintaining a comfortable level of exertion.

Step 6. Identify Mental Barriers to Exercise

Even if you know that you need to become more physically active, it may be difficult for you to get started. In fact, you may not be aware of all your reasons for not exercising. So before you set up your own personal exercise prescription, review your ideas and feelings about exercise. Make a list of all the mental barriers that could keep you from exercising.

For example, you might feel embarrassed about being overweight and ashamed of the way you look in shorts or sweatpants. Maybe you don't like to perspire, or you think that other people find the odor of perspiration repulsive. Perhaps you believe that the way you exercise or move will be criticized by others, or if you are a woman, you may think athletic women are unfeminine. This, of course, is not true.

Some clients tell us that they simply don't like to exercise. If this is true for you, discover the reasons. Search your memory for bad experiences. Did you feel clumsy or embarrassed as a child when you were physically active? Remember that you're different now, and it's never too late to start something new.

Step 7. Identify Medical Barriers and Warning Signs

Medical barriers include a bad back or bad knees, arthritis, and cardio-vascular disease. These disabilities don't have to keep you from exercising, but they may signal that some modifications need to be made in your exercise program.

If you have medical barriers, a doctor's approval and professional guidance will be important in helping you modify exercises to compensate for specific problems and establish the kinds of exercises that are safe for you.

Even if you don't have any medical problems, you may have wondered how to "read" a body signal that something is wrong. For instance, you may believe that if you're exercising correctly, you're bound to be short of breath or in pain. No pain, no gain. Not true.

The most practical way to monitor yourself and avoid injury is to pay attention to how you feel. Listen to your body. If you feel that you are working too hard, slow down. If you are stretching and it hurts, then you are stretching too far. Back off or stop. You should not experience pain with exercise. If you experience pain in your chest or dramatic shortness of breath, stop. These are warnings signs that should be evaluated by a physician.

In the long run, if you overdo it, if you put too much stress and strain on your muscles and joints, you may limit the time, frequency, and fun of your exercise, and, ultimately, your chances of success.

Step 8. Be Patient with Yourself

When you begin your personal exercise program, remember that this will not be a "quick fix." Weight loss is the result of regular exercise, and any successful long-term weight management program must include an exercise program. Research shows that initially, people who only exercise and do not diet do not lose as much weight as dieters who do not exercise. Over the long haul, however, exercisers are more successful in terms of improved body composition and loss of fat than people who only diet. Remember, exercise will be easier, more fun, and more natural as it becomes a part of your lifestyle.

Strategies for Maintaining Your Fitness Program

Step 1. Build Movement into Every Part of Your Life

To stay active, review all the ways you can incorporate extra movement into day-to-day activities, such as gardening, playing with the dogs, running with the kids, walking to work or a store. When you can walk, do it!

Step 2. Make Appointments to Exercise

Sit down every Sunday evening and schedule your exercise for the week. Be specific. For instance, write down that you will walk for forty-five minutes—from 7:00 to 7:45—on Monday, Tuesday, Thursday, and Saturday mornings. Or make a date to swim from noon to 1 P.M. on Monday, Wednesday, and Friday, and to walk from 10 A.M. to 11 A.M. on Sunday. Give yourself options. You may want to use a stationary bike on rainy or snowy days so you won't have to contend with the elements. Remember that an exercise appointment is just as important as any other business commitment, so don't cancel or postpone it.

Step 3. Decide What to Do and Stick With It

Don't worry about whether you'll still be exercising next year or the year after. Break the overwhelming future down into this week and next week, or simply into one day—today. If it helps, say to yourself, "I don't know about the rest of my life, but I will do the exercise I planned for today and worry about tomorrow tomorrow."

Step 4. Keep an Exercise Log

In the exercise log, write down your exercise and the time you spent doing it. Note your level of exertion, how you felt before the session, and how you felt afterwards. Develop a code: G = good, T = tired, E = energetic, and so on. It will be interesting to see your mood improve following exercise and to record the increase in your energy, endurance, and stamina.

An exercise log will offer you objective, tangible feedback. When you feel discouraged, look at your record of exercise and give yourself credit for progress. (See sample exercise log, page 310.)

Step 5. Find Exercise Partners or Exercise Alone

If you enjoy company, or if you are a social exerciser, find a partner or join an exercise class. Working out with a friend or in the company of other people may help you maintain your commitment to your program. Good places to look for exercise company include your local Y, recreation department, health club, pool, or aerobics class.

If you prefer to exercise alone, walking or biking may be perfect for you. Be sure your exercise program isn't neglected because of work or family pressures. Remember, you owe yourself up to an hour a day. Stick with it; you'll be glad you did.

How to Start Again

No matter how committed you are, there may come a point when you stop exercising regularly. It may be for reasons as uninspiring as the flu or as satisfying as an all-expense-paid trip to South America or Europe. Whatever the interruption, it disrupts your routine and you stop exercising regularly.

If you're coming back from a vacation or a business trip, the break can provide you with the impetus to restructure and recommit to your exercise routines. Don't expect to begin again at full capacity. Gradually but steadily work your way back into your full routines.

If you're coming back from an illness such as bronchitis or the flu, make sure that you are completely recovered before you start to work out again, otherwise you may prolong the illness. Wait until all fever, aches, and other signs of the illness are gone. When you're feeling better, you can begin by doing stretch and strengthen routines at home to keep your muscles toned and flexible, but don't overdo it. When you're almost well again, take short walks around the block. Start slowly when you begin working out, and do so for short periods of time until you work your way back up to your previous level.

An injury can be treated a little differently from an illness in that alternative forms of exercise may be substituted. For instance:

- If you have a knee injury, swim.
- If you have a lower leg or foot injury, try stationary bicycling, swimming, or rowing.
- If you have an upper leg injury, swim, row, or take walks for moderate lengths of time.
- If you have lower back pain, swim or bicycle.
- If you have a shoulder or arm injury, walk or bicycle.

After an injury or an illness, resume your workouts at half the normal pace, distance, and intensity. Build up to your regular levels in measured steps.

Whenever you resume exercising after any break in your activity that lasts for more than a few days, extend and concentrate on the warm-up period, and give special attention to stretching. Focus on unused muscles.

Carefully monitor your post-exercise recovery. You will know if you're working too hard, of course, if you feel exhausted. Such signals as an unusually rapid post-exercise resting heart rate, a low energy level, or muscle fatigue that feels quantitatively different from your usual post-exercise feeling, are warnings to decrease the intensity and duration of exercise. If you listen to it, your body will let you know when it is ready to resume a normal workload.

As you develop your exercise habit, you'll be able to take an occasional break easily in stride. Just don't let an occasional break become a stopping point.

With time and practice, your exercise program will bring rewards. Most importantly, you'll feel better, and you'll see other specific health benefits and personal changes as well. For instance, studies have found that an hour of exercise a day enhances intellectual performance. What this means for you is that as you become more fit, you'll also have more energy, become more accomplished with less effort, and have more fun in the process.

How to Use the Exercise Log

The purpose of the exercise log is to record and track your exercise activity. It will serve as a tangible chronicle of your efforts.

- Choose the aerobic exercise that best suits your lifestyle.
- Prescribe for yourself the proper amount of exercise based on your fitness level and experience. Consult the Exercise Progression Chart provided on page 301.
- Plan your exercise sessions for the week by making appointments with yourself. Use an engagement calendar or diary.
- When you finish each exercise session, record it in the weekly exercise log. Record the date, the time of day, the activity performed, the duration of time in minutes, and your comments on the exercise session. Be creative with your comments because they may contain future motivational factors for you. For example, you may feel "overwhelmed" at the end of an exercise session. This is a good signal to back off and check your exercise intensity level. If you are just starting or restarting your exercise program, you might want to record your exercise intensity level (target heart rate or ratings of perceived exertion) until you are comfortable with your level of exertion. You may want to record other pertinent information such as temperature and humidity or whether the pool was crowded. Use this section to help assess your exercise feelings and behaviors so that your exercise becomes a positive experience.

Exercise Log

Date	Time	Activity	Duration	Comments
MONDAY DATE:				
TUESDAY DATE:				
WEDNESDAY DATE:				
THURSDAY DATE:				
FRIDAY DATE:				
SATURDAY DATE:				
SUNDAY DATE:				

10

DFC Exercises

Creating an exercise habit takes time. You may be someone who has always said that when it comes to exercise, you'd rather do it sitting down. Even if your mind hasn't fully accepted the need for regular exercise, your body longs for it and will respond once you begin. Think of exercise as a morning shower. Sometimes you don't want to take a shower. It's a hassle, but you do it anyway. Sometimes you love the feel of the hot water, and other times you just do it and don't think about it. In the same way, exercise will become a habit. You'll feel the benefits. A shower gets you clean, but exercise will give you even more profound results.

Remember to Practice All Components of Physical Fitness

Remember that your muscles and tendons need to be stretched and warmed up to prepare them for the main conditioning phase of your workout. As we've said, usually a slow form of your aerobic exercise is an effective warm-up. Before the main conditioning phase of swimming, for instance, do warm-up laps slowly for five to ten minutes. If you are doing aerobics or fast walking, begin with five to ten minutes in a slow form. Often, when you are warming up, beginning to sweat is a good signal that you are ready to begin your main conditioning phase. Afterwards, don't forget the importance of cooling down and stretching.

Let's review the components of a good workout.

Warm-up
• Prepare your body for the upcoming workout.
• Reduce chances of injury.

- Stimulate the body progressively and moderately.
- Increase the blood flow to your working muscles.
- Increase your body temperature.
- Stretch appropriate muscles and tendons.

Aerobic, or Main Conditioning Phase
- Begin after a sufficient warm-up.
- Make sure muscles are warm.
- Work out at a comfortable intensity—between levels 11 and 15 on the perceived exertion scale, or at your target heart rate (see pages 293 and 292).
- Maintain a comfortable but vigorous pace for a minimum of twenty to thirty minutes when you are doing regular aerobic activities such as walking, swimming, cycling, jogging, dancing, or rowing.

Cool-Down
- Taper off for five to ten minutes after the completion of the main workout.
- Continue the main conditioning activity at a lowered intensity. Do not stop abruptly.
- Stretch for maintaining or even improving flexibility.

DFC Stretch and Strengthen Routines

The DFC stretch and strengthen routines that follow are part of a balanced physical fitness program. These routines are not aerobic, but are designed to tone and condition your body.

As you'll recall, the components of physical fitness are flexibility, muscular strength, muscular endurance, and aerobic fitness. While the primary focus of your aerobic activity is to increase and maintain aerobic fitness, the primary focus of these DFC stretch and strengthen routines is to increase or maintain flexibility, muscular strength, and endurance.

Most of your fitness concerns will be addressed by the aerobic activity that you pursue. If you're swimming, for instance, obviously you're going to stretch and strengthen a lot of muscle groups because so many are involved in that particular exercise. But, at the same time, your shoulder muscles might be tight at the end of the swim. If you're riding a bicycle, your leg muscles are going to get a good workout because they're the primary muscle group involved. However, you might also want to help tone and stretch your chest, neck, and arm muscles.

Just as you don't drink only milk, you shouldn't do only one exercise. Your body, like your life, needs variety. That's why we encourage you to do the stretch and strengthen routines on a regular basis as a way of focusing on those areas that your aerobic exercise might miss, as well as providing you with a balanced program.

This routine won't get rid of inches or fat, but it will firm up underlying muscles and produce visible and positive differences in your posture, body tone, flexibility, and range of motion.

When to Use the DFC Stretch and Strengthen Routines

Plan to do these routines when it suits you. The long routine takes approximately twenty to thirty minutes and can be done on its own at any time of day. You may choose to do it every day or every other day. The short routine, which takes five to ten minutes, can be done when time does not allow for a more complete routine.

Some DFC graduates, like Mark Loomis and Louise Borngard, do the long stretch and strengthen routine first thing every morning. They don't feel right unless they start their day by getting in touch with their bodies.

John Larsen, on the other hand, does the short routine right before lunch. On the days he doesn't play squash after work, he does the long routine to help him loosen up and enjoy his evening. Rita Caparelli says she likes to do the short stretch and strengthen routine after her walk. On the days she doesn't walk, she does the long routine because it helps her unwind and feel as if her body is in harmony.

Remember, there are no hard-and-fast rules. Your decision about when to do the stretch and strengthen routines should be based on your own time clock and lifestyle. Do, however, try to do some abdominal strengthening and some stretching of your leg and arm muscles every day. If you have been sitting at a desk, or working intensely, get up and stretch your hamstrings, your shoulders, your neck, and your lower back. You may avoid many years of lower back pain by taking just five to ten minutes a day to strengthen your abdominal muscles and stretch your back and legs. If you have strong abdominal muscles and if your legs are limber, you may save yourself hours of fatigue and pain.

The short routine can be helpful at the beginning of a warm-up if your muscles are tight, but it is particularly effective as part of your cool-down, when your muscles are still warm.

Tips for Stretching and Strengthening

Don't
- Force a stretch.
- Bounce.
- Rush.
- Compare yourself to others.
- Lock your knees.
- Hold your breath.

Do
- Work at a deliberate pace.
- Exercise correctly and comfortably.
- Give priority to form and technique.
- Listen to your body and work at your own pace.
- Stretch within your limits.
- Remember that most gains in stretching come after exercise when your muscles are warm.
- Stretch whenever you feel like it.
- Take charge of your body.
- Be careful if you have a history of back problems.
- Remember that relaxation and regularity are the keys to effective stretching.
- Concentrate on the muscles that you're stretching.
- Allow an adequate amount of time between each repetition of each stretch.
- Breathe comfortably.

Stretch and Strengthen Routines Long Version (20–30 minutes)
(pages 316–33)

Standing

1. Marching in Place (1–3 minutes)
2. Arm Circles

3. Shoulder Stretch
4. Half-Squats
5. Standing Thigh Stretch
6. Heel Raisers
7. Calf Stretch

Sitting

8. Seated Hamstrings Stretch
9. Seated Groin Stretch

Lying Down

10. Pelvic Tilt
11. Single Knee Pulls
12. Double Knee Pulls
13. Modified Sit-Ups
14. Full Stretch and Reach
15. Modified Push-Ups

Standing

16. Triceps Stretch
17. Shoulder Stretch
18. Neck Stretch

Short Version (5–10 minutes)
(pages 334–36)

1. Seated Hamstrings Stretch
2. Double Knee Pulls
3. Full Stretch and Reach
4. Standing Thigh Stretch
5. Calf Stretch
6. Shoulder Stretch

Do any additional stretches on muscle groups that are tight.

Long Version

1. Marching in Place

March in place by gently lifting your knees. Swing your arms, keeping your hands relaxed and fingers cupped. Do not clench your fingers or make a tight fist. Continue at a comfortable pace for 1 to 3 minutes.

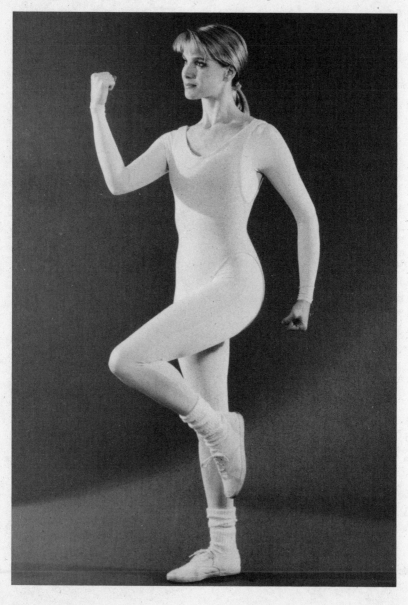

2. Arm Circles

Position:
Stand comfortably with your chin and jaw relaxed. Extend your arms to the sides at shoulder height, palms facing down.

Action:
Slowly circle arms forward in ten-inch circles.

Repetitions:
Circle 10–50 times forward, then 10–50 times backward.

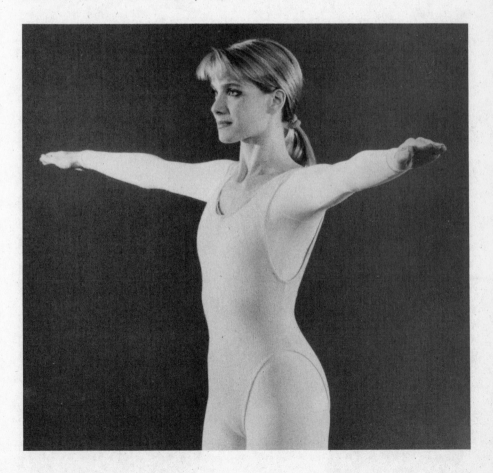

3. Shoulder Stretch

Position:
Stand with feet shoulder-width apart. Your knees should be slightly bent and relaxed.

Action:
Extend arms behind your back and grab one wrist at waist level. While maintaining an erect posture, gently lift your arms upward until you feel a mild stretch in your arms, shoulders, and upper back. Keep your legs flexed and DO NOT lean forward. Look straight ahead. Hold for 10–15 seconds.

Repetitions:
Grab your other wrist and repeat the action 2 to 3 times.

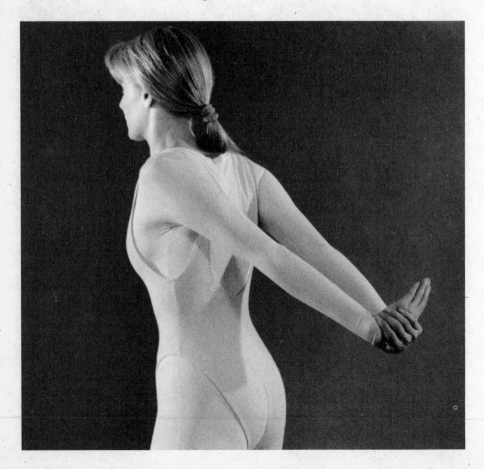

4. Half-Squats

Position:
Stand with knees slightly bent and feet hip-distance apart. Put hands on hips.

Action:
Squat or bend your knees slowly to a count of 5, contracting your thigh muscles and keeping your back straight. Pause for a count of 3–5. Do not let your heels come off the floor. Keep your head, shoulders, hips, and ankles in the same vertical plane. Slowly return to starting position.

Repetitions:
Repeat 3 to 5 times.

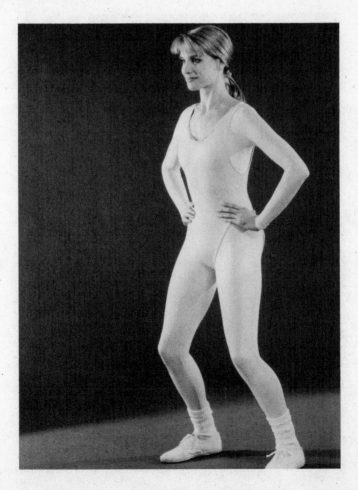

5. Standing Thigh Stretch*

Position:
Stand facing the wall, with your right hand resting on the wall for support.

Action:
Bend your left leg behind you. Slowly reach back with your left hand and grasp your left ankle. Gently pull your left ankle directly behind your left buttock. DO NOT force your heel toward your buttock. Hold 10–15 seconds. Carefully release ankle and slowly place foot on floor.

Repetitions:
Repeat action with right leg. Do each leg 2–3 times.

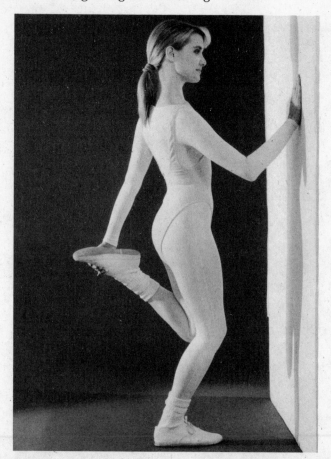

*DO NOT do this routine if it causes any discomfort in your knees or back.

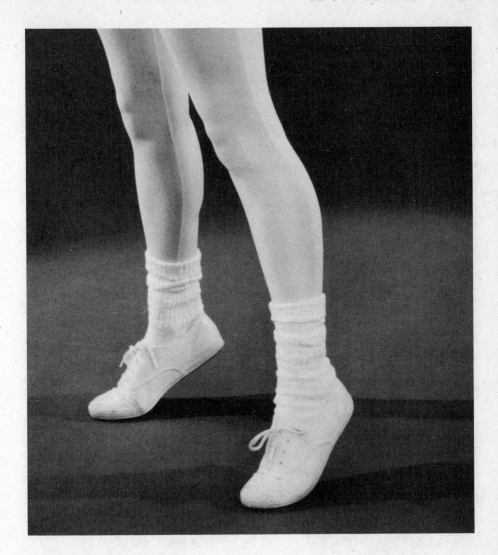

6. Heel Raisers

Position:
Stand with feet hip-distance apart.

Action:
Raise up onto your toes to a count of 2. Hold for 5 seconds. Slowly lower your heels to a count of 2.

Repetitions:
Repeat 10–15 times.

7. Calf Stretch

Position:

Stand arm's length away from wall. Place hands on wall at shoulder height. Do not look down.

Action:

Place your right leg behind you. Keeping the right leg straight and toes pointed toward the wall, press your right heel into the floor. Bend the left leg slightly. Slowly move your hips toward the wall keeping your weight on top of your hips, creating a stretch in the right calf muscle. Do not stretch to cause pain. Hold this position for 10–15 seconds. Return to standing position.

Repetitions:

Repeat action with left leg. Do each leg 2–3 times.

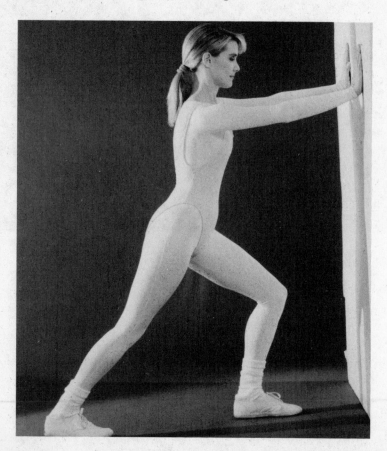

8. Seated Hamstrings Stretch

Position:
Sit with your legs straight in front of you with thighs relaxed, and with toes pointed up and relaxed.

Action:
Carefully reach for the position on the legs that gives you a mild stretch on the back of the legs. Keep your legs straight and relaxed. Keep your back straight and your head up. Look straight ahead. Hold for 10–15 seconds.

Repetitions:
Repeat 2–3 times.

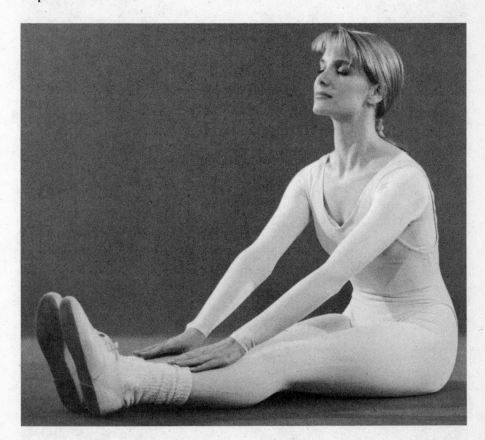

9. Seated Groin Stretch

Position:

Sit with the soles of your feet together at a comfortable distance from your torso, with your knees relaxed and out to the side.

Action:

With your hands holding both feet, pull your feet toward your groin. Keep your back straight and look forward. Hold for 10–15 seconds.

Repetitions:

Repeat 2–3 times.

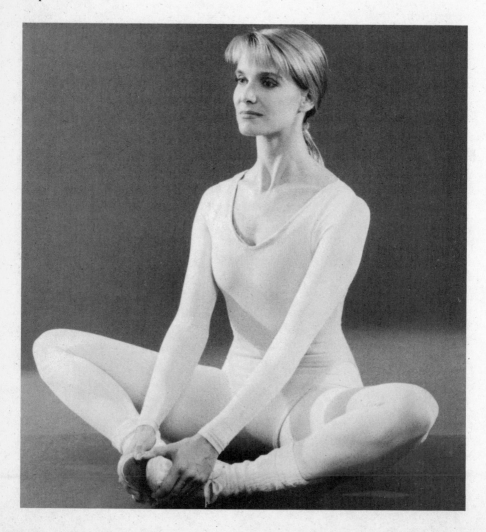

10. Pelvic Tilt

Position:
Lie on your back, knees bent and feet flat on the floor. Put your hands on your hips.

Action:
Contract your abdominal muscles. Press and flatten your lower back into the floor. Do not hold your breath. Hold the contraction for a count of 5, then relax.

Repetitions:
Repeat 5 times.

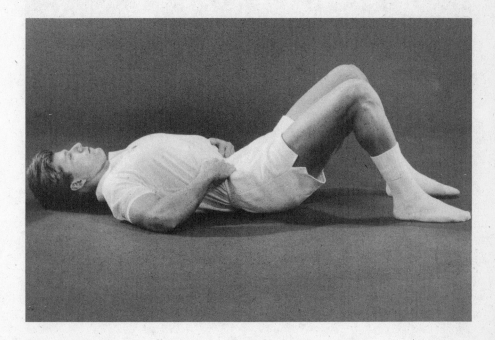

11. Single Knee Pulls

Position:
Lie on your back, knees bent and feet flat on the floor.

Action:
With both hands behind your right knee, gently pull leg toward you. Hold for 10–15 seconds. Release.

Repetitions:
Repeat with left leg. Do each leg 2–3 times.

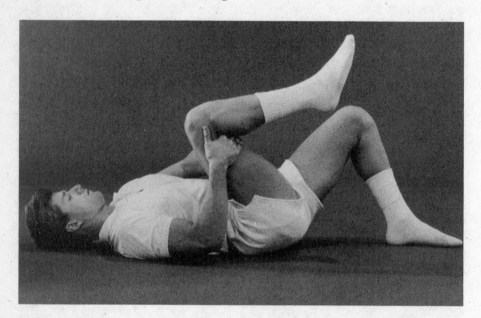

12. Double Knee Pulls

Position:
Lie on your back, knees bent and feet flat on the floor.

Action:
Holding knees with both hands, pull both legs toward chest. Hold for 10–15 seconds. Release.

Repetitions:
Repeat 2–3 times.

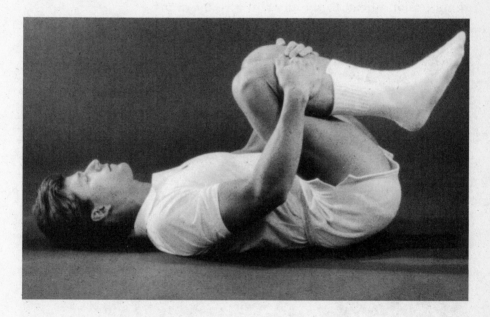

13. Modified Sit-Ups

Position:
Lie on your back, knees bent. Feet are flat on the floor, hip-distance apart.

Action:
With straight arms, reach between your knees, lifting your shoulders and head slightly off the floor, using *only* the abdominal muscles to do so. DO NOT use the neck and shoulder muscles. Do not lift the shoulders higher than a 45-degree angle. Do not hold your breath. Slowly lower shoulders and head to the floor to a count of 5.*

Repetitions:
Reach between the knees 5–25 times.

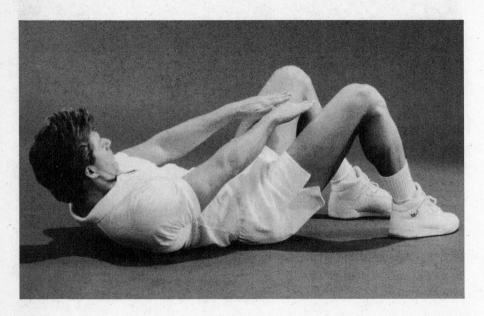

*This may be a difficult exercise at first, so you may want to do only the Pelvic Tilt (page 325) until your abdominals are strong enough to do this modified sit-up.

14. Full Stretch and Reach

Position:
Lie on your back, arms extended above your head on the floor and legs straight.

Action:
Reach with arms and legs in opposite directions. Keep your back straight. Hold to a count of 5. Do not hold your breath.

Repetitions:
Repeat 2–3 times.

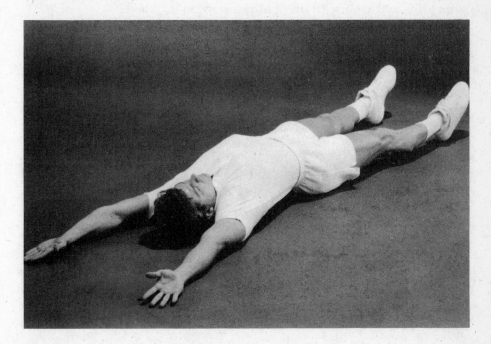

15. Modified Push-Ups

Position:
Face down on floor, support yourself with knees and feet 2–4 inches apart. Your hands should be shoulder-width apart. Your arms, too, should be relaxed, not locked. Create a slight "V" shape with your buttocks elevated. Hold your stomach in, and keep your head in normal alignment with your body.*

Action:
Slowly lower body, bending elbows, until face and chest are near the floor. Maintain a slight "V" position with your body. Slowly straighten your arms and return to original position.

Repetitions:
Repeat 5–25 times.

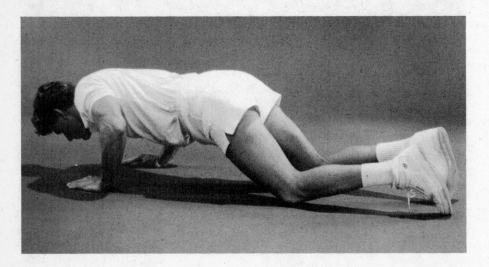

*Do not be discouraged; this may be a difficult strengthening exercise initially.

16. Triceps Stretch

Position:
Stand with your feet parallel and shoulder-width apart, knees and shoulders relaxed. Look straight ahead.

Action:
Reach with your right hand over and behind your head toward your upper back. Reach across with your left hand and hold your right elbow. Gently pull the right elbow inward as far as you comfortably can, pushing your right hand down your spine. Hold 10–15 seconds.

Repetitions:
Repeat with your other arm. Do each arm 2–3 times.

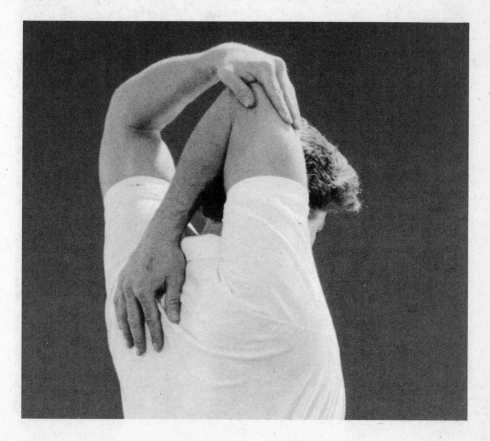

17. Shoulder Stretch

Position:
Stand with your feet parallel and shoulder-width apart. Keep your knees slightly bent and relaxed.

Action:
With your left hand, pull your right elbow across your chest toward your left shoulder. Hold 10–15 seconds.

Repetitions:
Repeat with your other arm. Do each arm 2–3 times.

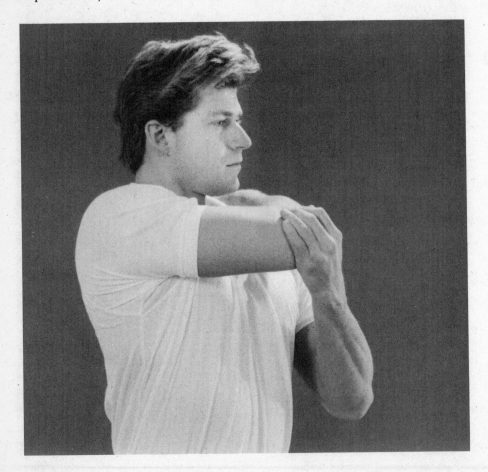

18. Neck Stretch

Position:
Stand with your arms at your sides, looking straight ahead.

Action:
Tuck your chin toward your chest so that you feel a mild stretch in the back of your neck. Hold this position for 10–15 seconds. Slowly raise your head.

Slowly bring your right ear toward your right shoulder, stretching the neck muscles as you do so. Hold for 10–15 seconds. Slowly raise your head to its upright position. Repeat on the left side and hold for 10–15 seconds. Again, slowly raise your head.

Repetitions
Repeat 2–3 times.

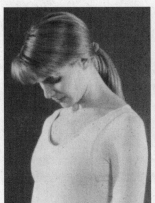 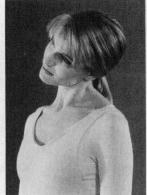 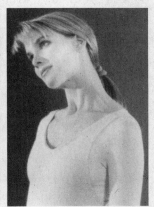

Short Version

1. Seated Hamstrings Stretch

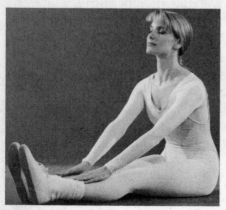

Position:
Sit with your legs straight in front of you with thighs relaxed, and with toes pointed up and relaxed.

Action:
Carefully reach for the position on the legs that gives you a mild stretch on the back of the legs. Keep your legs straight and relaxed. Keep your back straight and your head up. Look straight ahead. Hold for 10–15 seconds.

Repetitions:
Repeat 2–3 times.

2. Double Knee Pulls

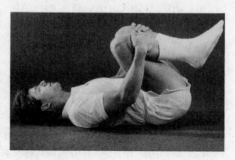

Position:
Lie on your back, knees bent and feet flat on the floor.

Action:
Holding knees with both hands, pull both legs toward chest. Hold for 10–15 seconds. Release.

Repetitions:
Repeat 2–3 times.

3. Full Stretch and Reach

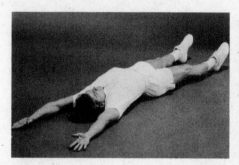

Position:
Lie on your back, arms extended above your head on the floor and legs straight.

Action:
Reach with arms and legs in opposite directions. Keep your back straight. Hold to a count of 5. Do not hold your breath.

Repetitions:
Repeat 2–3 times.

4. Standing Thigh Stretch

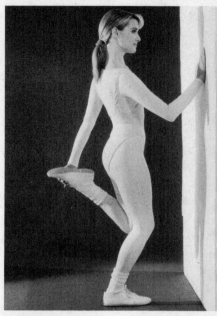

Position:
Stand facing the wall, with your right hand resting on the wall for support.

Action:
Bend your left leg behind you. Slowly reach back with your left hand and grasp your left ankle. Gently pull your left ankle directly behind your left buttock. DO NOT force your heel toward your buttock. Hold 10–15 seconds. Carefully release ankle and slowly place foot on floor.

Repetitions:
Repeat action with right leg. Do each leg 2–3 times.

5. Calf Stretch

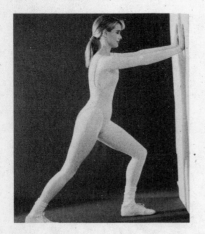

Position:
Stand arm's length away from wall. Place hands on wall at shoulder height. Do not look down.

Action:
Place your right leg behind you. Keeping the right leg straight and toes pointed toward the wall, press your right heel into the floor. Bend the left leg slightly. Slowly move your hips toward the wall keeping your weight on top of your hips, creating a stretch in the right calf muscle. Do not stretch to cause pain. Hold this position for 10–15 seconds. Return to standing position.

Repetitions:
Repeat action with left leg. Do each leg 2–3 times.

6. Shoulder Stretch

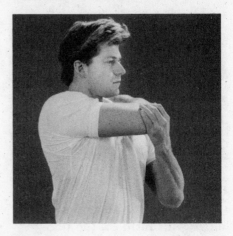

Position:
Stand with your feet parallel and shoulder-width apart. Keep your knees slightly bent and relaxed.

Action:
With your left hand, pull your right elbow across your chest toward your left shoulder. Hold 10–15 seconds.

Repetitions:
Repeat with your other arm. Do each arm 2–3 times.

How to Be a Success Forever

11

Recognizing Your Emotional Eating Patterns

While everyone occasionally eats for emotional reasons rather than for physiological needs, many overweight people rely on eating as a way of coping with their feelings. If you can identify eating patterns that you have developed in response to emotions rather than physiological hunger, you eventually will be able to modify those patterns and manage your weight more effectively.

There are many reasons why people use food for coping with strong feelings. When we were babies, food meant love. It was associated with being held, fed, and nurtured by our mothers. Thus, we find food soothing, and eating sometimes tends to give us a feeling of internal fullness when we feel emotionally empty.

Eating is also an easy outlet for emotions because food is so readily available. You don't have to call up and make a date with it if you are lonely. Food doesn't talk back to you if you are frustrated. It can't reject you, and unlike friends, it's always close at hand when you feel that you need it. Food serves other purposes as well. Foods high in sugar content provide a feeling of instant energy when you need a pick-me-up. Heavy foods, dairy products, and large portions can be relaxing. They can make you sleepy, or numb your feelings. Eating is also an activity that fills empty hours. The time you spend purchasing, preparing, and consuming food can distract you from problems and unwanted feelings.

Many people eat because they have difficulty admitting that they are angry or frustrated, or they have difficulty expressing those feelings. Other emotions expressed through eating occur when you are tense, stressed, or anxious (eating calms you down); disappointed, rejected, hurt, or sad (it soothes you); sexually unfulfilled (it provides feelings of gratification); happy (it helps you celebrate).

Chronic Problems of Emotional Eating

If you habitually overeat, emotional eating may be part of your lifestyle and not necessarily related to events on a day-to-day basis. You may have started overeating in this way when you were a child and continued the habit into adulthood. Linda Green, a DFC client, recalls that her overeating began at age nine, during her parents' divorce. Another client, John Garber, remembers how much pleasure he received from food as a youngster because mealtimes were the only times his father paid attention to him. Stephanie Wolfson says that her chronic problems with food began when she was a teenager trying to cope with her mother's alcoholism and their chaotic, disrupted household.

A crisis in your adult life, such as the death of a loved one, can also trigger overeating that turns into a chronic problem. Dottie Mason had never been overweight until after her husband of eighteen years had a heart attack and died. Dottie wasn't even aware that she ate for company during the long evenings that haunted her the first two years after her husband's death, but she did. She gained weight slowly, and the habit of eating from seven o'clock in the evening until she went to be bed became highly ingrained. Five years later, she was still continuing this pattern, and she didn't even realize she was an emotional eater. She'd simply developed a pattern of overindulgence. When Dottie came to the DFC, she was forty pounds overweight.

Ray West began overeating after five years of marriage. When he looked back over his eating patterns, Ray recognized, with the help of his therapist, that he had begun to eat as a way of distracting himself from the feelings of frustration he had about his marriage. He remembered that at one crisis point, he had talked to his wife about his dissatisfaction and had asked her to go into counseling with him, but she had refused. She said he was the one at fault for any problems in their marriage. She criticized him, and told him that he was the one who needed help. Ray felt frustrated, hurt, and confused, and had turned to food to distract him from those feelings. Fortunately, he now understands that he had been eating for emotional reasons.

We have found that many other people involved in unhappy and destructive relationships turn to food as a way of coping with dissatisfaction, tension, anxiety, anger, loneliness, or depression. Often they feel hopeless about changing the relationship. Sometimes they want out of the relationship, but they're scared and unsure about leaving. They eat to avoid their unhappiness and their frustrations with the situation.

A similar chronic pattern can occur if your job is unpleasant and frustrating. You may want out, yet be afraid of the consequences of leaving. You may want to change jobs, yet feel sure that no one would hire you because you're overweight. In cases like these, you may eat as a way to numb your feelings and mask your problems. With chronic emotional eating, you may not even be aware of having feelings. Eating takes the place of feelings and becomes a highly ingrained habit.

Acute Problems of Emotional Eating

With acute emotional eating, you don't have a day-to-day habit of coping with your feelings by eating, but you experience episodes of eating to soothe yourself. Your normal routine might be to eat three meals a day without snacking, but you may reach for food when you experience particularly strong feelings. When you feel exhausted at two o'clock in the afternoon, when your boss gives you an unrealistic deadline, or when you've had a disagreement with a co-worker, you may find yourself at the vending machine buying potato chips or candy bars.

A DFC client, Sarah Johnson, told us about one particular episode of acute emotional eating that she'd experienced. "I was looking forward to a three-day weekend with my husband," she said, "and I was all excited planning for it, thinking it was going to be really romantic and wonderful. We were going to a beautiful spot in the Poconos where we had wanted to go on our honeymoon. But when the weekend actually came, my husband was tired. He didn't want to play tennis and he didn't want to swim. The first night we didn't even make love, and on Saturday afternoon, he wanted to stay in the room to watch a baseball game on TV. I was so upset! I probably ate and drank 15,000 calories that weekend!"

A common source of acute emotional overeating occurs in response to a weigh-in. If the scale doesn't go down as you expected it to, you may turn to food as a way to deal with your disappointment. You feel frustrated because all of your efforts appear unrewarded. So you let go of your resolve and take larger portions at mealtime or eat higher calorie snacks. You know that overeating won't help you lose weight, but you feel justified in doing so because the scale treated you so unfairly.

It may be that when a crisis occurs to someone who is close to you, you deal with your anxiety over the event—and your inability to "resolve" it—by eating. Kate Evans told us that when her twenty-two-year-old daughter admitted that she had been using cocaine, Kate got so upset that she immediately went to the refrigerator and ate all the leftovers she could find. She felt so worried and tense—and so unsure of how she could help—that she turned to food as a way of trying to calm herself down.

Patterns of Emotional Eating

From the self-assessment of your emotional eating patterns and your nutritional habits (see chapter 3), you have already learned something about the ways you express your emotions through food. Our DFC clients have helped us to identify additional patterns of emotional eating, which we describe below. As you read through these descriptions, ask yourself if any of these patterns apply to you. Remember that none of these patterns are "bad." They are simply descriptions of observable behavior that lead to overeating. If the patterns can be identified, they can be successfully addressed.

The Driven Eater

You *have* to eat even when you're not hungry. You feel controlled by food. While you may be unaware of it, many times you use eating to remove the focus from troublesome feelings such as anger, sadness, loneliness, or rejection. You focus your attention away from the situation and on to the food. You may feel that you are "stuffing down the feeling" or "swallowing your anger" along with the food. This often leads to feelings of shame and depression. If this is your pattern of eating, food overpowers many aspects of your life.

The Planner and Organizer

You may be a person who plans and organizes the consumption of large quantities of food. You look forward to your eating event in almost the same way someone else might plan and look forward to a date. If you are one of the many people who follow this pattern, you often are very ritualistic and perhaps secretive when you do this. You may have fantasies about what to eat, where to get it, or how to prepare it. By becoming so absorbed in making detailed plans for your binge, you are able to avoid other feelings. Often these plans lead to an uncontrollably large eating binge in which you eat and eat and don't stop until you're in pain or until someone catches you in the act. This binge often occurs at night.

The Constant Eater

Many people maintain a continuous pattern of low-grade eating. If you are one of these people, you eat as an activity. You frequently take food breaks. Eating also accompanies many of your activities throughout the day, and you probably use food as a supplement to nearly everything you do. You often carry food with you "just in case" you feel hungry. This pattern is a preventive method that you use to avoid feeling or dealing with emotions, particularly intense emotions.

The Closet Eater

If this is your pattern of eating, you consume normal amounts of appropriate foods in the presence of others. However, when you are alone, you give yourself permission to "sneak eat" your favorite high-calorie items. Often this eating takes place late at night, when others have gone to bed, or during the day, when you are all alone. You feel that you are doing something wrong, but you enjoy it anyway, and perhaps enjoy it even more because there's a delightfully "sinful" aspect to it. Additionally, no one is around to judge or criticize you. Often closet eaters feel that their loved ones are overly critical of their weight, their eating habits, or their actions in general. They may eat out of a sense of revenge.

The All-or-Nothing Eater

A great deal of the time, you eat well-balanced, low-calorie meals. You feel "in control" when you are eating this way, and you see yourself as "good." At other times, you have an irresistible urge to eat whatever you want, when you want it. You set no limits: you may consume three candy bars, a pint of ice cream, some cookies, and a five-course dinner. At these times, you feel "out of control" and even helpless about your eating. You see yourself as "bad." All-or-nothing eaters are usually perfectionists who are unable to allow themselves a normal range of experiences and emotions. If this is true for you, you find certain emotions unacceptable. Making mistakes and being imperfect are also unacceptable to you. Eating is your emotional release and may be the only area in which you let yourself go. Even your food intake is perfectionistic: it's feast or famine.

With all of these patterns, eating has become a coping mechanism—a defense that works in the short run, but is unhelpful and destructive in the long run. We all need coping mechanisms; they're a natural part of life, and in that sense, emotional eating is like any other defense. Denial when a loved one dies, for instance, can be helpful on a short-term basis for coping with the pain. If after five years, however, you are still wishing that he or she would come back to life, then the denial is no longer helping you. It's getting in the way of your dealing with death and getting on with life.

The same is true for you if you eat when you're lonely, bored, depressed, guilty, angry, or anxious. If you eat when you need nurturance, love, or intimacy, you are using food as a buffer between you and your feelings. Eating takes the place of expressing your feelings or taking action in your life.

Food may seem to have magical control over you, but you are the person who has given food that power. You need to identify your emotional eating and those aspects of your life that are unfulfilled. You need to stop the avoidance process you've been using and allow yourself to see what other issues may exist in your life, as well as your options for dealing with them.

Strategies for Dealing with Emotional Eating

The following strategies may help you to identify your tendencies toward emotional eating, increase your awareness of your feelings, accept and understand various emotions, and deal with them in other, more constructive ways.

Step 1. Identify Emotional Eating Tendencies

In chapter 3 you assessed your emotional eating patterns. Now review your answers and list your areas of difficulty. Write down how you feel about your problems, and what you do when you're faced with them. Nina Halloran made the following list based on her answers to some of the questions in chapter 3. You can use it as a guideline for your own list.

I Eat When Feeling Hurt or Disappointed.

"My feelings are easily injured. I like to please everyone. When I sense that my friends are disappointed in me, I feel hurt and ashamed. I turn to food for comfort. It makes me feel better for a little while and then I forget the hurt."

I Eat When Feeling Bored or Lonely.

"When my husband is off with his friends playing golf and the children are out playing with their friends, I feel very lonely and I eat. I'm not used to having time on my hands. I feel selfish using my free time to read novels when there's always work to be done. I guess I allow myself to eat to fill the time and the emptiness I'm feeling. Maybe I would be better off reading!"

I Eat for Relaxation.

"There's nothing better than some potato chips and dip to make me feel relaxed at the end of a hard day. Is there another way to relax?"

I Eat in Secret and Then Feel Guilty.

"I guess I am a 'closet eater'! I would feel ashamed and embarrassed eating fattening foods in front of other people. What would they think?"

I Eat after a Conflict.

"I always grab something to eat whenever my husband and I have quarreled or even disagreed over something minor. I hate conflict, and I'll do almost anything to avoid it."

I Eat Out of Control.

"I guess I am a 'driven eater.' I do feel helpless about food a lot of the time. Once I start eating, I can't stop. Is it hunger or is it something else?"

Step 2. Keep a Record of Your Eating Episodes

Keep track of times when you eat in response to various emotional states. The following chart is an excerpt from the one-week diary Nina Halloran kept on her eating episodes. We recommend that you use a large notebook and organize it similarly.

It's easy to see that in several instances, Nina is an emotional eater. Her morning tea and cookies are probably used for relaxation after a

Nina's Record of Emotional Eating

Time	Food	Portion	Hungry?	Satisfied?	Situation	Emotions
6:30 A.M.	bagel, cream cheese	1 1 oz.	slight	little	rushing to get Jay & kids off to school	upset, hassled, frustrated
9 A.M.	tea & cookies	6 cookies	not sure	very	Alone at last!	relaxed
12:30 P.M.	salad bar	average	moderately	very	lunch w/friends	sociable
8 P.M.	turkey breast, mashed potatoes, gravy, broccoli	large	famished	little	family dinner	troubled, listening to Jay's problems & anxious, need to go to the store!
11:30 P.M.	ice cream	huge/kept going back for more!	unsure	very	alone	disappointed, lonely; Jay asleep before I got back from store.

346

difficult time getting her children and husband ready for the day. She receives very little satisfaction from breakfast, probably because she is attending to the needs of others, but feels very happy with her solitary eating. On the day recorded here, we see that she felt lonely and disappointed that her husband had gone to sleep without her, so eating a huge portion of ice cream at bedtime was her way of comforting herself. Unfortunately, eating was Nina's habitual way of trying to make herself feel good.

After keeping a record for a week, go over it carefully and look for patterns of emotional eating. Does your eating change on a day-to-day basis depending on your mood or the type of day you are having? Think about it: Are you eating as a release of tension or to soothe yourself? Do you eat large portions or high-calorie foods when you are experiencing a strong emotion?

Step 3. Observe Your Feelings

Often difficulties with emotional eating arise because of a lack of self-observation. A feeling may trigger an eating response so quickly that you eat even before realizing that you feel angry, sad, lonely, or anxious about something. The association between the feeling and the behavior (eating) is so strong, you may not realize that you have used food to cover up or avoid dealing with the feeling. If you habitually overeat, you may be numb about many of your feelings.

In order to break the association between uncomfortable feelings and eating, you first need to become more aware of your feelings. Some of the following techniques may help.

Pay attention to how your body reacts in emotionally stressful situations. If you are overweight, you may dislike your body so much that you've lost touch with it. It's important to get back in contact with your body because feelings are experienced *within* the body. If you have just had an encounter at work or at home that upsets you, pay attention. Do you have a tight stomach? This may be a sign of anxiety or fear. Is your jaw clenched? This may be a sign of anger. Do you have a lump in your throat? This may be bottled up feelings of sadness, hurt, or anger.

Talk about your feelings, using such words as *sad, mad, glad, scared, confused.* Are these emotions "positive" or "negative" to you? Do you think it's okay to have these feelings?

Take your "emotional temperature." If you are out of touch with your feelings, put a red dot on your watch, and every time you look at it, you'll know that it's time to assess your mood. It might be useful to record your feelings in a small notebook. Write down what you're noticing at the moment—whether it's anger, anxiety, sadness, loneliness, depression, confusion, comfortableness, calmness, or happiness.

Notice your feelings when you are overeating. Whenever you are eating between meals or to excess, ask yourself if you are hungry, or if you are responding to emotions.

Pay attention to other people's perceptions of you. If someone says that you seem irritable, fatigued, or depressed, don't immediately discount that impression; it may have some validity. If it confuses you, think about it later when you have time to be more objective.

To discover "negative" feelings in yourself, analyze and observe things you dislike about other people. Write down the names of six people you know fairly well. Next to each name, write down what you feel about them, including what you particularly dislike about their emotional responses. This exercise can help you to discover feelings that you value, don't value, or overlook in yourself. You can gain insight from your "outsight" and discover if you may be avoiding looking inward by focusing on other people. Sometimes you may discover that the qualities you particularly dislike in other people are actually qualities of your own.

Use bibliotherapy. In other words, read books! Today, a great number of self-help books are available, many of which deal with anger, assertiveness, interpersonal communication, and other emotional issues. They can be a wonderful resource. Often they give you "typical" situations and help you practice new approaches to dealing with old problems. Fiction and historical literature also describe people and how they deal with a variety of emotional conflicts in their lives.

Step 4. Acknowledge Your Feelings

It may be hard for you to acknowledge all of your feelings, especially if you were taught that certain feelings were "bad." For instance, you may have been taught the following:

"Don't have angry feelings. It's not polite to be angry. Rational human beings don't get angry."

"Don't have sad or hurt feelings. Don't feel sorry for yourself! You don't have any reason to be sad! You don't have anything to cry about! Boys and grown-ups don't cry!"

"Don't be lonely. You have no reason to be lonely! Go out and
make friends! Don't be self-indulgent."

"Don't have lustful or sexual feelings because they're 'naughty.' "

"Don't feel scared! Only wimps and cowards feel afraid of
anything!"

"Don't feel good about yourself. It's not okay to feel good about
yourself because that's vain, selfish, and conceited."

"Don't be an independent person. To win love, you need my
approval; you need to be dependent!"

The truth is, a wide range of emotions—including sadness, anger,
confusion, loneliness, fear, sexual excitement, vanity, and pride—are
quite normal. Acknowledging an angry feeling does not mean that you
would allow yourself to scream at everyone with whom you feel angry.

Starting today, give yourself permission to recognize a variety of feelings within yourself. You may find that you will be less judgmental of
others as you become less judging of yourself. If you feel that your
emotions are so intense or out of control that they have a deleterious
effect on your life, get professional help in addressing and solving these
problems.

Step 5. Plan Alternatives

Once you have identified your feelings and the eating response you have
to them, you can plan alternatives. The following list may be useful to
you, and you'll very likely be able to think up other options as well.

Instant diversions. Think of things you enjoy doing that are unrelated to
food—going to a movie, a museum, or a bookstore; shopping for household items or clothes; visiting a friend; going to the zoo or the library;
exploring a new part of town; going for a bike ride, a swim, or a walk;
reading a good book. You can do any or all of these immediate, noneat-
ing activities without any planning or previous notice. Make a list, and
post it by the refrigerator. When you get the urge to eat between meals,
look at your list and choose an activity. Then do it.

Relaxation. Find a quiet spot to rest, even if you only take five minutes
to do it. Shut the door, put your feet up, close your eyes, and relax.
Watch a fish tank, pray, or sit by the fireplace and watch the logs burning.

Sit in a chair with your legs elevated and a cool cloth on your face. Turn on music that you find relaxing. If you have more time, have a massage, sit in a whirlpool or a sauna. Learn the techniques of progressive muscle relaxation, and practice them instead of eating. You may also try yoga, hypnosis, or meditation. These relaxation activities are particularly helpful when you are tired, angry, or anxious.

Physical activity. Go for a brisk walk or swim, rearrange furniture, or hit some tennis or golf balls. You may want to plant flowers or a vegetable garden. Think about doing some of the things you pay other people to do, like mowing the lawn, raking leaves, or walking the dog. Physical activity burns calories, decreases boredom, curbs anger, and reduces physical, sexual, and mental tension.

New interests. If you eat because of boredom or loneliness, remember that it's never too late to learn new skills. Call the local parks and recreation center, the Y, or some other community center or adult school in your area for information about activities and classes. Try painting, take up golf or carpentry, take a flower-arranging class, or try your hand at photography. Learn to dance or to play a musical instrument. Go to a museum, a lecture, or a concert. Join a social club.

Social service activities. Many community service organizations need volunteer help. Conservation groups, political groups, social service agencies, groups working on problems of the homeless, environmental and animal protection associations, and many other organizations depend on volunteers to accomplish their tasks. Local hospitals, schools, and community organizations are often looking for people who are willing to contribute their time to tutoring, reading to the blind, visiting incapacitated or elderly people who need social contact, helping abandoned babies who need to be held and cuddled, becoming a Big Brother or Sister, or doing any number of other worthy projects. You have skills you can share that will benefit other people and make you feel good about yourself. Often when you become lonely or bored, you have lost a sense of your own power. These volunteer activities can stimulate good feelings about yourself and help you find fulfillment.

Now make a chart of your moods, your typical responses, and an activity that could interrupt the predictable cycle. Propose quick and easy solutions for yourself, such as walking around the block, window shopping, or buying yourself a book or a present. If it's not convenient to remove yourself from a situation, have a glass of diet soda, get up and comb your hair, or phone and talk to someone friendly as an alternative—anything to change the mood and make you feel good. The chart should look something like this:

Feeling	Situation	Typical Response	Proposed Alternative
Lonely	especially on weekends	I eat all weekend to keep from thinking about my ex-boyfriend	Do more socially; join a singles club; sign up for a bowling league; become more active in church or community activities
Bored	after work	I eat, grab anything!	Go for a walk or call a friend; go to museum; take up a new hobby
Anxious	usually late at night	I eat sweets	Self-hypnosis; hot bath with music; write in my journal
Angry	at my boss; at work	I smile, but inside, I am full of rage; I eat chocolate!	Take a 10-minute break; shut the door, turn on my radio, and relax

The most difficult task you face is to implement the changes you propose to break your habit of eating in response to emotions. Take one change at a time and implement it for one week. At the end of the week, evaluate what happened. If you were successful even some of the time, give yourself a nonfood reward—a new book, a new shirt, or flowers.

If you weren't successful, examine the situation. Was your standard unrealistic? Did you expect yourself to conquer long-standing feelings of loneliness by calling one friend at a time? You might need to modify your proposal and try it again. Take on the easier feelings first. Set your standards low and gradually increase them. When you are successful, you will feel more confident to tackle the difficult and more powerful feelings. Praise and reward yourself for the slightest improvements you make. Remember that the smallest improvements will accumulate and help you reach your goals.

Everyone experiences unpleasant or uncomfortable feelings. If your anxiety, loneliness, or anger occur with great intensity and high frequency and you can't seem to get a grip on them, you can always get help from a psychologist, a psychiatrist, a pastoral counselor, or a social worker. Each is trained to help people cope with the powerful feelings we all experience.

Remember that identifying emotional eating is the first step toward eating in a new and controlled way. You'll find that the strategies for changing your eating patterns will be successful if you keep working at them.

If the material in this chapter seems complex or new to you, read it again after a time of reflection. We've found that once our clients begin to implement strategies that address their emotional overeating, their understanding and coping ability expand in conjunction with their weight loss. We believe that the same will be true for you.

The next two chapters will add further practical insight into how to change destructive eating patterns by successfully restructuring your eating experience at home and at restaurants. You may be surprised to find that you can, in a very easy way, break down automatic associations with food that you have developed when you eat out or eat at home.

CHAPTER 12

Eating at Home: A Supportive Environment

Make Your Kitchen a Healthy Place to Be

Now that you know how to plan healthy, calorie-controlled meals, it's time to reorganize your kitchen to suit your new philosophy of eating.

Before getting down to business, think about the principles involved. In a supportive and controlled kitchen, you need to have supplies on hand only for those meals you have planned. You don't want a lot of high-calorie, high-fat temptations beckoning you during weak moments. You don't want food sitting out on a counter. The old adage "Out of sight, out of mind" is a good one to abide by when it comes to the food in your kitchen. Tempting and easily accessible food can too easily disappear into your mouth when you're not thinking.

Rearrange your kitchen when you are not rushed. Begin with the following suggestions *after* you've eaten a meal, when you are not hungry and therefore are more likely to get rid of unwanted and unnecessary foods.

Step 1: Get Rid of Tempting Foods

In the same way that you periodically go through your closets to get rid of clothes you don't wear anymore, go through your kitchen cupboards to get rid of unwanted and ultimately unflattering foods.

Don't eat the food as you remove it from your shelves. Instead, give away what you don't want or need. Churches, soup kitchens, homeless shelters, and the Salvation Army welcome boxes of cake mixes, peanuts, or other nonperishable food supplies. If you don't want to give away the food, throw it away.

Shelf by shelf, clean out your cupboards and get rid of all the food items that aren't part of your diet. What foods tempt you? Even if you're not eating them as you read these words, there are bound to be some items that tempt you at one time or another, whether it's Ritz crackers, chocolate chip cookies, Oreos, potato chips, peanuts, giant jars of peanut butter, or even unsalted sunflower seeds that can be eaten in an evening. As you go through your shelves, think about your menu plans. Think about the six food groups from which you're planning your meals. When you see food items that are not part of your plan, set them into a trash bag or box.

Do the same with the foods in your refrigerator and freezer, and don't be timid.

Step 2: Store Your Food for Success

Even when your kitchen is reorganized, bringing groceries home from a shopping trip provides a dangerous opportunity for nibbling. If you normally nibble while you put away groceries, it may make sense for you to sit down with a large glass of ice water or a diet drink *before* you put them away. This can help you to relax, review your plan, and dampen some "hunger pangs" before you attempt your task.

Put away all of your groceries; don't leave any of them sitting out. We recommend organizing them into categories according to their food groups. One shelf, for instance, can hold cereals and grains, while another holds canned fruits and vegetables.

The position of each item is also important. If you must keep tempting foods on hand, place them high up on shelves and in back of your storage areas where they will be out of sight and hard to reach. For example, you might have a strong urge to eat chocolate chips out of the bag, but the time lapse between wanting them and finding the bag on the top shelf behind the flour and other baking supplies might be enough for you to regain control. Storing items out of sight also eliminates the visual cue every time you open a storage area. Chances are that you will forget about the tempting food until you plan to use it.

Containers can also be used as strategic tools. Store in clear containers any staples that don't tempt you so you can see when they are getting low and can add them to your shopping list.

Store tempting foods in opaque containers, and label the containers with the contents and date you stored them. Place them in the back of the refrigerator or on a hard-to-reach shelf so that you won't be tempted.

Step 3: Keep All of Your Food in the Kitchen

Don't leave food in other rooms. There is no reason to keep a candy dish in the living room or a bowl of peanuts by the television. You may rationalize that the candy dish or the peanuts are for "company," but inevitably you have to rush to the grocery store to buy something else when company actually is coming.

Don't tempt yourself repeatedly by the sight of food. You do not need to eat constantly, and neither does anyone else. If you have company and feel that it's necessary to offer a snack, serve what you have on hand (fresh fruit with a yogurt dip can be a delicious snack). A constant supply of food is unnecessary and is detrimental to your success. We recommend that you throw away the contents of the candy jar. If you must keep snacks on hand for company, put the foods and the containers they are in out of sight, and set them out only after company has arrived.

Step 4: Put Other Family Members in Charge of Their Snacks

Let your family know that you don't want to eat alluring snack foods and you don't want them left out on the kitchen counter at any time. Tell them to take charge of the snacks they eat and to keep them in an out-of-the-way place, such as the back of the cupboard, in a basement pantry, or in a cupboard that you don't have to open every day. A perfect cupboard space for family snacks is one that's difficult for you to reach. An even better option is to simply ask your family members to help you by not having these foods in the house for a while, or to eat them outside the home.

Don't rationalize that you are keeping your favorite crackers or cookies around for your children or husband when it's really for you! If you feel that you must keep snacks, buy those that your family will eat but that are not exciting to you.

Step 5: Make Proper Utensils and References Accessible

No matter how limited a space you have, keep a food scale for weighing portions, particularly for items such as meats and cheeses. Looking at a piece of chicken and guessing that it weighs "about four ounces" won't do. While you may have become quite adept at eyeballing or estimating portion sizes, it's easy for your perception to become distorted. Check your accuracy!

Have several measuring cups and utensils on hand, and store some in containers that always call for certain portions. For example, keep a one-third cup measure in the oatmeal box, a half cup in the rice container or in other cereal boxes. We also recommend that you attach a measuring spoon to your oil bottles. None of us can be accurate in estimating one tablepoon of oil, and since one tablespoon of oil is 120 calories, it's critical to be accurate.

Be sure that your equipment is easy to reach. Using a wall grid to store pots, pans, measuring cups and spoons, and other utensils is helpful. If you don't have or want a wall grid, keep your utensils in a convenient cupboard close to your working area.

As for references, a large variety of caloric guides, nutrition texts, and cookbooks are available. As you reorganize your kitchen, set aside an area for specific cookbooks and calorie guides that you want to keep handy. Essentially you need the recipes for the week and a reference to help you with measuring equivalents or substitutes if needed. If you don't want to clutter up your counter, copy the recipes for the week and keep them in a small notebook along with your weekly meal planner.

Maintain Control While You Are Handling Food

Step 1. Choose the Best Time to Plan Menus and Shop

As you know from chapter 8, we recommend planning your meals on a weekly basis. It may be time-consuming initially, but in the long run, it saves time and calories. Remember to set a specific time each week for menu planning and grocery shopping.

Step 2. Choose the Best Time to Prepare Meals

An important step in planning ahead is determining when to prepare dinner. Think again about your schedule. Probably the most important factor to consider is when you are the least susceptible to temptation.

Four to six o'clock in the afternoon is one of the worst periods of the

day to prepare dinner because during this time you are probably exhausted and physically hungry, and maintaining control when you are
tired and hungry is difficult.

To eliminate unplanned eating while you're preparing food, consider
the following options for preparing dinner.

Option A: Make as much of the dinner as possible after breakfast in the morning.
Morning is the time when you are least susceptible to food cues. If you're
going to make a stir-fry for dinner, you can cut up vegetables in the
morning and put the meat in a marinade. You can even cook the rice and
refrigerate it. Then when you come home from work, all you have to do
is stir-fry and reheat the rice.

If you're going to bake chicken, you can wash it, take off the skin, and
prepare it before you go to work. You can cut up vegetables and put
them in a sealed container, wash the baking potatoes, and wrap them in
foil. Then when you get home, put the chicken and the potatoes in the
oven. Relax with a diet drink or go out for a walk or a bike ride while
the food cooks.

With morning preparations, you won't need to spend more than fifteen or twenty minutes in the kitchen during the dinner hour.

Option B: Prepare dinner the night before you plan to eat it. If your mornings
are too hectic, you can do a minimum amount of preparation for the
following night right after you have finished your dinner, when you are
no longer hungry. For example, if you were making tuna casserole, you
could cut up all the ingredients, mix them together, and refrigerate them
in a baking dish. When you arrive home the next day, you can pop the
dinner into the oven. Right before you sit down for dinner, put together
a salad.

Option C: Prepare batches of meals. If you don't mind spending a day or
a long evening in the kitchen, eliminate time spent in the kitchen during
the week by cooking large amounts of different foods, dividing them into
portions, putting them into containers, and storing them in the refrigerator and freezer. (Be sure to do this at a time when you are *not* susceptible to large quantities of food.)

Chapter 8 includes recipes for foods that are excellent for freezing,
such as Beef Loaf and Basic Tomato Sauce. Mark each package or container with the date stored, the day of the week you plan to use it, the

contents, and the calories. That way, during the week, all you have to do is pull out the container, heat up the contents in the microwave or oven, prepare a salad or a vegetable, and be ready to enjoy your meal.

The advantage of preparing frozen diet dinners yourself is that you control the ingredients. You can reduce the sodium content, increase fiber, and avoid additives and preservatives. These homemade dinners are not only less expensive than commercial frozen dinners, but they will better suit your tastes and increase your satisfaction.

Step 3. Deal With Food Cues While Preparing Meals

Does the sight of tomato juice trigger you to make a Bloody Mary to drink while you are preparing dinner? Do you stir and taste as you cook? Do you take a nibble of each item as you work on it, giving yourself the equivalent of one whole meal before you sit down to eat with the family?

If you are preparing dinner at a time when you are tempted to snack, keep a low-calorie beverage close at hand. Drink iced tea, seltzer with lime, or a diet soda. Sometimes even a glass of ice water with a squeeze of lemon or lime quenches your thirst and gives you pleasure while you work. Another strategy is to chew sugarless gum during meal preparation. The act of chewing will keep your mouth busy; but be careful with this habit, since for some people gum increases the desire for food.

You have to consciously break the habit of popping pieces of food into your mouth as you cook. The low-calorie drink will help, but you will also need to remind yourself that you don't want to put food into your mouth. Remember, for instance, that every extra ounce of cheese adds 100 calories to your day's intake.

Being organized and focused on goals also helps break the habit of nibbling before dinner, as does substituting activities. Rita Caparelli, who lost forty-five pounds on the DFC program and maintained that loss, says that she used to eat a whole meal as she prepared it. "I used to put away a whole wedge of cheese and a half box of crackers before I even thought about what to fix for dinner," she says. "Now I do it differently. I usually get everything ready for dinner right after breakfast. It takes me about fifteen minutes because I make simple dinners. I get my chicken trimmed or marinated, and wash the vegetables. Then I set out the skillet or pans, and measure the spices I'm going to use and seal them in a bowl on the counter so I don't have to take the time to get into the cupboards at dinnertime.

"After work, I usually change into sweatpants, have a diet drink, and go for a walk. When I come back, I watch the news on TV while I cook dinner. I feel good about it, and dinner isn't a problem anymore. It's just pleasant, and I end up feeling really successful every evening!"

Step 4. Create a Pleasant Atmosphere in Your Kitchen

Keep your kitchen clean and enjoyable. Do dishes after meals and keep your counters clean. Buy flowers, and if possible, set up a tape recorder or a radio so that you can listen to music while you prepare dinner. A pleasant atmosphere will help you to relax and will thus reduce your food cues. If you also eat in your kitchen, you'll have a nice place to sit, relax, eat slowly, and enjoy every bite.

Step 5. Divide Food into Portions as You Serve It

Prepare the exact amount of food that you need for a meal, including larger portions for your family. Make enough for leftovers only if you have a specific purpose for them included in your weekly meal planner. For example, bake an extra chicken breast Tuesday night if you are making chicken salad for lunch on Wednesday.

Use smaller-size dishware for smaller meals, particularly for breakfast and lunch, so that you don't feel deprived by what would appear to be skimpy portions on a larger plate. Use small glasses for beverages such as skim milk or juice, and measure the amount of liquid your glasses hold ahead of time so that you can count calories accurately.

Don't serve family style. It's too large a food cue, and there's no reason to expose yourself to it. Arrange individual portions on each plate in the kitchen. If family members want second helpings, let them go to the kitchen to get more. (Don't volunteer so you can nibble when no one is around.)

Step 6. Treat Yourself as if You Were Company

Don't wait for company to bring out the tablecloth or placemats. Make a ceremony out of eating. Set the table with flowers, good silver, and candles. You are special and you deserve the best. Whether you are eating by yourself or with children or other adults, your table should be inviting. Even a frozen dinner tastes better when it's served with some ceremony, out of its foil and on a nice place setting. Candlelight and soft music in the background can also help you to relax and enjoy your meal.

Your days may be hectic, but when you come to the table, take time for yourself. Focus on the activity of eating and savor each bite. Eat slowly, just as you would if you had company. Don't rush. Put a smaller amount of food on your fork, and chew it deliberately. Put your fork or spoon down between bites. The slower you eat, the more pleasure you experience with each taste, and the less likely you are to want second helpings. Also, by eating slowly, your stomach can signal your brain that you are getting full.

Step 7. Deal Successfully with Cleanup and Leftovers

If you eat alone and prepare exact portions, you don't have to worry about leftovers. But if you cook for other people, and if there is food left over, you need to maintain control. Think about your habits. Are *you* the food disposal in your home? Do you eat the last half of your son's English muffin when he's left it and run off to school? Do you eat the cold scrambled eggs another family member left on the plate? Nibbling leftovers when you are cleaning up or putting food away is just as easy as mindlessly nibbling 500 calories when you are preparing a meal.

If you are tempted during cleanup, ask your family members to clear the table. Ask them to scrape and rinse their own plates. Ask them to put away leftovers and mark them for their own snacks if they want them.

If you are the one clearing the table, beware. You may have been taught as a child that you should clean your plate because of all the starving children in the world, but those children won't be any better off if you eat the leftovers. If you don't have a purpose for the leftovers in your weekly meal planner, throw them away, feed them to your dog or cat, or give them to your neighbor's dog. It is better for you to throw away good food than to add to your weight and jeopardize your health and sense of well-being.

Remove Temptations from the Rest of Your House

Step 1. Limit the Number of Rooms and Places Where You Eat

It's very important to designate one, or at the most, two spots in the house as places where you can eat. The best place to eat is at the table—either the dining room table or kitchen table. Unless your family has its meals at the kitchen table, however, use your kitchen *only* for food storage and preparation. You can't help being tempted to eat when you are surrounded by food. Socialize in other rooms in the house; change the habit of talking with your friends and nibbling on snacks in the kitchen. Pour yourself and your friend diet sodas and go sit in the living room or on the porch.

Make a rule that you will avoid eating in rooms or in places other than the ones you designated. If members of your family snack in the living room or den, ask them not to do so in front of you.

You can eliminate hundreds, and eventually thousands, of unnecessary calories by making a rule to never eat while standing. Don't stand at the refrigerator and snack. Don't eat standing at the counter, and don't walk around eating. Many of us hardly notice the amount of food we eat while we're standing, yet the results of this unconscious and uncontrolled eating become visible over time. Gary Summers, a DFC client, learned this lesson the hard way. He loved ice cream, but he never felt he had the calories to spend on such a high-calorie choice. So instead of portioning himself out a small bowl and sitting down to enjoy it, he stood by the freezer and nibbled spoonfuls throughout the day. What Gary didn't realize was that he was consuming at least an extra 50 calories a day, which on a yearly basis adds up to 18,250 calories, or 5½ pounds in one year.

Step 2. Change Rooms and Routines to Break Down Food Cues

An important strategy for changing your eating habits is to interfere with automatic associations you have developed and to create new, food-free routines. If there are rooms in your house that are not associated with eating, for instance, spend more time in them. If you never eat in your bedroom, go there earlier in the evening and read, pay bills, or watch television.

Sometimes it's a good idea to rearrange your furniture to break down old associations and create new ones. If, for instance, you are used to eating at your desk, move your desk to a different location or to a different room in order to disrupt the association you have between sitting down at your desk and eating.

Be sure to plan substitute activities for the times you normally snack at home. One DFC graduate—whose food cue was the ubiquitous television food commercial—began to keep a needlepoint design on the table beside her when she watched TV. During commercials, she used her remote control to turn down the sound and worked on her needlepoint. She broke the association she had developed between commercials and eating, and she produced many fine needlepoint designs as well.

If you associate certain times of day with snacking, it can be helpful to create new routines. Many of our DFC graduates who are tempted to snack between 3:00 P.M. and dinner choose exercise as an alternative to eating. Exercise gets them away from food, and after they have worked out, they have more energy and motivation not to snack. Those who find that late-night eating is their problem time change rooms and routines. If they associate eating with watching television in the den, for instance, they instead read in the bedroom or listen to music in the living room.

When you have assessed the way you deal with food in your home, restructured and reorganized your kitchen, designated your "eating room," chosen the best time to prepare meals, and generally gained control over food in your home environment, you will be miles ahead of yourself in reaching your goal. You will truly be "master of the house" and on the way to a healthy destiny.

13

Eating Out and Enjoying It, Plus Party Plans

Eating Out

The good news is that even though you're on a diet, you can still eat out. In fact, we encourage you to eat out, and to have fun doing it! At the DFC, we believe it's essential for you to integrate new ways of dealing with food into your everyday life, and that includes social occasions. No matter how frequently or infrequently you go out, you'll be able to enjoy yourself and, at the same time, maintain your low-calorie plan by making good choices.

If you're like a majority of Americans, you're probably eating at least one of every five meals out already. And why not go out for business reasons, for convenience, to celebrate special events, or simply because you hate doing dishes? It's fun to try out new cuisines, or to eat well when you're traveling, attending a conference, or having a vacation.

At the Diet and Fitness Center, we take our clients to dinner at restaurants so that they can learn how to eat out and continue to lose weight—which they do! In this chapter, we will teach you strategies that can help you to eat out with calorie control *and* pleasure.

Step 1. Identify the Potential Problems

To remain within your caloric guidelines at a restaurant, you must increase your awareness of the potential problems of eating away from home. When you think about it, the problems of restaurant eating are as abundant as the food. Here are some of the common pitfalls.

• The menu looks so good! When you're scanning a vast number of inviting choices, it's easy to get carried away. Usually you won't know how the recipes are prepared, or how many calories they contain. Is the food cooked in oil and smothered in butter? Has cream been added? How much?

• The "freebies" add up quickly. A basket filled with breads and rolls is usually on the table. At some restaurants, crackers, cheese, peanuts, chips, or relish trays are abundant. With two saltines at 30 calories and cheese at 100 calories per ounce, it's easy to eat 300 calories before you've even ordered dinner. If you decide to eat a roll with butter, that's another 150 calories.

• Food cues are heightened when the senses are enlivened by enticing aromas, the sight of beautifully presented foods, the sounds of popping corks and ice clinking in glasses.

• The portions in restaurants are usually larger than necessary, and when you order a full-course meal the quantity can be overwhelming.

• Peer pressure from your friends may discourage you from controlling your food intake. Famous last words: "We're celebrating tonight! How can dessert or a few extra calories hurt!"

• Your mood may lead to overindulgence if you feel like celebrating and treating yourself well. On the other hand, you may also tend to overeat if you're nervous, upset, depressed, or angry.

• The timing of your restaurant meal may be later than you usually eat, and you may eat too much from simple hunger.

• The restaurant itself may be a problem, particularly if most of its specialties are rich and filled with high-calorie ingredients, or if it serves ethnic foods that mystify you in terms of their ingredients and calorie count.

• Calorie control is difficult when the expected eating routine begins with drinks and continues with appetizers, soup, salad, bread, entree, wine, dessert, coffee, and after-dinner liqueurs. It's easy to spend more than an entire day's budget of calories on such a meal.

• Alcohol, at 7 calories a gram, is almost as calorically dense as fat. Many DFC clients say that when they drink, they also tend to overeat.

• All-you-can-eat restaurants with buffet lines and second and third helpings provide temptations to gorge. The visual presentation of enormous quantities of food can be so overwhelming that it becomes difficult to make appropriate choices.

Step 2. Cope with the Problems

If you look at the potential problems as challenges, you can handle them more effectively. There are usually several workable strategies, and the ones you choose depend on your particular strengths and weaknesses and how you feel at the time. As you consider the following guidelines and options, remember that these techniques are fueled by your motivation to be successful.

- The menu will be no problem at all if you decide what you're going to eat before you go to the restaurant. One option is to go into a restaurant and never open the menu. You can ask for the fresh fish of the day (broiled, without butter), a baked potato, and a salad, and be set calorically and nutritionally. One DFC graduate told us that when she goes to a restaurant, she *never* looks at the menu. "When I read it," she says, "I'm seduced by the descriptions of the food, so I have a much better time if I just decide beforehand what I'll have and then stick to it." Other strategies might include calling ahead to find out what types of foods and specialties the restaurant serves, or selecting from the menu while paying attention to the estimated calories involved in the dishes you select.
- Freebies can be removed from the table if you're eating alone or with a like-minded friend. You don't have to tell the waiter that you're on a diet; some people ask for things to be taken from the table simply because they create clutter. If you decide ahead of time that you want a special item, put the appropriate portion on your plate and ask for the rest to be removed. If you're with friends and feel tempted to eat more, ask them to take what they want and send the rest away. Or ask your waiter to bring you a salad so you can eat while everyone else is munching on the freebies.
- Food cues will always be there. Preparing yourself for them by planning should reduce their effect. Also, if you go to the restaurant before you are extremely hungry, you will be better able to resist food cues. Simply sipping water and enjoying conversation with friends may distract you from the temptations.
- Portions usually are too large, but find out how large by asking about

their weight. This is something the chef knows. Your waiter, for instance, can tell you whether you'll be served a six-ounce steak or an eight-ounce steak. Even if a six-ounce steak is not on the menu, request it. You may be required to pay for the ten-ounce portion, but not eating those extra calories justifies the expenditure.

If you are a member of the Clean Plate Club, order an entree that allows you to eat the whole thing. If you're not very hungry, or if you know that sizes are much too large, order an appetizer as your entree or make a meal out of soup and a salad. If your dining partner has similar taste, consider sharing your order. Ask the waiter to divide the meal before bringing it to the table. If not, ask for a second plate and serve yourself the amount that you want. One of our clients at the DFC always asks for a second plate to be brought to her table so she has control over portioning the amounts she plans to eat. Remember to portion what you are going to eat *before* you eat it.

• Peer pressure needn't always be negative. It's a good idea to enlist the support of your friends when you're going out to eat. Ask them not to encourage you to eat foods you haven't planned. Tell them to reinforce the choices you make, or at the very least, to ignore them. Let your friends know that you enjoy the company and the atmosphere. Your fun is not dependent on eating anything extra. (If a friend urges you to overeat despite your requests, the next time that friend asks you to go out to dinner, suggest instead that you take a walk together or go to a movie.)

• Your mood affects everything that you do. Anticipate the difficulties you might encounter, and work through them before you go out. If, for instance, you're inclined to "reward" yourself with food when you eat out, prepare yourself to deal with that impulse. Remember that a dinner commitment is not written in stone. You may need to change your plans from time to time if your mood is likely to be a negative influence on your eating during a particular evening.

• Timing is a problem if you're eating at a later hour than usual. If you have the option, suggest the dinner hour yourself. If you don't have that option and you're going to be eating late, plan a mini-meal before you go to the restaurant. Set a caloric limit for the mini-meal (100 to 200 calories). Sometimes a small bowl of oatmeal, an apple, or half of a 200-calorie sandwich will take the edge off your hunger and help you to be moderate during the meal.

• As for the restaurant itself, make some decisions. Do you want American, French, Indian, Chinese, or Mexican? Choose a restaurant that allows you to plan your meal and that puts you in control. Consider whether a particular restaurant triggers you to overeat. Restaurants that don't serve à la carte may inadvertently encourage you to eat the whole dinner because you paid for it. If you know the restaurant and the menu, you'll be able to plan. For a new restaurant, call and ask about the food. Find out if there are any low-calorie items on the menu and whether special requests will be honored. Usually restaurants where food is made to order will be much easier for you than fast-food restaurants where all the food is prepared ahead of time or cooked according to formula. If you're going to a restaurant where you love the specialty, order it and enjoy it. If you're going to a fish house, for instance, and you love shrimp scampi, then plan to have it. Save calories on the extras—clam chowder, wine, bread and butter, and apple pie. If you go the other route and order something you really don't want, you may feel deprived, then binge when you get home because you were so "good" at the restaurant.

• Calorie control involves making choices based on caloric content of specific foods as well as being aware of appropriate portion sizes. In Step 3 you will learn how to estimate caloric values.

• If you enjoy drinking alcohol, plan for it. A reasonable goal is to drink seltzer before dinner and save the calories from cocktails for one or two glasses of wine during the meal. When you drink wine with the meal, you are also combating the problem of lowered resistance because you will be drinking slowly and will have food in your stomach. Another strategy is to alternate an alcoholic beverage with a nonalcoholic, low-calorie beverage. No matter when you decide to drink alcohol, determine how many calories you want to spend on it. Remember that alcohol has no nutritive value.

• At a buffet or in an "all-you-can-eat" situation, go through the line *without* a plate. Then sit down, drink a low-calorie beverage, and decide what you will eat when you go back through the line *with* a plate. Another plan is to go through the line and choose a variety of low-calorie items— for instance, green salad, carrot strips, and fruits without toppings—eat them, then go back for the entree you've chosen. Another approach is to take a small plate (a dessert plate instead of a platter) and go through the line only once, putting anything that you want on your plate. If this type of restaurant presents real problems for you, choose a different restaurant.

Step 3. Plan for Success

There are three key elements in planning any meal at a restaurant.

1. *Plan your calories.* Before our clients go out for a "restaurant experience" with a DFC dietitian, they spend quite a bit of time studying the restaurant's menu and thinking about what they are going to order. In order to maintain control in a potentially expensive caloric situation, it's important to go over your budget and remind yourself of how much "money" you have in the calorie bank to spend on that meal.

2. *Plan a "skeleton menu."* In planning for dinner or lunch, decide how to divide your calories into the categories of foods you enjoy. Have you been dying for a particular dessert or looking forward to a piece of veal? What are your priorities? If you have 500 calories to spend, which items will get the highest allocation? Is half of a dessert worth 200 calories, or would you be more satisfied with a glass of wine and a shrimp cocktail before dinner? Examine your priorities and decide how you want to distribute your calories—what part you want to go to an appetizer, what amount to your entree, what amount to some other food you enjoy. Concentrate on your favorite choices that will satisfy you, and decide which unnecessary calories you can omit in order to make your more preferred choices feasible. Look at the following sample dinner plan. As you can see, if you don't determine your priorities, the total number of calories can skyrocket.

Category	Portion	Choice Food	Calories
Alcohol	4 ounces	Wine	100
Freebie	5 (2")	Breadstick	150
Freebie	1 ounce	Roll	100
Appetizer	1 cup	New England clam chowder	200
Side Dish	small	Salad	30
Fat	¼ cup	Blue cheese salad dressing	320
Side Dish	10 ounces	Baked potato	250
Fat	1 tablespoon	Butter or margarine	100
Entree	6 ounces	Broiled fish, plain	210
Dessert	1 cup	Ice cream	300

TOTAL CALORIES: 1,760

When one of our clients looked at the skeleton menu, he decided the following priorities for himself: First of all, he wanted a glass of wine, but he decided to save it for dinner. He thought about whether he could afford clam chowder for 200 calories, but since he was having the wine, he substituted shrimp cocktail (for 150 calories) and saved the extra calories for a tablespoon of blue cheese salad dressing (80 calories) on the side to use both on his salad and on his baked potato. He wanted fish for dinner. By asking to have it broiled without butter, he knew he would save calories.

The result of his decision-making process was the following sample meal plan:

Food	Calories
4 oz. wine	100
Shrimp cocktail	150
Tossed salad (plain)	30
1 Tb. blue cheese dressing	80
½ 5 oz. baked potato	125
6 oz. broiled fish	210
TOTAL CALORIES:	695

3. *Write down chief problems and coping strategies.* Before going out to eat, review the problems you have encountered in the past. Think about the particular restaurant, event, and people involved. Where was your weak point? What triggered your overeating? Make a list of strategies for overcoming these difficulties, and take charge of your new restaurant experience. Decide which restaurant is best for you. What day, what time, and what company will help you stay in control and still have a good time?

Caloric Survival Skills—Applying the Plan

Regardless of how mentally prepared and motivated you are when you dine out, to be successful it's essential for you to have some idea of the caloric content of a number of different foods. The lists contained in the six major food groups (pages 93–106) will serve as a starter course in counting calories. In addition, consider these important points:

Without any added fat or sauces, an ounce of lean beef is usually about

60 calories; lamb, 100; poultry without skin, 50; seafood—fish and shell-fish, approximately 35, and baked potato, 25. When you add regular salad dressing to your greens, you are adding 60 to 100 calories per tablespoon. And if you add butter, oil, or margarine either for cooking or for eating with your fish or potato or roll, you're talking about 100 to 120 calories per tablespoon. For example, a six-ounce filet mignon grilled plain would be approximately 360 calories. If you had a brown sauce with the filet mignon, that would add at least 100 calories.

Keep the following average caloric values in mind when you begin to plan your restaurant meal.

Vegetables, ½ cup	
cooked	25
1 cup raw	25
Fruit serving	60
Egg (whole)	75
Lean beef	60 calories/oz.
Poultry, without skin	50 calories/oz.
Seafood (includes lean fish and shellfish)	35 calories/oz.
Cheese	100 calories/oz.
Baked potato, plain	25 calories/oz.
Pasta, plain	100 calories/½ cup
Regular salad dressing	60–100 calories/Tb.
Oil, butter, or margarine	120 calories/Tb.

The caloric values above for the nonfat items are values without any added fat or sauces. Most restaurants use fats in preparing their foods. If your food is sautéed, expect 100 to 300 additional calories from butter or oil. Sauces are also high in calories because they're predominately fat. Four tablespoons of hollandaise sauce, for instance, is 190 calories. Ask for sauces to be served on the side so you can portion the amount you wish to use, or eliminate sauces altogether.

To plan your restaurant meals, check the following sample restaurant meal. Use it for planning a meal before you go out, or use it at the restaurant. Make decisions about where to spend your calories—for instance, do you want an appetizer or a glass of wine?

Category	Food	Portion	Calories	Special Instructions
Alcohol	Wine	4 oz.	100	
Side dish	Tossed salad	small	30	No dressing, use vinegar
Entree	Fish	6 oz.	210	No butter or oil, broiled with lemon
Side dish	Baked potato	4 oz.	100	plain, margarine on the side
Freebie	Hard roll	1 oz.	80	plain
Fat	Margarine	1 tsp.	35	measure with a teaspoon or use one pat

Total calories: 555

My Restaurant Eating Guide

Category	Food	Portion	Calories	Special Instructions
___	___	___	___	___
___	___	___	___	___
___	___	___	___	___
___	___	___	___	___
___	___	___	___	___
___	___	___	___	___

TOTAL CALORIES:

Knowing How to Order

Restaurants today, familiar with people on special diets, are used to accommodating an individual's needs. When you're at a restaurant, don't be afraid to ask the waiter to have the meat or fish broiled, to bring oil and vinegar for your salad instead of salad dressing. Remember, you are the patron, and you are entitled to ask questions and make requests. Don't be intimidated by your waiter. Trust your own judgment and your own choices. Don't be embarrassed to ask that your food be prepared in a simple fashion without fat or butter. The real pros will never get impatient with your questions. They, too, are aware that low-fat foods are healthy, and that many Americans are cutting down on their dietary cholesterol, saturated fats, and calories.

"Okay," you may be saying, "how do I do it? What should I ask?"

Often, the menu will identify the ingredients in a dish and tell you how the food is prepared. For instance, "red snapper sautéed in white wine sauce, with red potatoes" tells you quite a bit. If the fish is sautéed in white wine sauce, you can ask what is in the sauce and whether butter is used for the sautéeing.

Most likely, the menu will contain many answers to your questions and point you in the right direction for your order. Most menus these days describe the mode of preparation, allowing you to choose among the alternatives. Foods prepared with a minimum of fat are "steamed," "broiled," "roasted," "poached," or "dry-broiled" (in lemon juice or wine). Vegetables are "garden fresh" and fruit served without sugar is "in its own juice." Some selections may even indicate that they're low in fat or cholesterol.

Be aware, however, that some low-fat, low-cholesterol preparations are high in sodium. Watch out for foods that are "pickled," "smoked," "in sauce," "in a tomato base," or "in broth." Unless otherwise specified, these foods probably will have a high sodium content.

Menu descriptions that signal foods high in saturated fats (and usually high in calories) should be taken as warnings written in red. Read these warnings as *"Stop!" "Stay Away!" "Beware of this food!"* These descriptions include: "buttery," "buttered," "in butter sauce," "sautéed," "lightly breaded," "fried," "panfried," "deep fried," "crispy" (which usually means fried in fat), "braised," "creamed," "in cream sauce," "in its own gravy," "hollandaise," "au gratin" (with cheese), "Parmesan," "cheddar cheese," "in cheese sauce," "escalloped," "marinated" (in oil), "stewed," "basted," "casserole," "prime," "hash," and "potpie."

If you have any questions about how the food is prepared, ask the waiter. Make it clear that you would rather have your meat, fish, or poultry broiled, baked, steamed, or poached rather than sautéed, fried, or deep fried. Ask that visible fat be trimmed from meat and that skin be removed from poultry. Ask that the kitchen limit your portion to four to six ounces of cooked meat, fish, or poultry. (If you don't want to ask this, judge the appropriate portion and leave the rest on your plate.) Ask that your vegetables be steamed (using no butter) instead of sautéed, and request a small- or medium-sized baked potato.

You can also request that
• the dressing or sauce be served on the side
• skim milk be served instead of whole milk
• the dish be prepared without added salt or MSG (monosodium glutamate)

• unwanted foods such as bread and rolls or french fries not be served
• the food be prepared with no added fat or butter

Be clear in your instructions. Request exactly what you want or don't want. Say, "I would like my fish broiled with garlic and lemon, and *no* butter."

If your food arrives and it has not been fixed as you requested, send it back and repeat your request. If you have asked that something extra, such as french fries or chips, *not* be served and the waiter brings them anyway, either ask that they be removed, or make sure you don't eat them by liberally sprinkling them with pepper or sugar to make them inedible.

Eating at Fast-Food Restaurants

There may be times when you long for a fast-food specialty, such as a Taco Bell taco, a Big Mac, a Wendy's sandwich, or Kentucky Fried Chicken. If so, you can plan for it. It is better for you to have a fast-food meal that you yearn for, but in a controlled manner, than to deny yourself and then binge.

The good news is that even at fast-food places these days, you can get low-calorie foods. Many of the fast-food chains are accommodating health-conscious Americans by adding salad bars offering a wide variety of vegetables and toppings. If you want protein, add beans to your salad and combine it with whole grain bread. Or order a baked potato and add fresh vegetables or yogurt topping from the salad bar. If you crave a burger, order the smallest size, then fill up on a diet drink and salad, or eat a piece of fruit that you brought with you. This way, you'll probably be able to stay within your calorie quota. To stay low-calorie, avoid double-decker burgers, milk shakes, french fries, and specialty sauces.

Away from the salad bar, you can count on most foods being high in sodium, fat, and calories. They're prepared quickly and eaten quickly. Nevertheless, they can contribute to your nutrient intake, and every now and then you may want to "afford" even the double-deckers with sauce. As a guide, we've included a few examples of fast-food choices that could fit into your 500-calorie dinner allotment.

Fast-Food Combos—500 Calories or Less!

McDonald's	Calories	Sodium (mg.)
Hamburger with bun	260	490
Garden salad, plain	91	100
Lite Vinaigrette, (½ pkg.)	25	150
Diet Coke, 12 oz.	4	70
TOTAL:	380	810

Optional:		
Medium apple from home	80	2
TOTAL:	460	812

McDonald's		
Chicken McNuggets (6 pieces)	320	510
Honey sauce (1 pkg.)	50	2
Side salad	48	45
Lite vinaigrette (½ pkg.)	25	150
TOTAL:	443	707

Taco Bell		
2 tacos	370	160
Diet drink, 12 oz.	4	70
TOTAL:	374	230

Wendy's		
Chili, regular serving	240	990
Salad bar, 2 cups greens, 1 cup raw vegetables	45	25
1 Tb. Italian dressing	60	150
1 oz. Cheddar cheese	110	250
TOTAL:	455	1,415*

Pizza Hut		
2 medium slices cheese pizza, thin	370	840
2 cups greens, 1 cup raw vegetables	45	25
1 Tb. Italian salad dressing	60	150
TOTAL:	475	1,015

*Note that this is approximately half of the recommended daily sodium intake.

Parties and Other Special Occasions

Any social event at which food is served, whether a cocktail party, dinner party, dance, banquet, or holiday celebration, presents potential difficulties in terms of unplanned eating. Without giving a single thought to what you're eating, it's not at all difficult to take in a thousand calories or more within a couple of hours as you take a sample from each tray of hors d'oeuvres that passes your way, accept another glass of champagne or other drink, and make one or two repeat visits to the buffet spread.

Most people feel that they must eat and drink in order to enjoy a party. That may be true for you, but remember, you don't have to eat and drink without a plan. A plan puts you in control, and will make you a lot happier about yourself and about the way you enjoyed the party.

Two General Plans for Special Occasions

Plan One: Drink only noncaloric beverages that will be readily available. Seltzer, club soda, and Perrier water have the fizz and bounce of a carbonated drink, and they don't make you feel deprived. For a slightly different taste, ask the bartender to add a lemon or lime wedge to your seltzer. You can drink as much as you like of these beverages and still feel as if you are having "a drink" while you are consuming zero calories. You'll be able to maintain your three-meal eating plan and stay within your caloric guidelines. You can plan to have a glass of wine with your dinner if you want to budget alcohol into your meal.

Plan Two: Decide to increase your low-calorie diet by a specific caloric amount—say, an additional 100 to 200 calories—for the occasion. Write this caloric allowance in your food diary. Although you won't know the actual foods that will be served, at least you'll have a plan for the amount of calories you can spend. When you get to the party, look over what's available, then decide what you will eat and how much. Later you can record what you ate in your diary.

If you want to save calories from lunch or dinner and use them at a late-evening social activity, you can do so. As you know, we don't usually approve of "saving" calories, and we don't approve of snacks. But incorporating your activities into your diet plan is different from planning a snack every night. When Jacqueline Kennedy Onassis was First Lady, she used to eat only an apple for lunch on the day of a state dinner. Although she didn't seem to have any weight problem, she was clearly planning ahead for the overload of calories she knew she would have at the evening's banquet. Also, you can be sure, she tasted all of the food on her plate, but she didn't eat every last crumb. We don't advocate only an apple for lunch, but we do think that you can plan to add an extra 200 calories to your diet for a special occasion, assuming that such special occasions don't occur on a weekly basis.

Eating at the Homes of Friends

When you're invited to dinner by close friends, let them know that you're watching your calories and ask them not to be troubled if you eat lightly. If you're not comfortable telling your hosts that you're dieting, simply decide when you see the food how much of it you can afford to eat.

Before dinner, when drinks and appetizers are served, we suggest that you have a diet soda or a glass of club soda, Perrier, or seltzer. If you want a cocktail, ask that the drink be mixed with water, juice, low-calorie soda, or seltzer rather than with presweetened mixes. A spritzer—wine with seltzer—is usually a good choice.

Remember, it's okay not to eat the appetizers unless they're low in calories. Be pleasant but firm in your refusal. If you are inclined, say that you're saving your appetite for dinner.

If dinner is served family style, look at what is available before you put the first serving on your plate. Decide what you want the most, and serve yourself small portions. If you don't want something, simply pass the dish. If your dish is prepared for you, look at your plate before taking a bite and decide how to spend your calories. You may want to take at least a taste of each food so that you can compliment your friend's efforts.

If your host is serving, ask for small portions. You might say, "Would you give me half of the amount that you gave to Ron?" A small portion also allows you to eat it all rather than to leave food on your plate. If, however, you're served a large portion, let food remain on your plate.

When you can, skip sauces, gravies, fried foods, and high-fat items such as dips, spreads, butter, nuts, and creamed foods. If your host is serving you, ask if he or she would mind putting your sauce on the side. If you're serving yourself, either skip the sauce or put a very small amount of it on the side. That way you can dip into the sauce, taste it, and comment on it, but you don't have to consume it all. If you're served salad, ask if you can have yours without salad dressing or with lemon or vinegar. If you are eating at the home of a very close friend, you may want to bring your own low-calorie salad dressing.

Eat slowly. Don't feel that you have to finish every bite you are served. Leave what you don't eat on the plate, and don't apologize. Comment on what you enjoyed most about the food. If your host insists on offering you seconds, refuse politely but firmly. You don't need to say that you are on a diet and can't eat more. It's best to say that you have had enough to eat and to look and act as if you mean it. Often well-meaning friends will undermine your efforts if you give them the opportunity by saying, "No, thanks," with a wistful tone of voice that translates, "Please, encourage me to eat more."

Going to the Movies

For many people, going to the movies is just no fun without popcorn. If this is true for you, air-pop your own popcorn at home and take it along, or buy popcorn without butter at the theater. Air-popped popcorn from home, however, is a better choice simply because it has fewer calories (80 for 3 cups), while three cups of movie popcorn without butter is 140 calories because it has been cooked with oil.

Holiday Eating

The most dangerous season for dieters runs from Halloween or Thanksgiving to New Year's. A popular response to holiday binging is the New Year's Eve resolution: "Starting tomorrow, I will turn over a new leaf! I will lose weight!" Hundreds of thousands of diets begin every year on the first day of January.

We strongly encourage you to approach the food-centered holidays armed with the same strategies you use the rest of the year. Just because your eating has gotten out of control over previous holidays doesn't mean it has to this year. Don't let the season weaken your resolve and your commitment to the healthy patterns you've begun. You can still have fun! Simply be realistic, and continue to *plan* when and what you are going to eat. Anticipate the influences on your usual meal pattern. Consider the parties, dinners, brunches, and lunches you'll be attending. Think about the dinners you'll be giving, whom you'll be inviting, the food gifts that will be given and received, and the meals you'll miss due to a hectic schedule. You may decide that it is not necessary to attend every party to which you receive an invitation.

Decide in advance how you want to budget your calories for the holidays. If you are on a low-calorie diet, a temporary increase in calories can allow you to taste or eat certain foods that make the holidays special for you. If you're on a 1,200-calorie diet, you may want to expand your diet to 1,500 calories for the holidays. Sometimes you may decide that it's easiest and most realistic to *maintain your weight* over the holidays, not to lose weight.

Never skip meals during the holidays. Continue to eat three meals a day. If you're going to want to eat at a party, decide ahead of time how many calories you will spend while you're there. Allow extra calories for this event, and keep within your budget at mealtimes.

Going into the holidays, bone up on the number of calories in your favorite holiday treats. A few old favorites include the following:

Holiday Foods	Calories
Champagne, 4 fl. oz.	100
Cheese, most kinds, 1 oz.	100
Cookie, 2 ½ in.	60–100
Sugar cookie, one small	60
Eggnog, ½ cup	175
Fudge, 1 sq. in.	90
Nuts, 1 oz.	170
Pecan pie, 1 in. slice	430
Plum pudding	300
Pumpkin pie, 1 in. slice	300
Smoked salmon, 3 oz.	150
Stuffing for turkey, ½ cup	260

The same principle that applies to the particular dishes you love in good restaurants also applies to these holiday foods and drinks. If you want to have a special holiday treat, plan for it. Incorporate it into your budget.

As for holiday food gifts, you don't need to keep (and eat) every item that you receive. Pass food gifts along to a neighbor or give them to a charitable organization. Another option is to freeze a cake or cookies for a future party. This saves you from future preparation time and the temptation that can come from preparing high-calorie foods. It may be a good idea to tell your close friends that you would appreciate it if they didn't bring you holiday cookies or fruitcake this year. Tell them that their friendship, not their delicious desserts, is what's important to you.

If you are accustomed to making baked food gifts for others and overindulging as you prepare them, reconsider this practice. If you must give food gifts, make them healthy, such as a basket of fresh fruits or freshly baked whole wheat breads. If you are not committed to the notion of food gifts, change your focus and give the gift of a special book, a plant, or something else that can be enjoyed and appreciated in a different way.

Make meals over the holidays that include some of your favorite low-calorie recipes. This way you have plenty of opportunities to indulge, not bulge. Also, during these busy holiday times, consider making simple, quick meals. You can have a low-calorie frozen dinner and add a small salad, fruit, or vegetable. Not every meal needs to be a major event. If you are entertaining or preparing special meals for the holidays—whether it's a big Christmas, Easter, or Passover dinner—look at the recipes. Decide how you can substitute lower calorie ingredients. (See page 279 on how to modify recipes.) This will allow you to enjoy family favorites and holiday specials while you are cutting down on calories, sodium, and fat.

Traveling

When you are traveling, maintain direction over what, when, and how you eat. Because you often can't control where you eat, simply maintaining your weight or losing weight while traveling requires extra effort and forethought.

When you're planning a trip, evaluate your options. Do you have an approximate idea of when you'll be eating each day? Keep in mind that you want to eat according to a specific caloric level that includes a variety of foods in reasonable portions. Try to keep to a schedule of eating at regular times. Often travelers skip or delay meals and then overindulge because they are so hungry when they finally sit down to eat. Also continue your exercising while traveling. If your regular exercise routine is not possible, walking is a healthy and advisable option.

Some information about your route and means of travel will allow you to plan ahead and make choices about your menu.

On a plane. Most airlines offer a variety of "special" meals on long-distance trips. Call your ticket agent or airline and ask them to tell you the options. You can usually order one of the following meals: low-calorie, low-salt, kosher, vegetarian, diabetic, or seafood. The low-calorie meal is usually a fresh fruit plate or a chef's salad. Often there is a choice of a hot seafood dish or a cold seafood salad. By ordering one of these meals, you save one-third to one-half of the calories of regular airline food. Besides, the substitute meal is often tastier because it is usually fresh. We know someone who always took his own brown-bag lunch along on the plane. This, too, is an option.

On the road. When you set out on your trip, take a brown-bag lunch along for the first day. Most highway restaurants have limited low-calorie food choices, so packing your own lunch saves calories. You can keep soup in an insulated thermos, fruits and salads in a cooler. You may even want to picnic along the way. If you stop for breakfast or lunch, choose low-calorie selections. For breakfast, a good choice is a poached egg (75 calories), one slice of dry toast (80 calories), and 4 ounces of juice or ½ cup of fruit (60 calories). For lunch, order a turkey sandwich without mayonnaise and eat an apple you have brought along to supplement your meal. Use tomato and lettuce on your sandwich, and/or mustard to add moisture and flavor.

Use your knowledge of the calories in fast foods. Portions offered at fast-food chains are consistent throughout the United States, so you can plan a fast-food meal.

On board ship. On a cruise ship, plan your total calories and the number of times during the day that you will eat. Many ships offer "lighter" menu options, and some follow the guidelines set by the American Heart Association. Choose fresh fruits and vegetables and fresh seafood when they're available. Prioritize the meal or meals in which you really want to enjoy and taste a variety of foods. For example, decide to maintain a low-calorie breakfast and lunch and have a high-calorie dinner every evening that makes you feel satisfied and in control.

Be wary of dessert buffets at midnight and the trays of snacks served during cocktail hour. One DFC graduate who currently is at goal weight decided that she and her husband would continue taking extended vacations three to four times a year, but that they would avoid cruises. For her, the availability of food twenty-four hours a day on the cruise ship was too much of a constant temptation.

If you still choose a cruise, take advantage of your opportunities to exercise. Walk, swim, and go to the dances in the evenings. Exercise keeps you feeling fit and enhances your motivation to control your calories.

In your hotel. Be wary of the continental breakfast! You don't need the rolls and biscuits, butter and jelly that are served. Fresh fruit, one slice of bread, and coffee is lower in calories. Also, avoid the candies the staff so often place on your pillow at night. Many large hotels feature a selection of low-calorie choices if not a special menu. Ask the concierge about selections. Because so many travelers request low-calorie and low-fat diets, hotels are accommodating these needs. Consider buying your own food for breakfast or a light lunch.

In a foreign country. Find out as much as you can ahead of time about what foods will be available, and learn how to ask for what you want. Remember that no matter where you are, your goal is to eat a controlled amount of nutritious, low-calorie food. Fresh fruits, vegetables, and breads are delicious in all parts of the world. New cuisines can mean new possibilities for your day-to-day menu. Even if your choices are all high-calorie ones, you can always eat smaller portions.

When you get down to it, eating out is fun. Socializing, traveling, and partying don't have to ruin your resolve or your figure. As time goes on, new strategies for enjoying yourself and your activities become automatic substitutes for your old habits of overeating in social situations. As you look and feel better, you'll have more energy, and you'll find it increasingly easy to control what you put into your mouth—no matter where you are.

14

How to Be a Success Forever

Imagine that you have been exercising and eating properly for at least a year. When you look in the mirror, you see a body that makes you happy. You are thinner and more attractive, and you feel like a new person. You are proud of yourself and your efforts.

Often at this point, you imagine that you'll never be overweight and out of shape again. You have the feeling that you have arrived, that you'll stay this thin and healthy forever and will never again revert to your old habits of overeating or being sedentary. Like many others, you may think that now you no longer have to pay attention or keep track of your calories and your exercise. This is the kind of attitude that invites a relapse.

Stop and think. Now that you've come this far, you have to work to maintain your success. You have to keep counting calories, you have to keep planning your meals, and you have to keep on exercising. You must continue to write down what you eat, to weigh yourself, and to meet your emotional needs through ways other than eating. Although you will have developed many healthy habits and incorporated them into your new lifestyle, you must continue to pay attention to your behavior to prevent a relapse.

Weight management requires consistent attention and continued effort. The term *weight management* suggests that it is a process, rather than just a result or an end. At the DFC, we tell our clients that an important part of the process is to expect temporary setbacks when you are working on your weight. Setbacks are a normal and inevitable part of any lifestyle change. Of course, people generally don't like to hear about setbacks. They are often shocked, upset, frightened, concerned, or depressed by the possibility, afraid that a setback only leads to disaster, and that they'll never be in control again. That kind of thinking can be traced to perfectionistic ideas and an incomplete understanding of the process of change.

It's important to have realistic expectations regarding the nature of progress. Shut your eyes and imagine that you are climbing a mountain. You have ropes attached to you, and you are trying to get to the top. You have to get there to save your own life. You've come a long way, but the climb is steep now, and you're making slow progress. The terrain is rocky and the going is tough. Suddenly, you lose your footing and slide back a few feet. At this point, are you going to throw off the ropes and say, "Oh, to hell with it! I can't make it to the top anyway!" Or are you going to work to regain your footing and begin to climb again?

No one gets to the top of a mountain simply by putting one foot in front of the other and never slipping or needing to pause along the way. We've worked in this field for a long time, and we've never seen anyone lose weight in this fashion either. People who are successful lose some weight, gain a little, lose more. If they believe in themselves and keep working at it, they eventually reach their goals and work to stay there.

Most people can do pretty well changing their diet and lifestyle for a certain period of time. But when they stop doing well, when they confront a crisis, that's when problems arise. That's the point when they either throw off the ropes or decide to keep climbing. Learning how to handle the times that you don't do well is key to long-term, lifelong success in managing your weight. Begin by understanding the concepts of failure, success, setback, and relapse.

Failure

You may think that you have failed at a diet if you gain weight or go on a binge. But experiencing a lack of control or deviating from your plans for any given time is not failure. *Failure happens only when you give up and allow yourself to be defeated.* Failure is saying to yourself, "What's the use? I can't do it! This proves I'm always going to be a fat person, so there's no use trying anymore." Failure is wallowing in self-pity and feelings of inadequacy and guilt instead of actively solving the problems confronting you.

We want you to redefine failure so that you do not feel desperate when you experience normal human fallibility. Consider this new definition.

Failure is NOT
- Gaining weight.
- Going on a binge.
- Neglecting your exercise for a week.
- Forgetting your meal plan and eating between meals.
- Eating a whole pizza.
- Eating out of control for a week, or even for a month.

These are setbacks—not failures—that you can experience and still be successful, thin, and healthy.

Often when people fail, it's because they get into what we refer to as "the Ostrich Syndrome" and do not confront their behavior. They say, "Oh, it's only five pounds; that's no big deal." Instead of taking a problem seriously, they pretend that if they don't notice the problem, it will go away. They stop weighing; stop writing down what foods they eat; stop looking in the mirror; stop exercising or going to weight control classes. They tend to rationalize their behavior until they've regained all the weight they lost and can't deny reality any longer.

Success

You are being successful if you have realistic expectations about the nature of progress and take one day at a time. Success is not giving up in the face of discouragement. It's expecting setbacks and taking them in stride. It's having the ability to say, "I didn't do so well today. But I did well last week and I'll do well again, starting now." Success is giving yourself credit, appreciating the progress you've made, and reminding yourself that you can continue to make changes in your life.

To be successful, you must avoid negative thinking. The successful person refuses to generalize from one negative episode. Success is being able to follow a period of overeating or underexercising not with self-punishment, but with a period of controlled eating or realistic exercise plans. It is knowing that your calories will balance out over time, that your exercise patterns will become more regular, and that you will be able to maintain your weight or to continue losing weight.

You are being successful when you confront your behavior instead of avoiding it. This means not playing games by saying "This doesn't count," or "I'm doing so well that I can eat whatever I want," or "I'm in pretty good shape so I really don't need to exercise this week."

When you actively solve your problems, without either waiting for magic or wallowing in guilt, self-pity, or feelings of failure, you are making progress. You are making positive gains if you are conscious of the choices you make ("I bought these donuts because I wanted to eat them") rather than giving excuses ("I bought these for the kids"). Being positive about yourself is a key ingredient of success.

Setback

As we've said, progress in any major effort to change your habits is bound to be irregular and will involve setbacks. In weight loss, these setbacks can be temporary experiences of gaining weight, losing control of what you're eating, eating in an unplanned way in response to stress, or stopping your exercise regimen. Setbacks can occur when you stop weighing yourself or keeping your food diary, when you don't plan your meals ahead of time, or when you plan to walk one day or use the bike and don't do it. This can happen for an hour, a day, or an extended period of time.

Coping with a setback can be a useful learning experience. Remember that a setback is a single, independent event that can be avoided in the future. One setback doesn't have to lead to another. But the sooner you regain control following a setback, the easier it is to avoid relapse.

Relapse

A relapse occurs when you don't recover from a setback because it frightens you, you're depressed and guilty about it, or you're denying or rationalizing it. A relapse can be defined as an extended setback—one that occurs when you give up, don't do anything about it, and throw in the towel. Relapse is what we try to help you prevent and avoid.

Strategies to Help You Recover from Setbacks

Your setbacks may be small or large. You may have overeaten at a party, or you may have had an eating binge that continued for three days. You may have missed your aerobics class on Monday, or you may have stopped exercising for two weeks.

While everyone has an occasional setback, few people feel confident about their ability to recover from one. Recovery can be particularly difficult if you equate success with being in perfect control at all times and interpret even one slip as failure. This attitude can result in a further weakening of control and loss of self-confidence.

For many years, researchers have tried to understand what triggers relapses in people who stay in control for a long time and then lose it. They have seen that often, within sixty to ninety days after successfully establishing a program to control weight, alcoholism, drug addiction, or gambling, many people slide backward. The people who lose control, relapse, and then give up do so in large part because they have negative thoughts concerning the setback. The reaction to, rather than the occurrence of, a setback determines long-term progress.

People can make the same mistakes, but it's the way that they respond to the mistakes that makes all the difference in their continued success. Let's look at how two women who lost weight under the DFC program dealt with setbacks. Each had lost about twenty-three pounds over six months, then faced a high-risk situation.

Darlene's mother underwent surgery for a brain tumor, and Darlene, who lived nearby, began to juggle her job, time with her children, and trips to the hospital. She slipped into an old pattern of focusing on everyone else's needs and neglecting her own. Not surprisingly, Darlene began eating without careful thought and planning. As a result, she gained ten pounds during the initial period of her mother's illness. This was definitely a setback.

When Michelle, her husband, and their three children moved from St. Louis to Atlanta, Michelle felt totally disoriented. With the dramatic change in her routines and her surroundings, she abandoned food planning and stopped watching her calories. She stopped her morning walks and ate excessively and heedlessly to suppress her anxiety about being in a new city, her loneliness, and her exhaustion from the move. She gained eight pounds.

Both women, who had lost weight successfully up to that time, were alarmed and upset by their weight gain. They had been doing so well, and suddenly they were out of control. The weight gain was beginning to be noticeable. Their clothes felt tight and uncomfortable. How did they react? Was their progress doomed?

Michelle had a typical relapse. Negative thinking dominated her reaction to the weight gain. "I blew it; I knew it wouldn't last," she said. "How could it?" For Michelle, the setback was the beginning of the end. She felt so terrible about herself that she continued to overeat. She rationalized her overeating by saying that it made her feel less lonely and anxious. Defeated and out of control, she ate with abandon and resumed all her old eating habits. She consoled herself with the thought that she could go back on her diet and exercise program once she began to make new friends.

Darlene, on the other hand, although initially devastated, knew that she must replace her negative thoughts with a more positive and realistic assessment of the problem. "I've gained ten pounds," she said, "but I'm going to stop this and start right *now* getting back into good habits. If I start now, it will save me a lot of work. If I don't, I'm going to make it harder for myself and I'm going to feel even more defeated. I forgive myself for doing this! It's not the end of the world.

"I gained ten pounds, but before that, I had lost twenty-three," Darlene told her best friend. "I'm still thirteen pounds ahead! I'm not going to let those ten pounds keep me from where I want to go!" In spite of her busy schedule, she set aside forty-five minutes a day for herself, starting that same day. She used the first twenty minutes for a brisk walk and the rest of the time for relaxation and planning strategies to get her through this difficult period.

To be successful, develop skills like Darlene's that help you regain your self-confidence and recover from setbacks as soon as possible. Remember, there is no magic. Controlling your weight requires effort and active problem solving. Here are some strategies that we've found helpful.

Step 1. Confront Your Behavior as Soon as Possible

While it may be tempting to pretend that a setback did not occur, it is useful to confront your behavior so that you can continue your progress. When you avoid weighing yourself after a setback, or when you decide to skip your support group or Overeaters Anonymous meeting, you are avoiding dealing with the consequences of your behavior. You are also depriving yourself of an opportunity for self-awareness.

Be up front about what you've done. Don't make excuses. Instead, get right to the heart of it. Acknowledge the problem and decide what you can do to correct the situation. The sooner you intervene following a setback, the better off you are. The timing is critical here. If you have a setback on Monday and say, "I've already blown it for the week, so I might as well wait until next Monday to start again," you are asking for a relapse.

Be aware of your tendency to minimize the significance of your behavior. If you say to yourself, "Oh, hey, I only regained five pounds, that's nothing!" or, "I only skipped exercise twice this week, that's not much," or "It was only 650 extra calories; I don't have to worry about that!" or, "It's only for tonight; I won't do it again!" you're in trouble. The same is true if you tell yourself you can put off working on the problems. Denial and rationalization are just as dangerous and disruptive for you as the negative thoughts that involve hopelessness and guilt.

Don't be horrified by your behavior; don't deny, minimize, or avoid it. Instead, confront it by

1. Acknowledging to yourself that you deviated from your plans and strategies.
2. Recording the deviations (the extra calories, the missed exercise) in your food diary.
3. Identifying factors that contributed to the setback so that you can learn from the experience and minimize its recurrence.

Step 2. Identify Destructive Thoughts and Reactions to the Setback

Your attitude following a setback determines your future success. Most people tend to react to setbacks either with guilt and hopelessness, or with denial and rationalization.

Excessive guilt, self-hatred, hopelessness, or feelings of failure can prevent successful recovery from a setback. Usually these feelings lead to passivity and avoidance, or to further unplanned eating and loss of control. Similarly, punishment and self-deprivation are self-destructive responses to setbacks. Skipping meals and fasting not only make you feel worse, but they also continue an unhealthy, irregular pattern of eating. Punishing yourself with extra exercise—you'll swim a hundred laps instead of twenty—similarly sets up negative feelings about exercise that are likely to interfere with long-term motivation.

Some other negative thoughts and attitudes:

Exaggeration. When you're on a plateau, it's easy to exaggerate the situation. The pounds aren't not coming off, so you think you'll never be successful at losing weight.

Tunnel vision. All you can see is the scale, or the unplanned food that you ate. You've got blinders on. Your whole life is made up of the pounds you gained or the binge you had. You don't see the positives—you've lost more pounds than you have regained and you've maintained your exercise program. Focusing on the setback and negating progress are destructive.

Domino effect. Your setback is seen as the first domino to fall, which means that all future efforts are going to have the same outcome. You say to yourself, "I ate brownies yesterday, I have to eat brownies again today, and I'll eat cake tomorrow!" You allow one setback to start a negative cycle. It doesn't have to be that way.

All-or-nothing thinking. You think, "As long as I'm not being perfect, as long as I blew it, I'm bad." Your attitude lacks perspective; it paints the picture black or white and doesn't allow for being human, for allowing yourself a slipup or a mistake.

Step 3. Replace Destructive Thoughts with Constructive Ideas

Practice affirmative statements out loud. Tell yourself:

> "I did it before, I can do it again! I did well last week, I can do well again next week."
> "Everyone has setbacks. I won't allow this to keep me from being successful."
> "I don't have to be perfect to succeed."
> "I will take one day at a time."
> "I love myself, and I will take good care of myself."
> "I am making progress despite this setback!"
> "I'll continue to lose weight and to get in better shape despite this setback!"
> "Eventually I will reach my goal weight and maintain it as long as I keep working at it."

If you judge yourself negatively, remember that controlling your weight is not a moral issue. Replace words and phrases that are judgmental and make you feel bad about yourself. Don't say, "I was bad, I'm a bad person." Say instead, "I overate," or "I had some unplanned eating." Don't say, "I'm a failure." Say, "I'm 3,000 calories over my weekly maintenance level."

Step 4. Recall Previous Successes

Up until the setback, you were probably feeling good about your progress. Don't allow disappointment over the setback to interfere with your progress. The unplanned eating or the neglected exercise happened after a lot of good effort on your part. Examine your successes. How much weight have you lost? How has your body changed? Be specific. Look at your weight loss chart or your "before" pictures. Remind yourself that even though you have gained four pounds, you are still lighter than you were before. Compare the size of your present dresses or suits to your previous clothes. Call up your supportive friends and ask them to tell you about the positive changes they have seen in your appearance and behavior.

Remember that progress is doing anything better than what you were doing before. If you are used to gaining ten pounds a year, then losing ten pounds this year is an achievement. Not only did you lose ten pounds, but you also didn't gain the usual ten pounds. Eating four cookies a day is progress if last week you ate eight cookies a day. Changing your shopping habits is progress, even if you slipped up and overate yesterday. Feeling more positive about your ability to be successful is progress. Even learning how to cope with this setback is an achievement. You are changing, and you will continue to do so.

Step 5. Reevaluate and Modify Your Goals

You may feel overwhelmed at the thought of going back to your full program of exercise and food intake goals after a setback. If you do, start small. Look again at your goals, then modify them. Set small, easy-to-accomplish goals following a setback, and allow yourself to feel good about them. If, for instance, before the setback you were walking sixty minutes a day, six days a week, planning your food a week in advance in your food diary, and not snacking, it may seem too much to immediately resume your old schedule. Make a new plan. Walk thirty minutes five times a week. Set aside fifteen minutes each night for planning menus for the following day, limit your snacks to 100 calories, and throw out problem foods. If you had given up bread and butter, but during your setback ate half a loaf of bread and a quarter pound of butter, your new goal may be to have two slices of bread a day and no butter or to avoid buying bread and butter because they are too tempting. When you achieve these goals, you create the momentum to set larger ones, and eventually—sooner than you think—you are back to where you were before the setback and ready to continue your program.

Step 6. Re-create a Controlled Environment

Remember that a controlled environment is one that is planned, organized, and scheduled. Make time for such priority events as walking. Reduce your food cues by getting rid of problem foods or making them inaccessible. Think ahead. If you are going to be home alone, don't bake brownies. Instead, go to the movies, go swimming, or go to a dance-exercise class at the gym. Plan, purchase, and prepare low-calorie foods, and make your environment conducive to maintaining your plans. Remind yourself that you are going to eat a controlled number of calories a day and that you're going to exercise regularly.

Take time to review some of the successful strategies you used before. Think of some of the supportive things you did for yourself, and plan to do them again. Think of your needs. Take time for self-reflection and maintain your awareness of the tasks you need to do to control your weight.

When you were working well at the program, did you keep busy and stay away from food? Did you reduce your outside responsibilities? Did you spend time with people who were supportive and understanding? Did you seek help from experts on weight management, and did you believe in your ability to change? You can do all of these things again. You can deal with stress, anxiety, or boredom through means other than eating. Make a list of the environmental and behavioral strategies that will help you to regain control, and begin using them immediately.

Two of our clients, Tom Martin and Sue Benedict, made lists that are models for recovering from a setback. They each restructured their environments to support their renewed efforts. These are the lists they worked with to keep their footing and to cope with temptations. Notice that both Sue and Tom made a commitment to three to seven days of highly structured living to get them back on track. Neither intended to live this rigidly for the rest of their lives.

Sue's List
- Throw out peanut butter, crackers, and ice cream.
- Tell my family that I need their help and cooperation this week because I'm in trouble!

- Use DFC menus to make a shopping list of healthy foods to buy this week.
- Ask my husband to do the grocery shopping this week and to purchase only the items on the menu, no problem foods!
- When he comes home from shopping, I'll prepare salad ingredients and veggies so that they are available as needed. If I *have* to put something in my mouth, it will be a carrot or a celery stick.
- I'll spend afternoons away from home to avoid snacking. I'll arrange to meet Linda at the health club for afternoon aerobics on Monday, Wednesday, and Friday this week.
- I'll avoid watching TV at night this week. I'll go to Overeaters Anonymous meetings for the next three nights, and then I'll work on my needlepoint upstairs in the bedroom.
- I'll go to bed by 10 P.M. to avoid all-night snacking.
- I'll say no to all requests for my free time this week that could make me feel overtired or stressed.
- I'll ask Beverly to meet me at the park for a walk at 7 A.M. for the next three days.

Tom's List
- Refuse dinner dates and other social engagements for four days.
- Buy enough low-calorie frozen dinners and diet sodas to get me through this week.
- Throw out peanuts and potato chips left over from the party.
- Work eight-hour days this week. No ten- to twelve-hour days! Even though I have a lot of work to do, I need the time for myself.
- Call Joe. He's doing well on his weight management program and he always encourages me to keep going.
- Avoid spending time with Fred this week. He's a bad influence on me. I always drink and eat too much when I'm with him.
- Ride the exercise bicycle at work for twenty minutes at lunchtime for the next four days.
- For recreation, arrange to spend the next three nights playing squash at the YMCA with Ted and Jim. Ask them to meet me at the office and we'll go there together.
- Buy newspapers in the morning. When I stop at the convenience store on the way home, it's hard to avoid buying a snack.
- Once a day for the next three days, look at my "before" pictures to remind myself of how well I've done.

- Reread the DFC handouts and my short- and long-term goals tonight. I need a refresher.
- Call my therapist at DFC if I'm not back in control by the end of this week. I'll put it on my calendar so I won't forget.

Step 7. Adhere Strictly to Your Plan Until You Have Firmly Reestablished Healthy Patterns

Regaining control of your behavior is easier to do within the context of a highly structured environment than in a chaotic one. Once a setback occurs, it's usually necessary and appropriate to be fairly rigid regarding your behavior and the structure of your environment. Set your plans into action *immediately,* and stick to them so that you can regain control of your behavior and renew your confidence in your ability to succeed.

The first three days of this highly structured plan are the most difficult. Most people report feeling in greater control once they have followed a structured program for three to seven days. Once you have reestablished your healthy patterns of eating, exercising, menu planning, and calorie counting, however, you can allow yourself some flexibility because you are self-aware and in control. If you receive an unexpected dinner invitation, for instance, you can accommodate the change of plans without losing control of your eating.

Step 8. Take Each Setback Seriously

If another setback occurs within a short period of time, pay closer attention to what you are doing. If your setbacks occur close together, think about how you can reduce the risks of overeating. Deal with each setback using the strategies we have described, and recognize that this time you may require several weeks of continuous, rigid structure in order to feel completely back in control. Seek outside support to keep yourself from developing a full-scale relapse.

Step 9. Get Help and Support from Professionals or from a Support Group

It is *never* necessary to regain all of your weight before you seek help! Too many people wait until they have a full-scale relapse before they seek support or advice. They don't think they need professional help unless they regain twenty pounds or more. Sometimes, too, feelings of shame or embarrassment keep people from going after the help they need. They feel that since they've failed at their efforts, they don't deserve help, or that it's useless anyway.

It's always helpful to get advice from weight management experts, especially during difficult times. Groups such as Weight Watchers, Overeaters Anonymous, and hospital outpatient programs have been useful to many people who have returned home after being at the Duke University Diet and Fitness Center.

Crisis calls to friends or people from your support group can also help you regain control after occasional setbacks. Some people like to maintain regular, ongoing telephone contact with a therapist, an ally, or a fellow dieter as a way of maintaining progress. Of course, visits to a weight-control program like ours also help to reinforce positive behavioral changes, develop new levels of self-awareness, enhance feelings of self-confidence, and contribute to successful long-term changes.

Step 10. Believe in Yourself and Trust the Process

Research shows that dieters who believe in their ability to control their weight are more successful than those who do not. If you feel at some deep level that you will never be successful, then you won't be as likely to use the strategies we suggest to enable yourself to recover from setbacks. Don't set yourself up for failure.

No matter how hopeless it seems, it *is* possible to achieve long-term weight management. Think of the other things that you have done that have been difficult. If you went to college, or went through job training, you might have had a bad exam along the way. But you probably didn't drop out because of it. You kept going. Think of people you know who have been successful at losing weight in spite of setbacks. Remind yourself that you are no different from them. You are involved in a process of change, and if you work at it one day at a time, you too will be successful.

Prevent Future Setbacks by Anticipating High-Risk Situations

Identify the types of experiences that put you at risk for a setback. Once you are aware of potential problems, you can prevent many setbacks.

If you are apt to say, "I don't know what happened! I don't know why I gained back six pounds already," you need to become more aware of what's related to your loss of control. Setbacks don't occur out of the blue. They are, in fact, predictable. If you work at it, you will understand when you are at risk. Perhaps it will help you to look at the predictable risks for the average American population of dieters.

Many people assume that overweight people deviate from a program to change their lifestyle only when they are experiencing negative feelings such as boredom, depression, or loneliness. They imagine the person sitting home alone with no companionship is the one who starts overeating again. In fact, some research on dieters who experienced setbacks indicated that 32 percent of the setbacks resulted from negative emotional states such as anxiety, loneliness, sadness, and frustration, whereas 43 percent resulted from positive emotional states such as happiness and joy. Eating in these cases was often a way of sharing love or celebrating. It was seen as part of having a good time. Another 10 percent of the setbacks related to conflicts in personal relationships. Dieters ate in reaction to an argument or an event involving another person. Social pressure accounted for another 10 percent of the setbacks, and 5 percent were related to negative physical states such as sickness.*

In addition, setbacks also commonly occur in relation to disappointment over a lack of weight loss, changes in normal routine, or fatigue and stress. You need to plan strategies that will enable you to cope successfully with these situations.

Disappointment over a lack of weight loss. Inevitably, weight changes are irregular and slower than you would like. You're also bound to hit plateaus or periods of time when, even if you are eating correctly and exercising consistently, the scale doesn't show the weight loss you expect. This can be very frustrating, but don't feel that your efforts are useless. If you continue your program, eventually you will lose more

*See B. S. Rosenthal and R. D. Marx, "Determinants of Initial Relapse Episodes Among Dieters," *Obesity and Bariatric Medicine,* 10 (1981): pp. 94–97.

weight. It may take longer than you want, and you may feel upset from time to time with your tortoiselike rate of progress, but it is normal. Remember, the tortoise won the race, and you can, too.

A change in your normal routine. Any change in your daily pattern—whether it's good, bad, or indifferent—is likely to put you at risk for a setback. Therefore, if you know a change is going to occur in your life, plan to accommodate it and maintain control.

Earlier, we talked about the setback Darlene suffered when she took care of her mother and neglected herself. If Darlene had anticipated the risks of that situation, she could have avoided the weight gain. The way you can avoid a similar setback is to pay attention to the situation. Say to yourself, "Okay. This is a high-risk situation, and I need to develop a plan to deal with it. I know I'm not going to plan and prepare for my meals when I'm running back and forth from the hospital. How can I cope?" Take steps that will work. Do what's necessary—whether it's hiring a cook for two weeks, eating at a restaurant where you can get broiled fish every night, making a brown-bag dinner to take along, or buying a batch of low-calorie frozen dinners to eat at home. The important point is that more often than not, you can avoid the setback if you anticipate it and plan ahead.

Feeling fatigued, pressured, or upset. Be alert to these potentially high-risk states. You are better equipped to avoid a setback if you say, "I'm tired today—which means I'm at risk for overeating and underexercising—so I need to develop strategies to cope." Your strategies might be as simple as taking a nap after work, going to bed early, or not watching television because it tempts you to nibble.

The earlier you make yourself aware of these situations, the more immune you will be to those series of minor events that trigger overeating. Let's assume, for instance, that (1) you are tired; (2) you are upset over an altercation with your boss; and (3) you are watching a food commercial on television that shows a juicy hamburger (which you love), french fries, and a chocolate malt. Alarms should go off, but, instead, you remember that you should call your friend. You go into the kitchen to make a phone call. While you're there, you reach into the cupboard and start eating crackers. You see the peanut butter and you put it on the crackers, then pour yourself a glass of beer.

The problem here is not that you had the crackers, peanut butter, and beer. The problem is that you started the day feeling tired. Early in the day you should have been alert to the risk of overeating and then planned a strategy for dealing with your fatigue. Ditto for your altercation with your boss.

Plan how you are going to deal with your high-risk situations. Recognize that they can be compounded:

- Feeling lousy because you have a cold and your boss wants you to stay late to work might be enough to trigger buying a candy bar (or two).
- Coming home exhausted from work, feeling low because your spouse just criticized you, and heading out the door to eat at your favorite Mexican restaurant together spell trouble.

Develop strategies for dealing with high-risk situations. Avoid being around food, call a friend, go for a walk, be with other people. Recognize and be assertive about your needs. Take a low-calorie snack to work so that if you have to stay late, at least you'll be munching on celery instead of on high-calorie foods from the vending machine. Tell your spouse that you want to go out to eat tomorrow night instead of tonight so that you can stay in control.

If today is the day you normally do the food shopping but you're feeling stressed, think about rescheduling this chore. Otherwise, you may be tempted to put something in your cart that will be too much to resist. In any case, don't allow your feelings to trigger a setback. Take action as soon as possible and anticipate mastering the problem.

Reaching Your Goals and Staying There

When you look more like you want to look—when you feel healthier, sexier, and more attractive—many aspects of your life are affected. Because of your transformation and the changes in the way people react to you, you may experience culture shock. You have left part of the person you were behind you. Sometimes the surprise of getting what you wanted becomes a source of trauma. If you're not aware that these responses are normal and natural, and if you don't learn how to deal with them, you can regain the weight you lost.

Living with success isn't always as easy as it might appear. Change of any kind is never easy, even when it's a change for the better. Many changes take time to get used to. They involve feeling uncomfortable with new situations. There's no way to know exactly what the changes will be, or how you will react to them. But you have to adjust emotionally to the new experiences you have as a thinner person.

In order to get a handle on some of the problems that could cause you to sabotage yourself, you need to learn strategies for dealing successfully with some of the underlying issues that could make it difficult for you to maintain the healthy patterns you have established.

Step 1. Set and Maintain Realistic Expectations about How Weight Loss Will Affect Your Life

People often believe that losing weight will change their lives and make everything better. You might expect, for instance, that once you lose weight, life suddenly will be wonderful. All of your difficulties will be solved, and you will have tremendous self-confidence. Your marriage will be better, you'll get a job promotion, and you'll become a great athlete. You'll have a better social life and more intimate relationships. If you have blamed your weight as the source of your problems, you may think that once the weight is gone, all your life's difficulties will disappear. Of course, this is unrealistic thinking. Weight may be the source of certain problems you have experienced, but other issues in your life may have been masked by your weight. Learning to live in your new body and to deal with old emotional issues often takes time. There is no magic powder to sprinkle on problems to make them disappear.

To avoid falling victim to unrealistic expectations, be aware of them, and reframe them as something more attainable. Among other things, you may expect to meet someone special and establish a relationship, but don't set that up as the only reason to lose weight. Also, new activities require practice and patience. Although you have seen thin people who are excellent skiers, they aren't excellent because they are thin. They are excellent skiers because they have taken lessons and put in the time and energy to develop their skill.

Any number of disappointed expectations can trigger you to overeat again. Be aware of them—and wary of them. You may think you need to throw yourself into situations where you can prove yourself, but start slowly and don't put too much pressure on yourself. If you haven't had a lot of social experiences, go slowly. Don't put yourself into high-pressure scenes that make you feel defeated. Singles bars and dances are not usually the best places to gain confidence. Instead of asking someone new for a date for the whole evening, ask him to go to a museum with you for the afternoon or for a walk in the park. Get a cup of coffee together, or have a drink after work.

Begin working at new, "thin" activities *before* you have lost all the weight you want to lose. Play tennis, wear shorts, or go out dancing with friends. Apply for a new job, or ask someone you like for a date. You need the experience as you are losing weight. At the same time, explore your feelings and reactions to these new experiences. Just as you have learned to do with eating and exercise, set small goals for yourself in terms of these new experiences and strategies. Practice them. Rehearse them. Achieve the small goals, and then gradually set new and larger goals as you build your skills and confidence.

Step 2. Become Aware of Issues that You May Have Been Avoiding

Some people who are overweight have used food to numb their feelings. They eat to keep from expressing their anger or to protect them from their own sexuality. They may eat to mask feelings of inferiority or vulnerability. Perhaps they are in an unhappy marriage, and a focus on food diverts their attention from facing the situation and having to act on it. They may eat and gain weight as a means of rebelling against someone who is trying to control them, particularly if that person dislikes their being overweight.

If you have masked other issues in your life, or used fat as a defense, it's time to become aware of issues that you've been avoiding.

Larry Miller, one of our clients, had always been shy and uncomfortable around women. When he first came to the DFC, he expressed his belief that he was shy because he was sure that women would make fun of his body. During the year it took him to lose sixty pounds, Larry rode a bicycle to work every day and lifted weights at a local health club. He got into good physical condition. As a result, he looked good in his clothes and out of them. But he was still shy and afraid of sexual interactions. When he found himself staying away from the gym and starting to overeat again, he sought out a therapist and began to work on understanding the source of his embarrassment and the issues early in his life that had led to his adolescent weight gain and fear of his sexuality.

Another of our clients, Florence Tracy, was generally aggressive in her relationships. People tended to avoid her because she was argumentative and abrasive. After she lost forty pounds, she had to confront her personality and come to grips with the fact that she was avoided for reasons other than weight.

After losing fifty-five pounds, Mary Nichols, another client, looked a lot like Dolly Parton. Although she had been married for a number of years, she didn't know what to do when her friends' husbands started flirting with her. She was uncomfortable with their attention and was upset that she actually enjoyed it. Unconsciously, Mary started putting back her weight. When one of her friends asked her why she was eating so much, she said she had no idea; she just felt compelled to eat as many cookies as she could get her hands on. In fact, Mary's marriage was very unhappy. Since her husband was always telling her that she repulsed him physically, she had thought that losing weight might make things better between them. He didn't treat her any better once she was thin; if anything, he was more abusive. In truth, she was terrified of getting a divorce and facing life on her own. An abusive relationship seemed better than nothing. Eventually, with the help of a friend, Mary began to see a counselor and to confront her problems. Today, eight years after her weight loss, Mary is still maintaining her weight. She's been divorced for three years, and is currently having fun dating and building a new career as a stockbroker in New York City.

Step 3. Examine Your Fear of Success

If fat has been a defense against your sexuality, against getting close to other people, against feeling good about yourself, or against competing with others, it is very easy for you to sabotage yourself. Don't let this happen. Face your fears. Understand them, and be kind to yourself. Know that you can handle the changes. They will be gradual, and you can learn to cope with them.

It can be fun and enlightening to use what psychologists call a "double-chair technique" to confront the two parts of yourself—the part that wants to be successful and the part that is afraid of success. Set up two chairs, and role-play each part. When you switch chairs, switch roles. Have these two parts of yourself communicate with each other. Let them battle it out. This results in a greater understanding of your conflicting feelings, and you'll experience your real feelings about success. Do this more than once. Watch how the arguments change and develop.

Step 4. Identify Ways in Which You May Feel More Vulnerable

If you have been overweight all of your life, then being thin is bound to make you feel different. Even though you probably prefer being thinner, most likely you will feel more insecure initially as a thin person simply because you are not used to your new form and size or to the way people respond to you.

You may find that you feel awkward and strange in your new and smaller body, and you may feel less protected than you did when you were large. At a lower weight, some people report that, initially at least, they feel average and mediocre. They were used to "standing out in a crowd" and being noticed when they were large. Now they feel that they blend in and have to be special or unique in some other way in order to get attention. For many people, especially men, being large is unconsciously equated with feeling powerful and important. Losing weight makes them feel vulnerable, unimportant, and less authoritative.

Fortunately, the feelings of vulnerability and awkwardness will decrease over time, and you will begin to feel safe and less tempted to eat your way back into being heavy. With the experience of living life as a thinner person, you will gain confidence and eventually feel secure again.

Step 5. Anticipate a Lack of Support from Some People

It's important to think ahead to how your family, friends, even strangers may react to you when you lose weight. People may not respond the way you want. There's always the aunt or associate who will say, "You look sick!" or "You look too thin!" Friends who used to pig out with you may say, "You're no fun anymore!" Some people will tell you that you looked more attractive before, while others reinforce your self-doubts by saying, "You've never kept the weight off before. How long do you think it'll be before you balloon up again?"

While some of these comments may be well intentioned, they can upset your motivation to continue your success. A friend or loved one might say, "You should really gain some weight!" or, "Oh, you're so thin, it won't hurt you to have some ice cream!" Or, "Look at you! You *need* an extra serving!" You know the detrimental effects of using food as a reward or pretending that calories don't count, and you don't need this advice.

Remember that you have not lost weight to please or displease others.

The truth is that usually people who react this way are threatened by your new appearance. Friends may feel that you won't want to spend time with them anymore. Or they may not like to see what they perceive as competition for dates or attention. Even your spouse can be threatened by your more attractive appearance and be afraid that you are going to leave him or her for a "better" person. Don't let random comments or even outright hostility deter you from maintaining your weight.

If some of your old friends can't accept and support who you are, eventually either they'll come around or you'll find new friends who will support what you have done for yourself.

Sometimes you may feel misunderstood and undermined by others because they react too positively to your weight loss. Some people may be so lavish with their praise that you start wondering how horrible you looked to them before. People may say such things as, "I never knew you could look so good!" Or, "You look so great, I never would have recognized you!" Or, "Is it *really* you?" Such comments can make you very uncomfortable.

Other friends may offer now to set you up with dates, as they did with Carl Warneke. At first Carl was flattered, but later, when he thought about it, he was furious. "They never set me up on dates before!" he said. "I'm the same person now that I was then, but they were just ashamed of me before!" He resented his friends and felt that they hadn't ever fully accepted him before.

Acquaintances at work or at school may be so excited about your weight loss—or so interested in how to do it themselves—that they will bug you incessantly with questions about how you did it. This may make you feel like a freak who is required to give testimony to having proved the impossible possible! You may also find that people expect more of you now that you are thinner. People may start telling you that it's time you got a new job or a new relationship. Again, this may make you feel misunderstood. You are the same person, and you may not yet want to make other major changes in your life.

Recognize who is supportive and who is not. If close friends and loved ones lecture you when you have a setback, or attempt to police your behavior by saying such things as, "Don't forget to exercise," or "Do you *really* want to eat that piece of pie?" let them know that your efforts, not theirs, are what will ensure your success.

Tell people what you want from them. Be as specific as possible in your requests. For example, say, "I'd prefer it if you'd ask me how I'm feeling rather than how many pounds I've lost." Or, "Could you please not offer me any dessert or candy? If I want it, I'll ask for it myself." Avoid vague, general requests such as, "I'd like you to be more supportive." Also avoid indirect or critical comments such as, "So-and-so is so lucky that he has a wife who really understands his situation." It is unfair to others and potentially self-defeating to expect them to know automatically and precisely how to respond to you. Be patient with their attempts to be helpful to you. Just as you may experience setbacks in attempting to change your lifestyle, others may occasionally lapse into previously used unsupportive tactics. Remember that they also are learning, and that their habits may be as hard to change as your own. Show appreciation for their efforts, and remember that any long-term change requires time, patience, and effort.

Step 6. Keep Tracking Your Feelings

Are you feeling more vulnerable, sexy, sensitive, irritable, scared, or moody? If you're noticing new feelings, don't be surprised. Remember that all feelings are okay, and that you are bound to experience emotions and sensations you didn't have before. Your discomfort is perfectly normal. Stick with it and allow for it. Know that it's going to take time and patience to learn how to handle these new feelings.

Step 7. Continue to Look at Your Body

Look in the mirror every day so that you become familiar with the new you. This is you—not somebody else. As we said before, it sometimes takes many months or even a year or longer before the image you have of yourself as a thin person fits the image you have of other thin people that you see. This type of body-image distortion is normal if you have lost a lot of weight, especially if you have lost it quickly or have neglected to look into the mirror during the time you were losing weight. Ask friends to take pictures of the new you and study the photos to get used to your new image.

Step 8. Talk to Other People Who Have Lost Weight

People who have experienced weight loss and subsequent changes can be very understanding of what you are going through. Self-help groups, such as Overeaters Anonymous, can be particularly supportive. Sharing your feelings and experiences also can help you to identify what's happening to you and to adjust to your new situation.

Step 9. Mourn the Loss of Your Old, Fat Self

Many people who lose a great deal of weight feel as if they have lost a friend. This can happen to you even though you are excited about the changes you have made. If you lose a great deal of weight, you may need to mourn the loss of your old, fat self. Have a ceremonial burial of your fat self—bury an article of your "fat" clothing, write a eulogy, and grieve the loss of your fat friend. A burial or another method of dealing with your grief can provide you with a tremendous sense of relief and closure. You'll soon get over the loss of your former self, and learn to live with and enjoy your new self.

Other losses that may need mourning are the loss of the struggle to shed pounds and the loss of excuses you used to have as a fat person. Often people who reach their goals feel a void in their lives. Their "project" of losing weight is over and they don't know how to cope with that feeling of loss. Sometimes, too, they miss not having excuses for disappointments. When they were heavier and things didn't go their way, they could blame it on being overweight. If you find yourself mourning either of these losses, allow yourself a grieving time. Then realize that it's time to bury the negatives. Set new challenges for yourself, look for new adventures, even small ones, and take pleasure in your good health and energy.

A Final Word

Now it's time to congratulate yourself on what you've learned about yourself and the changes necessary for becoming a more healthy and fit person.

Remember that you have started a program that can work for you for the rest of your life. Keep setting goals, planning nutritionally balanced meals, practicing portion control and calorie control. Keep moving and exercising.

Anticipate difficult situations, and stay alert to all of the changes in your life. Every day ask yourself: Am I going to encounter any high-risk situations? Am I prepared to deal with them? Make continued success a high priority. Set aside time for relaxation, self-reflection, and, of course, more planning. Evaluate yourself weekly and monthly, and remind yourself that you are working for progress, not perfection.

When you need to, go back and review the particular chapters in this book that help you maintain your motivation to be a healthier and happier person, and remind yourself of useful strategies. Don't be too hard on yourself. Give yourself constant positive feedback for all your successes.

Last but not least, enjoy eating. Food is an essential part of being alive, and you can incorporate the best of it into a satisfying lifestyle. Above all, believe in your ability to continue learning and changing. You have the power, and all the tools you need, to enjoy a long and healthy life!

Index

All of the information in the
four-week program of diet and fitness,
included in this book has been developed from
THE DUKE UNIVERSITY MEDICAL CENTER
DIET AND FITNESS CENTER
residence program at
Durham, North Carolina.

To receive further information
regarding the program or answers
to any questions please contact
the Center directly:

DUKE UNIVERSITY
DIET AND FITNESS CENTER
804 West Trinity Avenue
Durham, NC 27701
(919) 684-6331

20.00 ✓
20.00 ✓ Dan
40.00

36⁰⁰

40.00
30.00